Medical Mini Review Series in Gastroenterology and Hepatology

Efficient Refresher for the Busy Clinical Gastroenterologist

Volume 2

Edited by

A.B.R. Thomson and N. Chande

www.giandhepatology.com

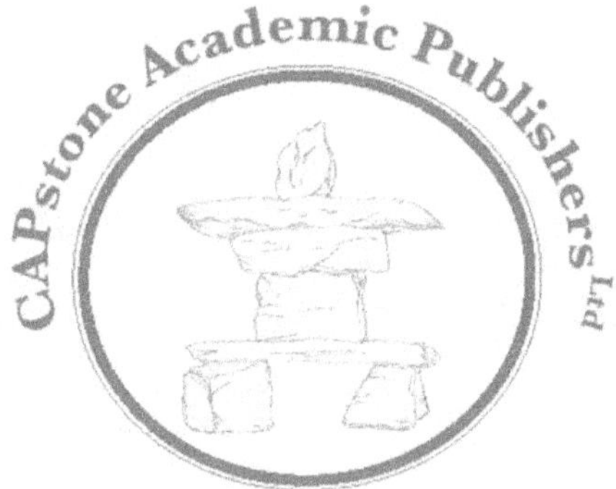

CAPstone (Canadian Academic Publishers Ltd) is a not-for-profit company dedicated to the use of the power of education for the betterment of all persons everywhere.

"The Democratization of Knowledge"

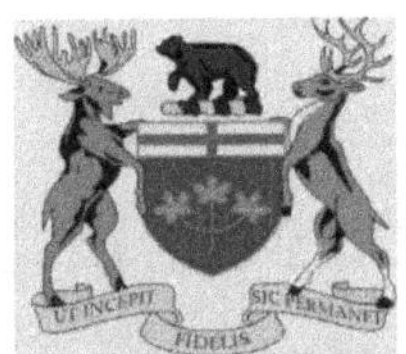

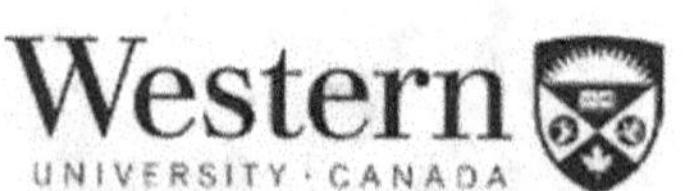
Western
UNIVERSITY · CANADA

MINI UPDATE

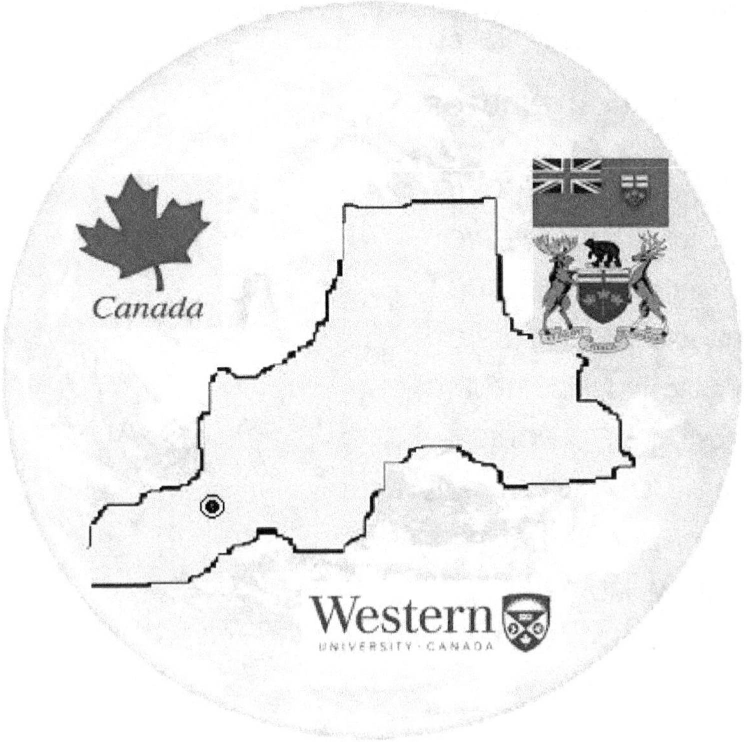

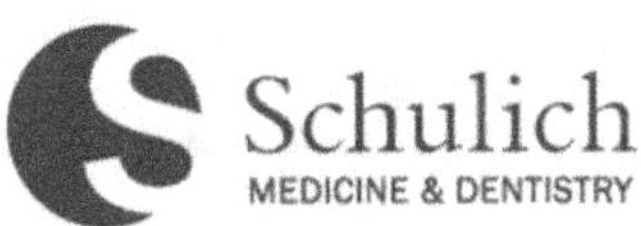
Schulich
MEDICINE & DENTISTRY

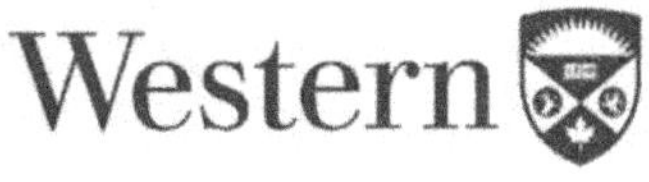
Western

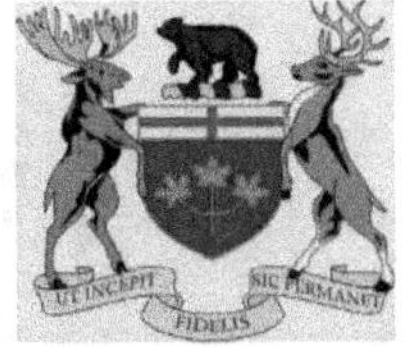
UT INCEPIT
FIDELIS
SIC PERMANET

MINI UPDATE

The editors wish to thank the trainee and staff contributors who maintain the excellence of the Division of Gastroenterology at Western University.

LIST OF CONTRIBUTORS

Aljawad M, MD, FRCP(C)

Beaton M, MD, FRCP(C)

Chande N, MD, FRCP(C)

Levstik M, MD, FRCP(C)

McIntosh K, MD, FRCP(C)

Mosli M, MD, FRCP(C)

So J, MD, FRCP(C)

Thomson ABR, MD, PhD, FRCP(C)

Wells M, MD, FRCP(C)

Wilson A, MD, FRCP(C)

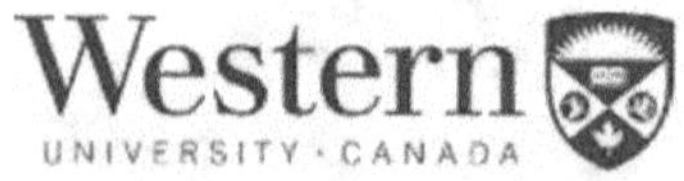

EDITOR BIOGRAPHIES

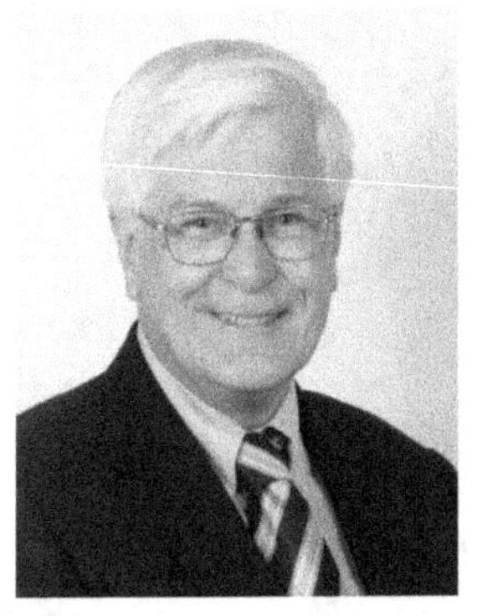

Dr. Alan Thomson has been President of the Canadian Association of Gastroenterology, a member of the Bockus Society, two-term Governor for Western Canada for the American College of Gastroenterology, winner of the prestigious University Cup in 2001, a recipient of the Gold Medal in Medicine of the Royal College of Physicians and Surgeons (Canada), Chief Royal College examiner in Gastroenterology, Director of the Division of Gastroenterology, three-time Teacher of the Year at the University of Alberta, Award for Excellence in Mentoring Graduate Students and Postdoctoral Fellows, and awarded Distinguished University Professor. Dr. Thomson is a Distinguished Emeritus University Professor, University of Alberta, and is currently an Adjunct Professor at Western University.

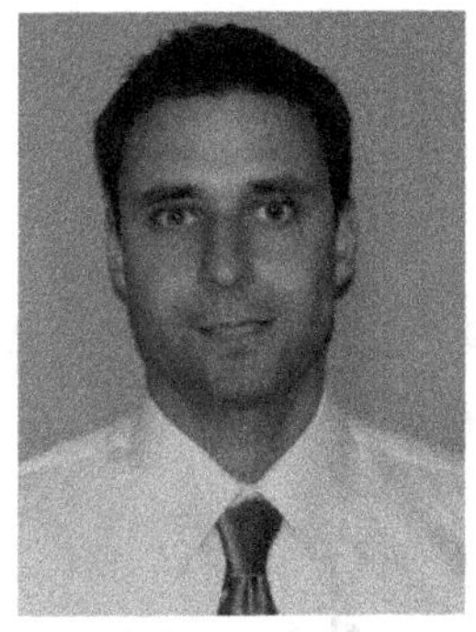

Dr. Nilesh Chande is an Associate Professor of Medicine in the Division of Gastroenterology at Western University, London, Ontario, Canada. He is the Director of the Gastroenterology Training Program and has interests in inflammatory bowel disease, general gastroenterology, and medical education.

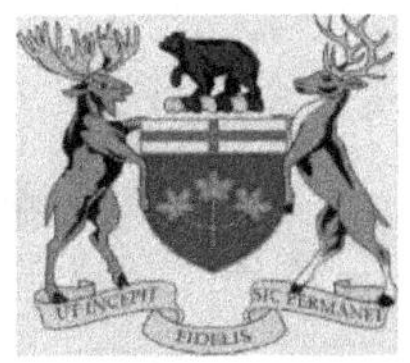

As physicians, learning is life-long.

This book is dedicated to our trainees and

To the patients whom they will care for,

And care about.

Alan Thomson

For Shannon and our children who keep my mind on the important things in life.

Nilesh Chande

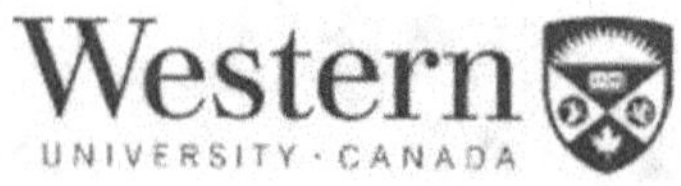

MINI UPDATE

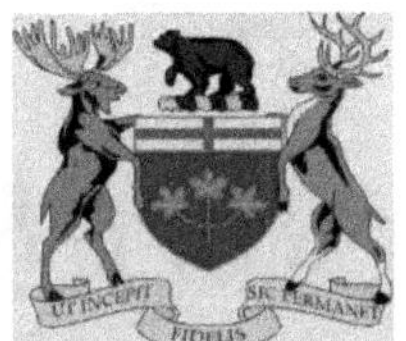

MINI UPDATE

TABLE OF CONTENTS

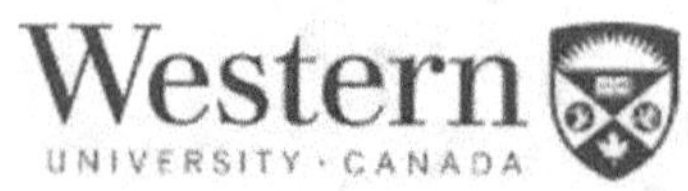

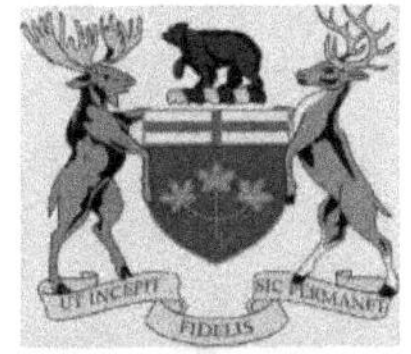
UT INCEPIT
FIDELIS
SIC PERMANET

MINI UPDATE

BACKGROUND

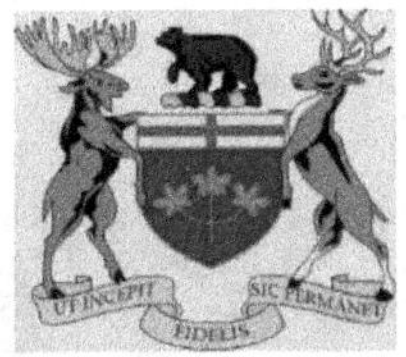

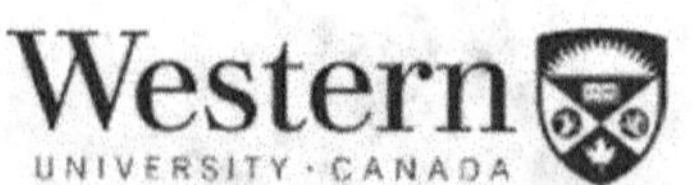
Western
UNIVERSITY · CANADA

EMBRYOLOGY OF THE GI TRACT

Keith Mcintosh

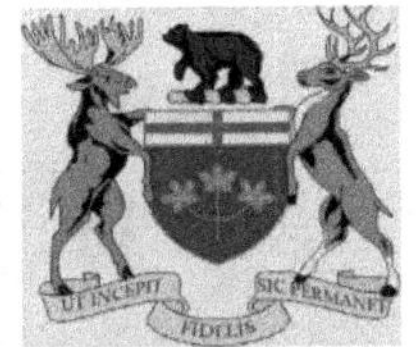

EMBRYOLOGY OF THE GI TRACT

Overview

- Primitive Gut Formation
  - Germ layers
  - Divisions of the Gut
  - Mesentery
- Parts of the Gut and Associated Malformations
  - Esophagus
  - Stomach
  - Liver
  - Pancreas
  - Small Bowel
  - Colon

Germ Layers

- **Ectoderm:** skin,nervous system, hair
- **Mesoderm:** skeleton, muscle, connective tissue, heart, spleen, kidneys
- **Endoderm:** digestive tract, lungs, thyroid
- Forms the epithelial lining of the digestive tract & gives rise to parenchyma of liver and pancreas
- Muscle, connective tissue and peritoneal components of the wall of the gut
  Derived from splanchnic mesoderm

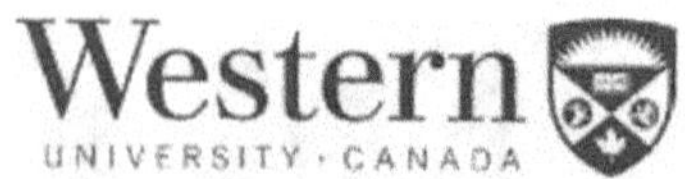

EMBRYOLOGY OF THE GI TRACT

Divisions of the Gut

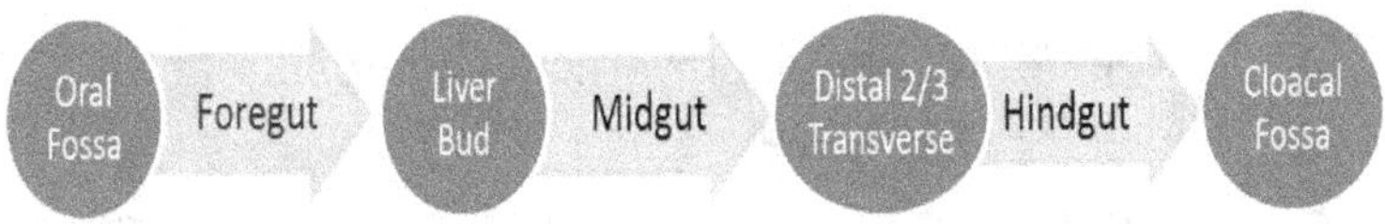

The Primitive Gut

- Starts at 3rd - 4th week of gestation
- Folding of a portion of endoderm-lined yolk sac into a tubular structure
- The cephalic and caudal parts of the embryo form blind ending tubes, the **foregut** and **hindgut** respectively
- The middle part, the **midgut**, remains temporarily connected to the yolk sac by the vitelline duct

Derivatives of Primitive Gut

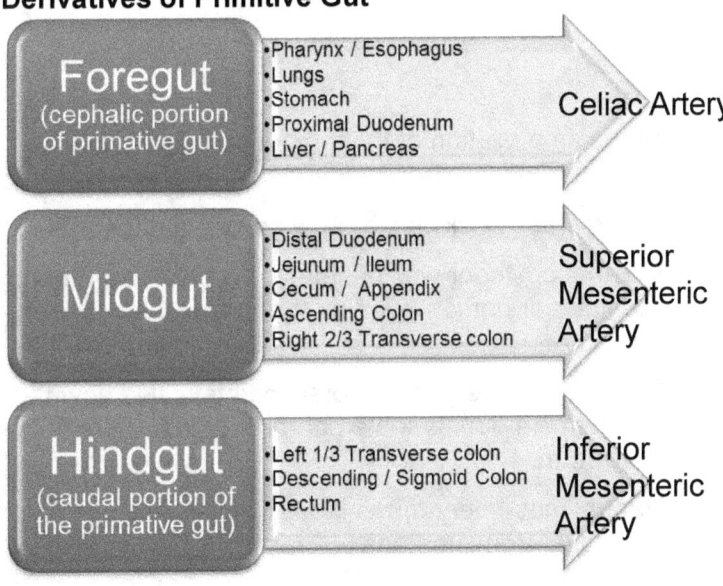

Foregut (cephalic portion of primative gut)

- Pharynx / Esophagus
- Lungs
- Stomach
- Proximal Duodenum
- Liver / Pancreas

Celiac Artery

Midgut

- Distal Duodenum
- Jejunum / Ileum
- Cecum / Appendix
- Ascending Colon
- Right 2/3 Transverse colon

Superior Mesenteric Artery

Hindgut (caudal portion of the primative gut)

- Left 1/3 Transverse colon
- Descending / Sigmoid Colon
- Rectum

Inferior Mesenteric Artery

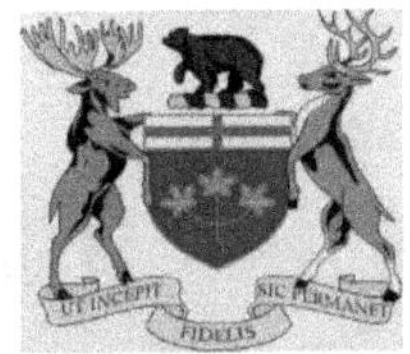

Esophagus

- At week 4, respiratory diverticulum appears at cranial part of foregut
- **Tracheoesophageal septum** gradually partitions into the trachea and esophagus
- Esophagus elongates with the descent of the heart and lungs

Developmental Anomalies

- Tracheoesophageal Fistula
- Atresia
- Stenosis
- Congenital Hiatal Hernia (esophagus fails to elongate properly)

Stomach

- Starts as a dilation of the foregut in the 4th week of development
- Rotates 90° clockwise around its longitudinal axis
- Original posterior wall of stomach grows faster than the anterior portion, forming the **greater** and **lesser** curvatures
- Dorsal mesentery in the rotation gets pulled down and forms a double leafed apron called the **greater omentum**
- Ventral mesentery forms **lesser omentum** extending from stomach to liver

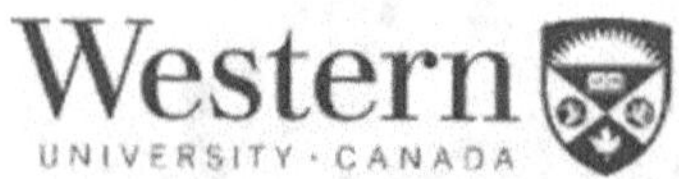

Stomach Developmental Anomalies

- Pyloric Stenosis
  - Circular musculature of stomach in region pylorus hypertrophies
  - Narrowing of the pyloric lumen, obstructing passage of food

Duodenum

- Formed from the terminal part of the foregut and the cephalic part of the midgut, just distal to the origin of the liver bud
- Due to stomach rotation, the duodenum takes on a C-shaped loop
- Duodenum presses against dorsal body wall (with pancreas) and dorsal mesentery fuses and obliterates with peritoneum
- Thus duodenum is fixed in a retroperitoneal position except for duodenal cap with retains its mesentery
- Arterial supply is by both celiac and superior mesenteric arteries

Liver and Gallbladder

- Starts as a **hepatic diverticulum** or **liver bud**
- Consists of rapidly proliferating cells that penetrate the **septum transversum**
- The connection between the duodenum and liver bud lengthens and narrows to form the bile duct and a ventral outgrowth on the bile duct forms the gallbladder

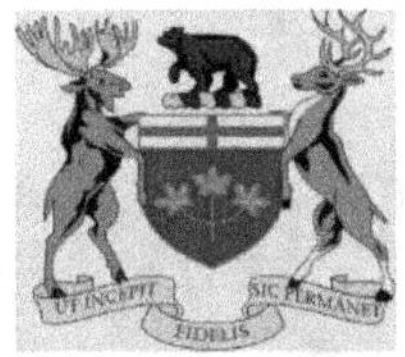

- Liver is covered in peritoneum, except for cranial surface adjacent to diaphragm which is bare

Liver Developmental Anomalies

- Accessory Hepatic Ducts
- Duplication of the Gallbladder
- Extrahepatic Biliary Atresia
- Intrahepatic Biliary Duct Atresia

Pancreas

- 2 endodermal buds from lining of duodenum: **dorsal** and **ventral** pancreatic bud form the pancreas
- Ventral bud forms the uncinate process and the inferior part of the head of pancreas
- Dorsal bud forms the rest of the pancreas
- **Main pancreatic duct** is formed from the distal dorsal pancreatic duct and the entire ventral pancreatic duct
- An **accessory pancreatic duct** may persist and drains at the **minor papilla**

Developmental Abnormalities

- Pancreas Divisum
- Annular Pancreas
- Ectopic Pancreas

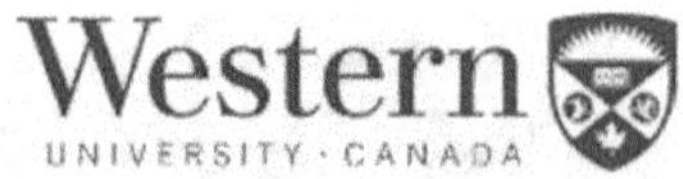

Pancreas Divisum

- TheFailure of the dorsal and ventral buds to normally fuse
- Very common – seen in 5-10% of people
- Usually is asymptomatic
- Don't need to treat unless pancreatitis develops
- Usual treatment: Sphincterotomy

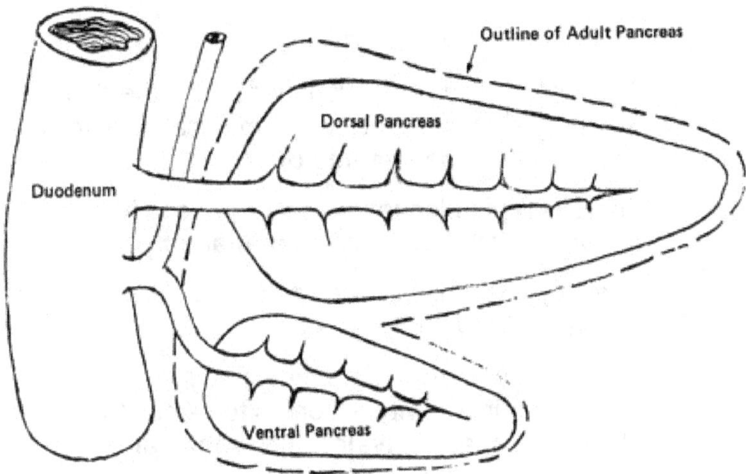

Annular Pancreas

- The ventral pancreas splits and forms a ring around the duodenum
- This can lead to duodenal stenosis and obstruction

Ectopic Pancreas

- Aka: Pancreatic Rest

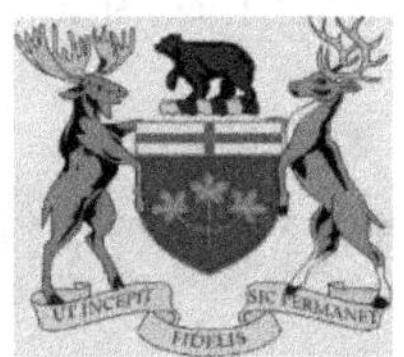

- Can be anywhere from distal end of the esophagus, to the tip of the primary intestinal loop
- Most frequently it lies in the mucosa of either the stomach and in Meckel's Diverticulum
- Usually asymptomatic
- Can cause pancreatitis, bleeding, ulceration, and obstruction

Midgut

- At 5 weeks, midgut is suspended from the dorsal wall by a short mesentery communicating with yolk sac by way of the **vitelline duct**
- There is rapid elongation of the gut resulting in the formation of the **primary intestinal loop**
- The loop extends into the vitelline duct and remains in connection with the yolk sac
- Due to rapid growth of the intestine the intraabdominal cavity becomes too small to contain all the loops, and **physiologic umbilical herniation** occurs at about the 6th week
- The primary intestinal loop rotates 270° counterclockwise around an axis formed by SMA
- Rotates 90° when herniated and 180□ back in the abdominal cavity
- During rotation, elongation of intestinal loops still occurs resulting in a number of coiled loops of jejunum and ileum
- By the 10th week, herniated loops begin to return to the abdomen

Abbreviation: SMA, superior mesenteric artery

Midgut

- At about the 6th week, the **cecal bud** forms at the caudal end of the primary intestinal loop
- Once back in the abdomen, it lies temporarily in RUQ
- It descends to the R iliac fossa, placing the ascending colon on the R side of abdomen
- The distal end of the cecal bud forms a diverticulum, the **appendix**

Mesenteries

- Double layer of peritoneum that enclose an organ and connect it to the body wall

- **Ventral Mesentery**
  - Only in the region of stomach and duodenum
  - Forms lesser omentum between stomach and liver
  - Forms falciform ligament between liver and body wall
- **Dorsal Mesentery**
  - Extends from distal esophagus to distal hindgut
  - Forms greater omentum in region of stomach
  - Forms mesentery proper of the jejunum and ileum

Intestinal Mesenteries

- Jejunum and ileum retain free mesenteries
- Ascending and descending colon mesenteries press and fuse with posterior abdominal wall, thus anchoring them in these positions

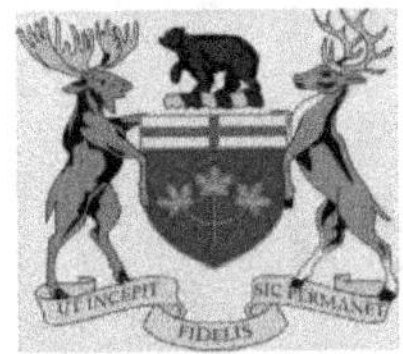

- The cecum and sigmoid colon retain free mesenteries
- Transverse colon mesentery fuses with posterior wall of greater omentum, but maintains its mobility

Midgut Abnormalities

- Omphalocele
- Gastroschisis
- Meckel's
- Volvulus

Omphalocele

- Herniation of abdominal viscera through an enlarged umbilical ring that is covered by an amnion
- Result of failure of the bowel to return to abdomen after physiologic herniation
- Occurs in 25 / 10^5 births, and has a 25% rate of mortality
- Half of infants have chromosomal abnormalities
- Omphalocele is associated with other severe congenital malformations

Gastroschisis

- Herniation of abdominal contents through the body wall directly into the amniotic cavity
- Usually lateral to umbilicus, through an area weakened by the regression of the umbilical vein

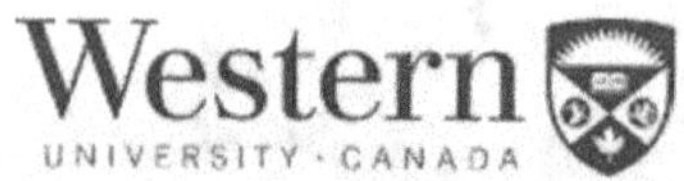

- Viscera are not covered by peritoneum or amnion and bowel may be damaged by exposure to amniotic fluid
- $10/10^5$ births, may be associated with cocaine use
- Not associated with chromosomal abnormalities, and survival rate is excellent

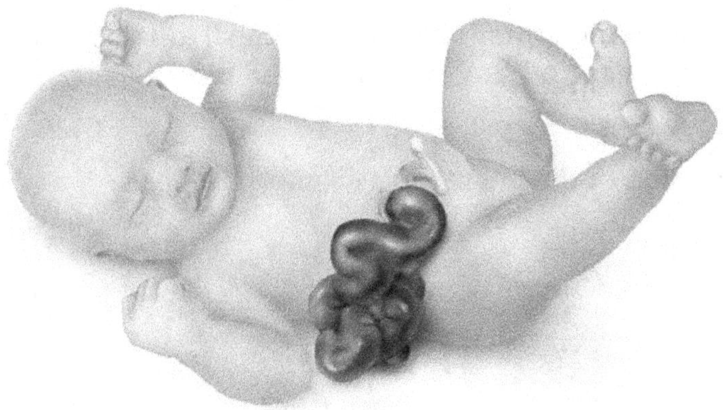

Meckel's Diverticulum

- Occasionally a small portion of the **vitelline duct** persists forming a small outpocket in the ileum, called a **Meckel's Diverticulum**
- Rule of seven 2's
  - 2% of population
  - 2% symptomatic
  - 2 years of age
  - 2 feet from IC valve
  - 2 inches long
  - 2x as likely in males
  - 2 types of ectopic tissue are common: gastric & pancreatic

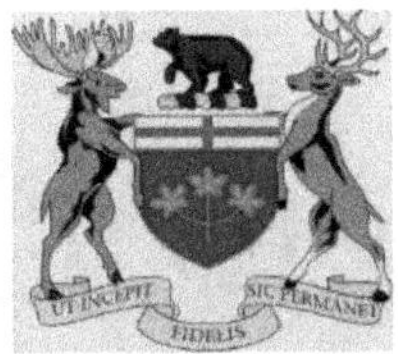

Malrotation & Volvulus

- Abnormal rotation of the intestinal loop may result in twisting of the intestine, **volvulus**, which can lead to compromise in the blood supply, ischemia and obstruction
- **L-sided colon** can result when primary intestinal loop rotates only 90°
- **Reversed rotation of the intestinal loop** occurs when the primary loop rotates 90° clockwise

Malrotation of the Intestine

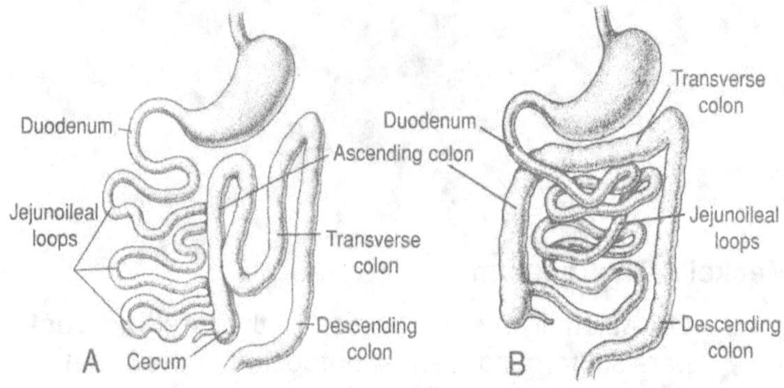

Hindgut

- Gives rise to distal transverse, descending, sigmoid & rectum
- Hindgut endoderm also forms the lining of bladder & urethra via the **allantosis**
- The hindgut terminates at the posterior **cloaca**, which forms the primitive anorectal canal
- The **cloacal membrane** is ectoderm derived and ruptures creating the anal opening at the 7th week

- Proliferation of the ectoderm closes the caudal most region of the anal canal, but it recanalizes by the 9th week

Anus

- Upper 2/3 of anal canal is endoderm-derived (columnar) mucosa.
- Drains through the superior rectal vein, a branch of IMV (inferior mesenteric vein, a branch of the portal vein)
- Lower 1/3 is ectoderm derived (stratified squamous)
- Drain through middle & inferior rectal veins (systemic circulation)
- The junction of the endoderm- and ectoderm-derived portions two is the **dentate or pectinate line**

Hindgut Abnormalities

- Rectoanal atresias & fistulas
- Imperforate anus
- Hirschsprung disease

Imperforate anus

- No anal opening due to a lack of recanalization of the lower portion of the anal canal

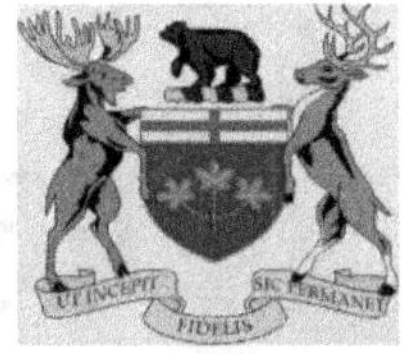

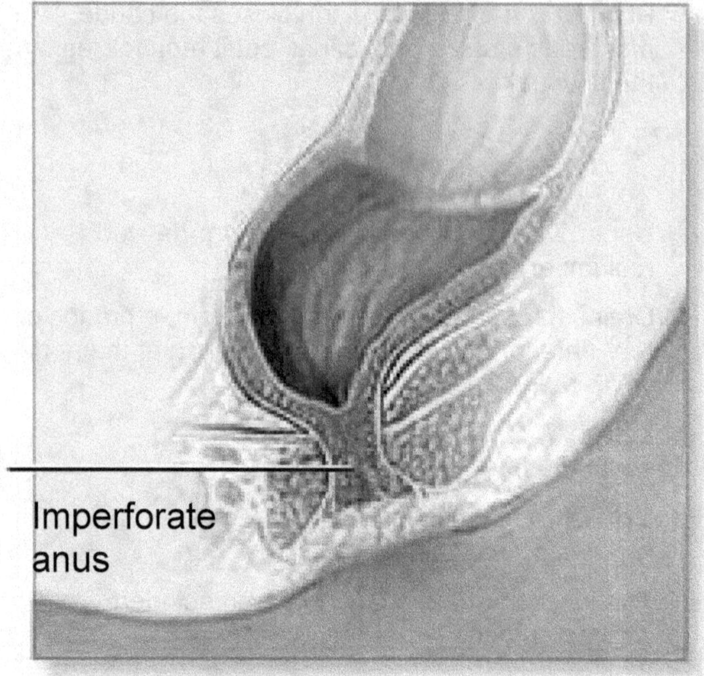

Hirschsprung disease

- Congenital megacolon (aka hirschsprung disease) is due to an absence of parasympathetic ganglia in the bowel wall
- Ganglia are normally derived from neural crest cells
- Mutations in RET gene, a tyrosine kinase receptor involved in crest cell migration, is thought to play a role
- Rectum is usually involved, 80% extend to sigmoid colon, 10-20% extend to transverse colon, & 3% involve the entire colon

ESOPHAGUS

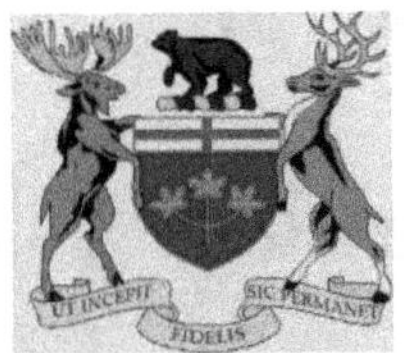

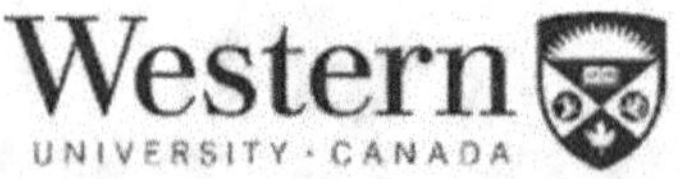
Western
UNIVERSITY · CANADA

Management of Barrett Esophagus and Treatment of GERD

Keith McIntosh

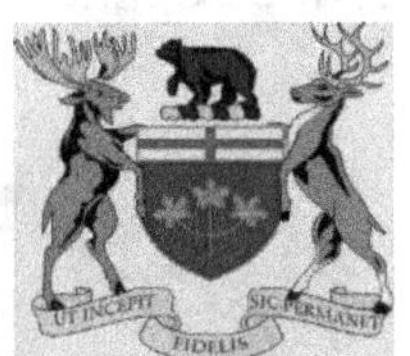

MANAGEMENT OF BARRETT ESOPHAGUS AND TREATMENT OF GERD

- Introduction

  - BE is defined as intestinal metaplasia of the distal esophagus, in which normal squamous epithelium is replaced by columnar epithelium.
  - Compared to the risk in the general population, the relative risk of adenocarcinoma among patients with BE was 11.3 (95% CI, 8.8-14.4), with an annual risk of esophageal adenocarcinoma of 0.12% (95% CI, 0.09-0.15).
  - This risk is much lower than the previously reported figure of 0.5%.
  - Detection of low-grade dysplasia on the index endoscopy was associated with an incidence rate of ~500 / 10^5 person-years.
  - The incidence rate among patients without dysplasia was 100 / 10^5 person-years
  - The progression of BE to ECa is 0.09% per person year, (not 0.5%)

Source: Nvid-Jenson et al. NEJM 2011; 365: 1375-1383 and Wani S, et al. Gastroenterol 2011; 141: 1179-1186.

  - SSIM (subsquamous intestinal metaplasia) can be detected in some patients with BE following long-term treatment with PPIs, and either before or after endoscopically ablation therapy.
  - SSIM may exist in the absence of endoscopically visible columnar epithelium characteristic of BE, or may coexist with endoscopically visible BE.
  - SSIM possesses unique biological properties compared with surface epithelium.

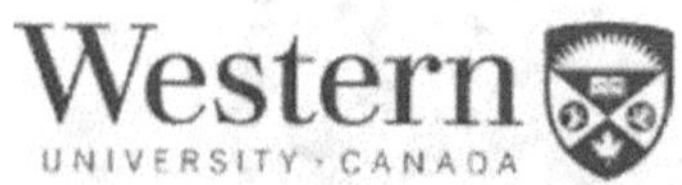

SSIM = Distinct biological properties from BE and normal squamous epithelium:

- Reduced rates of crypt proliferation
- No aneuploidy following PDT
- ↑ KI-67, COX-2, BCL-2 (than squamous epithelium)

Abbreviation: SSIM, subsquamous intestinal metaplasia

Source: Yachimski P, et al. Clin Gastroenterol Hepatol 2012; 10: 220-224.

➢ Molecular biology

- Barrett epithelium (BE) is suspected. Give 4 molecular tests which may suggest the presence of dysplasia.
  - DNA aneuploidy
  - Ki67 (proliferation) – increased expression on immunohistochemistry
  - Oncogenes – cyclin D1, TGFα, EGFR, Rus, B-catenin
  - Tumour suppressors genes
  - Anti-apoptosis genes
  - Anti-senescence markers - telomerase

Printed with permission: Flejou JF. *Best Pract Res Clin Gastroenterol* 2008; 22(4): pg. 680.

➢ Genetics

- Give the differences in the genetics of Familial Barrett esophagus (BE), hereditary diffuse gastric cancer (HDGC) and Tylosis Palmaris

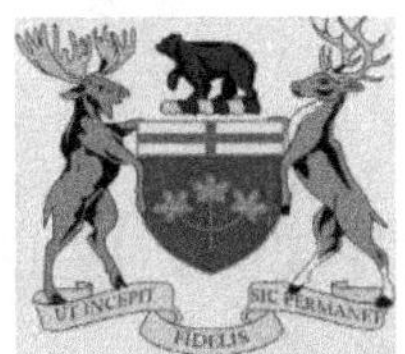

Genetics	Familial Barrett esophagus	Hereditary diffuse gastric cancer	Tylosis Palmaris
○ Pattern of inheritance	– Proposed autosomal dominant with incomplete penetrance	▪ Autosomal dominant	Autosomal dominant
○ Chromosome	– Unknown	▪ Chromosome16q22	Chromosome 17q25
○ Genetic basis	– Linkage analyses ongoing	▪ Mutations in E-cadherin/CDH1 gene	Downregulation of cytoglobin gene
○ Cancer risk	– ~ 30% risk of adenocarcinoma	▪ 70% of lifetime risk of diffuse gastric cancer	40-95% lifetime risk of squamous esophageal cancer
○ Clinical strategies	– Consider family history in assessment of GERD	▪ Genetic testing for CDH1 ▪ Endoscopic surveillance ▪ Prophylactic gastrectomy	Endoscopic surveillance

Abbreviations: BE, Barrett esophagus; GERD, gastroesophageal reflux disease; HDGC, hereditary diffuse gastric cancer

Printed with permission: Robertson E, and Jankowski J. *Am J Gastroenterol* 2008;103: 445.

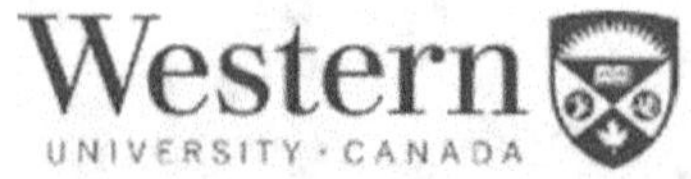

MANAGEMENT OF BARRETT ESOPHAGUS AND TREATMENT OF GERD

- Terminology

The terminology of early neoplastic lesions in Barrett esophagus (BE), using Riddell's and Vienna classification, and clinical consequences

	Terminology
Category 1	Negative for dysplasia
Category 2	Indefinite for dysplasia
Category 3	Low grade dysplasia
Category 4	4.1 High grade dysplasia; 4.2 Non-invasive carcinoma (carcinoma in situ) ; 4.3 Suspicion of invasive carcinoma
Category 5	Invasive neoplasia; intramucosal carcinoma; Submucosal carcinoma or beyond

Abbreviation : BE, Barrett esophagus

Adapted from: Flejou JF. *Best Pract Res Clin Gastroenterol* 2008; 22(4): 679.

- Endoscopy – Barrett esophagus
  - Even with the new high-frequency mini-probes, the accuracy of endoscopic ultrasound (EUS) in distinguishing T1sm (submucosal disease) is only 75-85% (Scotiniotis IA, et al. *Gastrointest Endosc* 2001:689-96.)
  - The multiband mucosectomy devise may be superior to the injection/CAP EMR (endoscopic mucosal resection) method for high grade dysplasia in Barrett epithelium, in terms of procedure time and cost (Pouw RE, et al. *Gastrointest Endosc* 2008; 67:AB75).

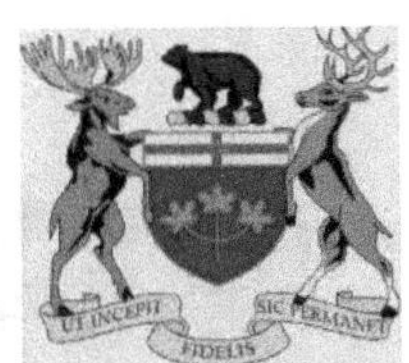

MANAGEMENT OF BARRETT ESOPHAGUS AND TREATMENT OF GERD

- Radiofrequency ablation (RF) with the Hab ablation system give a >90% cure rate for low and high grade dysplasia (LGD, HGD), in flat, non-nodular BE tissue (Waye JD, et al. Gastrointest Endosc. 2010;71(3):551-6.)
- Low pressure spray cryoablation using liquid nitrogen gives premise for modular and non-nodular HGD and early esophageal cancer (Johnston MH, et al. *Gastrointest Endosc* 2005: 62: 842-8)
- The morbidity of esophagectomy includes strictures (20-40%), leaks (3-39%), left recurrent laryngeal nerve paralysis (3-16%), gastroparesis, regurgitation of gastric contents, and mortality of 2-10%.
- Photodynamic therapy (PDT) with porfimer-Na, when exposed to non-thermal red laser light, yields singlet oxygen which results in ischemic necrosis in metaplastic and dysplastic BE
- The complications of PDT include stricture in 40% (8% severe), chest pain, mediastinitis, pleural effusion, chest pain and vomiting
- The 5 year survival rate for EMR alone, or EMR plus PDT for early stage esophageal cancer is 97%, and minimally invasive endoscopic therapies may be comparable to esophagectomy for early stage esophageal cancer (ASGE Technology Committee. *Gastrointest Endosc* 2008: 11-18.; Das A, et al. *Am J Gastroenterol* 2008:1340-5.)

Abbreviations: EMR, endoscopic mucosal resection; EUS, endoscopic ultrasound; HGD, high grade dysplasia; LGD, low grade dysplasia; PDT, photodynamic therapy; RF, radiofrequency ablation

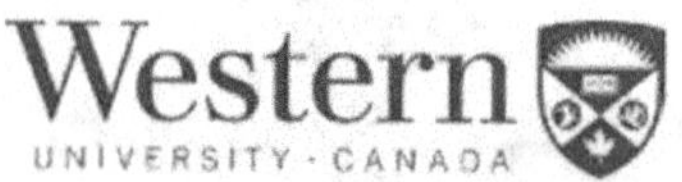

- Pathology

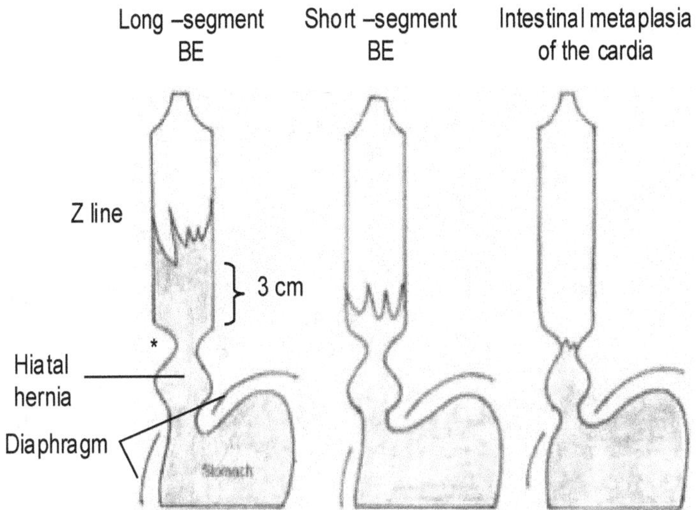

- Patients with long segment or short segment Barrett esophagus have salmon-coloured mucosa extending up into the tubular esophagus
- Biopsy shows intestinal metaplasia with goblet cells
- If intestinal metaplasia with goblet cells is found at a normally located zig zag line (Z line), the patient has intestinal metaplasia of the cardia, which confers a lower cancer risk.

*End of tubular esophagus and beginning of stomach.

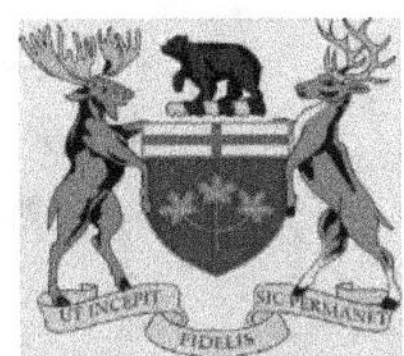

T and N staging of high grade dysplasia and esopgageal cancer

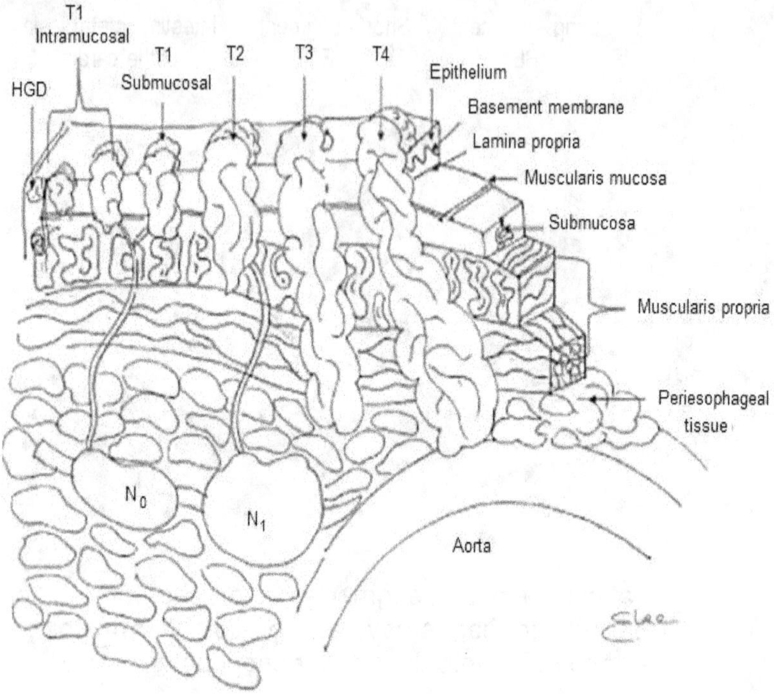

T1 Intramucosal
HGD
T1 Submucosal
T2
T3
T4
Epithelium
Basement membrane
Lamina propria
Muscularis mucosa
Submucosa
Muscularis propria
Periesophageal tissue
N_0
N_1
Aorta

Abbeviation: HDG, high grade dysolasia

Adapted from: Mayo GI, Figure 7, page 31.

"We have the intelligence; we often have all of the technologies. But do we have the collective capabilities?"
Sir David King

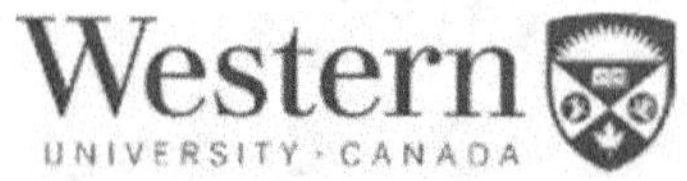

MANAGEMENT OF BARRETT ESOPHAGUS AND TREATMENT OF GERD

- Decreased incidence of Dysplasia with Use of PPIs

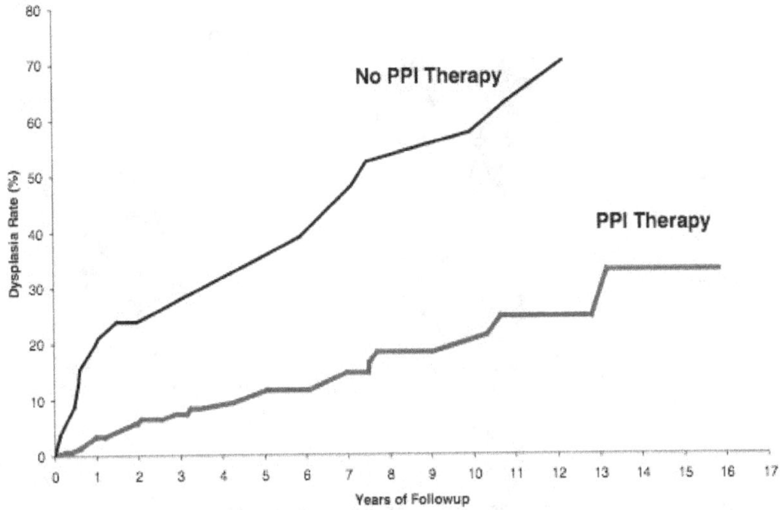

Printed with permission: El Serag HB et al. Am J Gastroenterology 2004; 99:1877-1883.

- Incidence of Dysplasia / Adenocarcinoma in Barrett Esophagus

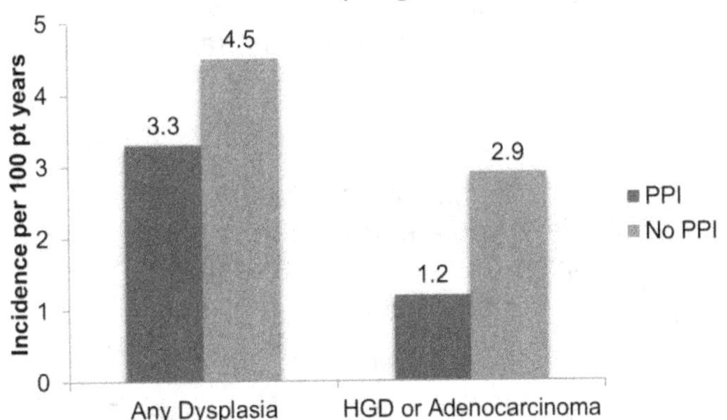

Printed with permission: Nguyen DM et al. Clin Gastro Hepatol 2009;7:1299-1304

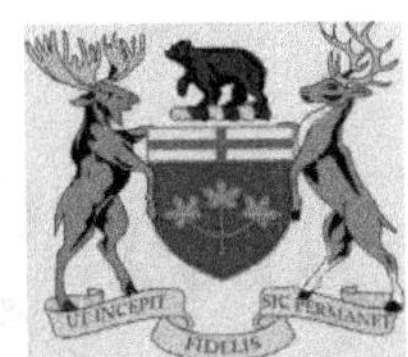

MANAGEMENT OF BARRETT ESOPHAGUS AND TREATMENT OF GERD

- Rate of Adenocarcinoma in BE by Treatment Type

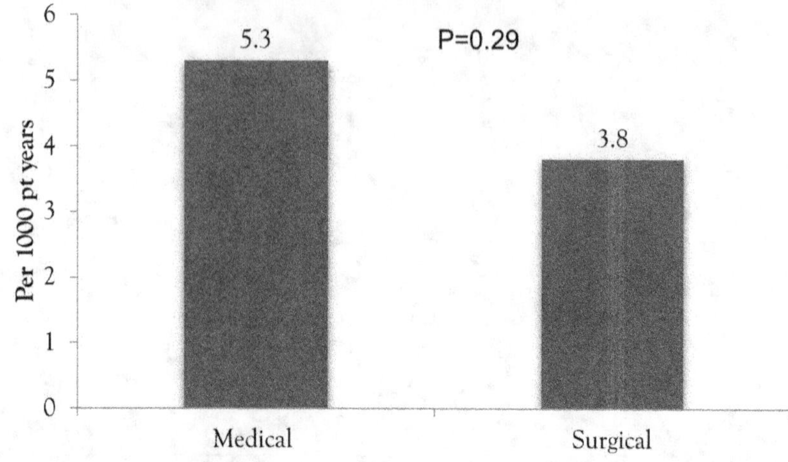

Printed with permission: Corey K et al. Am J Gastroenterology. 2003; 98:11 2390-4.

- Surveillance
  - 2 Major questions:
    - Does Barrett Esophagus reduce survival?
    - Does Surveillance decrease mortality?

" .... surround yourself with the best people. If you are one of the smartest people in the room, its's time to find another room."

Rick Mercer

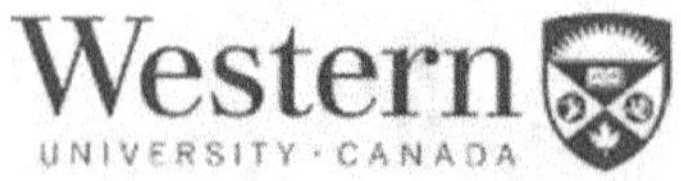

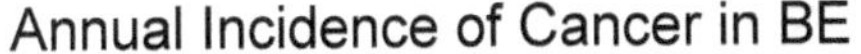

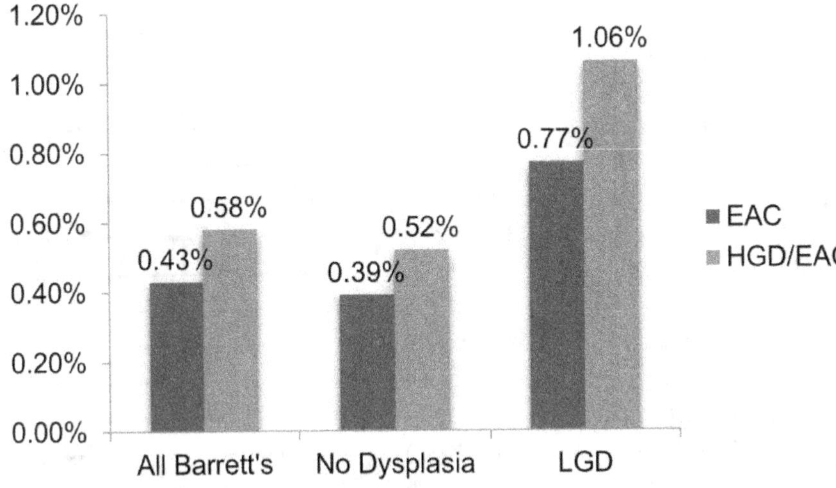

Printed with permission: De Jonge PJ et al. Gut 2010; 59:1030

Annual Incidence of Cancer with LGD

- Incidence of HGD and EAC in Patients with BE have LGD

Diagnosis	No. of incident cases	Incidence rate (%/y) (95% CI)	Mean (SD) time to development (y), range
HGD	21	1.6 (1.05–2.46)	2.86 (4.22), 0.18–10.07
EAC	6	0.44 (0.2–0.98)	4.41 (1.49), 3.34–7.05
HGD/EAC	24	1.83 (1.23–2.74)	3.08 (2.57), 0.18–18.67

Printed with permission: Wani S et al. Gastroenterology 2011; 141:1179-1186

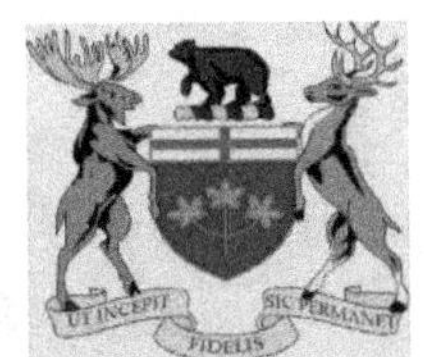

Barrett Esophagus: Mortality

Study (year)	Incidence rate (95% CI)
Spechler (1984)	2.9 (0.1, 15.9)
Cameron (1985)	1.1 (0.03, 6.3)
Robertson (1988)	0.0 (0.0, 18.5)
Miros (1991)	6.9 (0.8, 25.0)
Iftikhar (1992)	2.2 (0.05, 12.1)
Drewitz (1997)	1.2 (0.03, 6.7)
Katz (1998)	3.6 (0.4, 12.8)
MacDonald (2000)	4.8 (1.0, 13.9)
Eckardt (2001)	0.0 (0.0, 5.0)
Conio (2001)	1.7 (0.04, 9.5)
Rana (2001)	4.8 (0.6, 17.3)
Conio (2003)	2.7 (0.6, 8.0)
Anderson (2003)	1.6 (0.8, 2.8)
Hage (2004)	3.0 (0.8, 7.7)
Dulai (2005)	1.1 (0.2, 3.2)
Solaymani-Dodaran (2005)	5.0 (2.7, 8.5)
Gladman (2006)	0.9 (0.02, 5.2)
Cook (2007)	2.5 (1.3, 4.2)
Moayyedi (2008)	4.4 (2.8, 6.5)
Overall	3.0 (2.3, 3.9)

1 2 5

Fatal EAC incidence rate per 1,000 yrs

Printed with permission: Sikkema M et al. Clin Gastro & Hepatol 2010; 8:235-44.

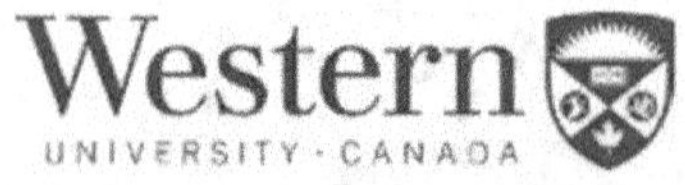

- Mortality for Barrett Esophagus

Mortalty in BE patients: causes of death in patients with BE

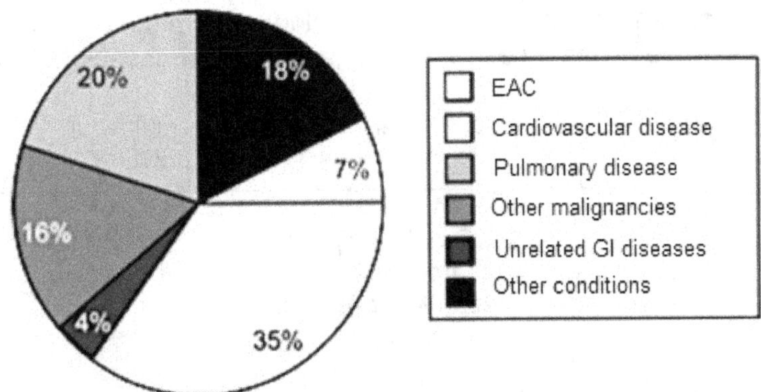

Printed with permission: Sikkema M et al. Clin Gastro & Hepatol 2010; 8:235-44.

Important observations

- Low rate of progression to HGD / Adenocarcinoma
- BE has a risk of adenocarcinoma and mortality, although this risk is likely substantially less than previously thought (1 per 1000 patient years)
- Most mortality in BE patients is due to other common diseases as patients are often elderly

- Surveillance
- Give who is at high risk for Barrett esophagus?
  - GERD symptoms > 10 yrs, 3 times per week, severe symptoms
  - Family history of BE

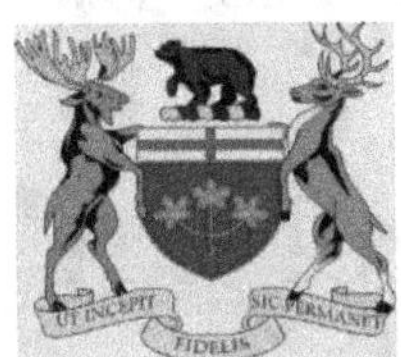

MANAGEMENT OF BARRETT ESOPHAGUS AND TREATMENT OF GERD

- Give an outline of suggested recommendations for endoscopic surveillance of persons with Barrett esophagus (BE).

American College of Gastroenterology recommendations for surveillance by esophageal gastroduodenoscopy (EGD)

Dysplasia	Documentation	Follow-up EGD
○ None (metaplasia)	2 EGDs with biopsy (4 quadrant, q 2 cm, separate jars), confirm by two expert pathologists	3 - 5 years
○ LGD	Repeat EGD with biopsy, when erosive esophagitis healed, confirm by two expert pathologists, confirm with #3 EGD plus biopsies to exclude HED/EMC	q 1 year until no dysplasia
○ HGD – Focal (<5 crypts)	Repeat EGD with biopsy to rule out cancer/document HGD expert pathologist confirmation	q 3 months
○ HGD – Multifocal (>5 crypts)	Radiofrequency ablation, PDT, cryosurgery, EMR, esophagectomy in surgical candidate	

Abbreviations: BE, Barrett epithelium; EGD, esophageal gastroduodenoscopy; EMR, endoscopic mucosal resection; EUS, endoscopic ultrasound; GERD, gastroesophageal reflux disease; HGD, high grade dysplasia; LGD, low grade dysplasia; PDT, photodynamic therapy

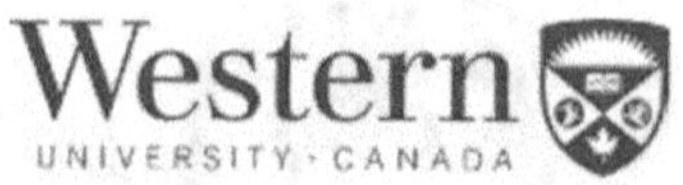

- Endoscopic therapy

Does surveillance alter outcome in BE

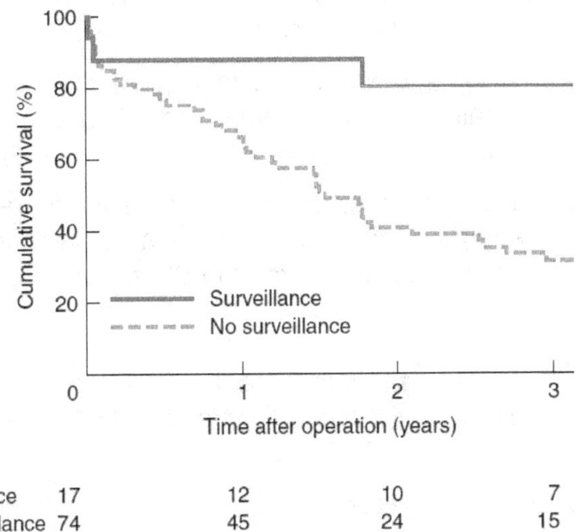

Postoperative survival in patients who did or did not have endoscopic surveillance for Barrett esophagus

Printed with permission: Fountoulakis A et al. Br J Surg 2004; 91:997-1003.

Characteristics	Survival (months)	Univariate P value	Multivariate HR (95% CI)
○ No EGD	7		1
○ EGD	11	0.001	0.66 (0.47-0.93)
○ No BE	7		1
○ BE	15	0.001	0.45 (0.25-0.80)

Printed with permission: Cooper GS et al. Am J Gastroenterology 2009;104:1356-1362

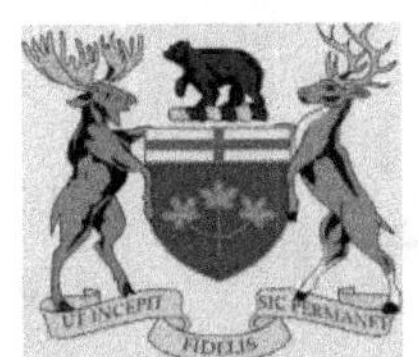

Conclusions on BE and surveillance

- Observational studies have demonstrated that surveillance detects earlier stage cancers, and may have improved survival
- This is subject to significant lead time bias so it still remains unclear whether surveillance is beneficial at all
- "It is **not possible** to make meaningful recommendations regarding the optimal intervals between endoscopic procedures" AGA Positon Statement

➢ Treatment

- Give 6 endoscopic therapies for Barrett esophagus (BE) with high grade dysplasia (HGD) or early mucosal cancer (EMC).
  - Nd: YAG laser
  - Argon plasma coagulation (APC)
  - Photodynamic therapy (PDT) with porfimer or 5-aminolevulinic acid (5-ALA)
  - Radiofrequency ablation (RFA)
  - Cryotherapy
  - Endoscopic mucosal resection (EMR)
  - Endoscopic submucosal resection (ESR)
  - Esophagectomy in surgical candidate

Abbreviations: 5-ALA, 5-aminolevulinic acid; APC, argon plasma coagulation; BE, Barrett esophagus; EMC, early mucosal cancer; HGD, high grade dysplasia.

Printed with permission: Curvers WL, Kiesslich R, Bergman JJ. *Best Prac Res Clin Gastroenterol* 2008; 22(4):687-720.

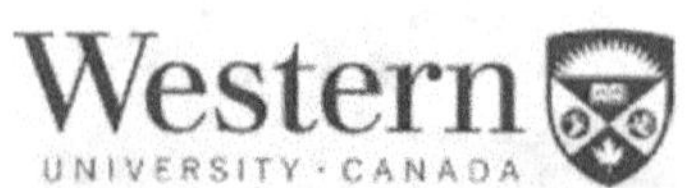

- Give the management of antiplatelets and anticoagulant use before / after EMR.
  - General
    - Avoid aspirin and all nonsteroidal anti inflammatory medications for the next 2 weeks
    - Advise patients to monitor for symptoms of overt gastrointestinal bleeding, consider prophylactic deployment of hemostatic clips to secure hemostasis, although this is unproven.
  - Warfarin
    - Stop Warfarin 5 days before the EMR
    - An INR level less than 1.5 is used as an arbitrary cut off value to proceed with EMR
    - Resume Warfarin 24 hours after the procedure with the usual daily dose
    - Check INR levels 1 week later to ensure adequate anticoagulation
    - In patients deemed to be at high risk of thrombosis, Warfarin cessation is bridged with low molecular weight heparin
  - Clopidogrel
    - Discontinue Clopidogrel 7 days before endoscopy
      In patients with high risk cardiac conditions, cessation of Clopidogrel is performed after discussion with the cardiologist; this may entail deferring the EMR, where feasible, until a suitable time period after the insertion of coronary stents

Abbreviation: INR, international normalized ratio

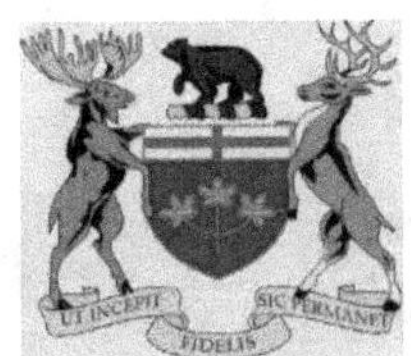

Printed with permission: Namasivayam et al. Clin Gastro Hep 2010;8:743-754.

- Prevention

ASA / NSAIDS for Prevention of Adenocarcinoma in BE

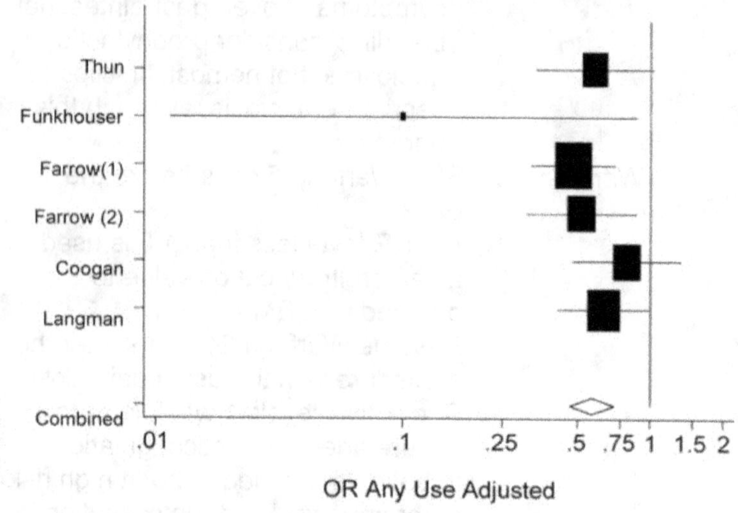

Printed with permission: Corley D et al. Gastroenterology 2003;124:47-56

Conclusions on BE and medical treatment of GERD

- Reflux symptoms with PPI therapy to ensure symptom relief and endoscopic healing of esophagitis.
- Treatment with PPI in BE may reduce the risk of dysplasia
- Consider ASA in GERD patients who would otherwise warrant treatment for cardiovascular reasons

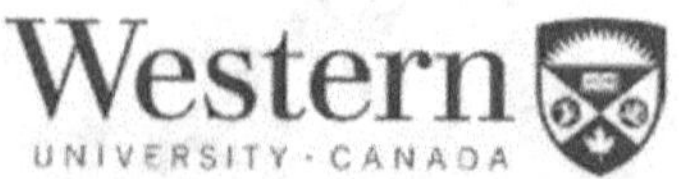

- Unanswered Questions
  - No controlled studies looking at BID vs. OD dosing of PPIs
  - If there are no symptoms or signs of reflux, do you still need anti reflux therapy?

Management options of High Grade Dysplasia

- Endoscopic Therapies:
  - Ablative techniques: Cryotherapy, APC, RFA, PDT
  - EMR
- Esophagectomy

Abbreviations: APC, argon plasma coagulation; RFA, radiofrequency ablation; PDT, photodynamic surgery; EMR, endoscopic mucosal resection

Radiofrequency Ablation (RFA)

- Balloon-based circumferential array of closely spaced electrodes to deliver radiofrequency energy to esophageal mucosa
- Also a smaller endoscope-mounted RFA catheter ablation device for focal ablation

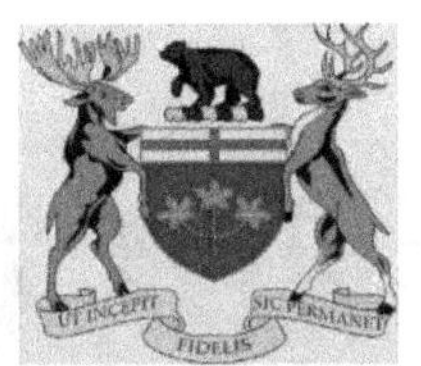

- Efficacy

Two- and Three-Year Outcomes of the AIM Dysplasia Trial

	CE-IM (entire cohort)		CE-D (HGD cohort)		CE-D (LGD cohort)	
	n	%	n	%	n	%
Year 2	99/106	93	50/54	95	51/52	98
Year 3	51/56	91	23/24	96	32/32	100

CE-IM and CE-D, allowing for interim focal touch-up RFA.

Printed with permission: Shaheen et al. Gastroenterology 2011; 141:460-468

Photodynamic therapy (PDT)

- Uses photosensitizer which in presence of light produces cytotoxicity
- Porfimer (Photofrin) IV approved by FDA. 5-ALA may be coming
- Typically use red laser light at 630 nm with a balloon diffuser
- PDT – Efficacy
  - 208 patients with HGD followed up 3.5 years
  - Complications: Strictures developed in 36% of PDT patients

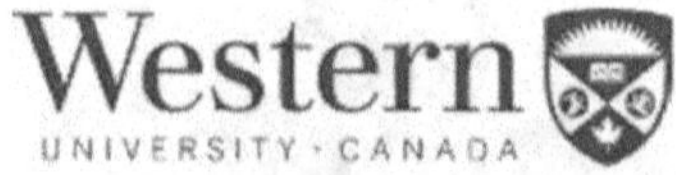

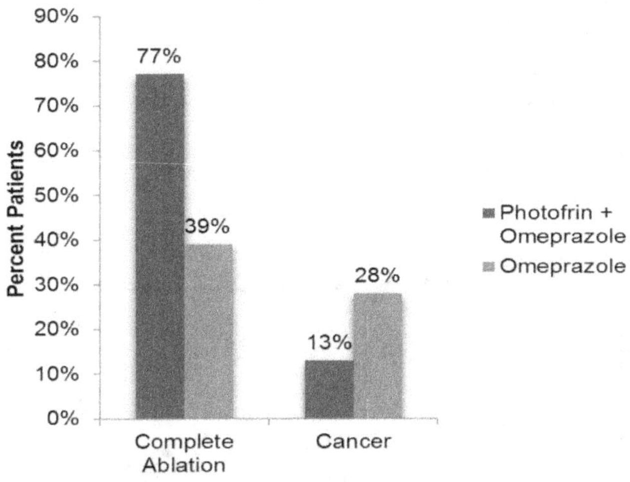

Printed with permission: Overholt BF. Gastrointestinal Endoscopy 2005; 62:488-98

Endoscopic Mucosal Resection (EMR)

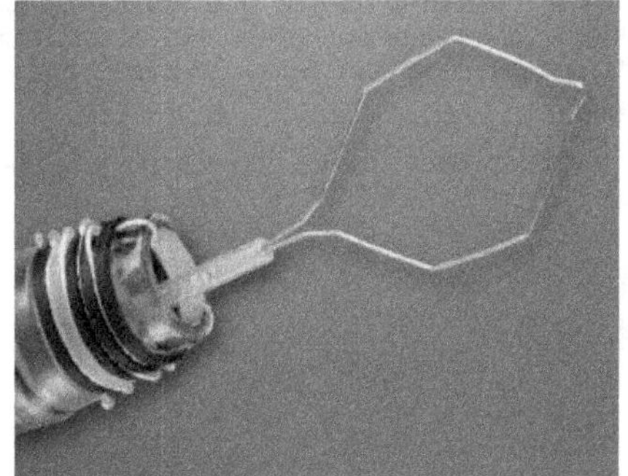

- Diathermic snare or endoscopic knife is used to remove Barrett metaplasia down to the submucosal
- Get a large tissue specimen that can be used to assess depth

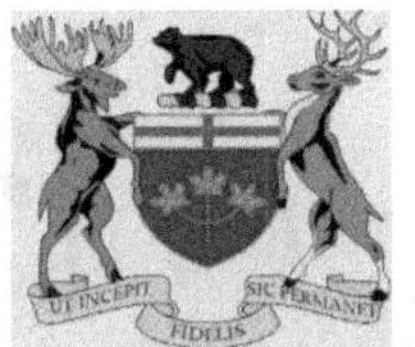

MANAGEMENT OF BARRETT ESOPHAGUS AND TREATMENT OF GERD

of involvement and adequacy of resection

- EMR – Efficacy

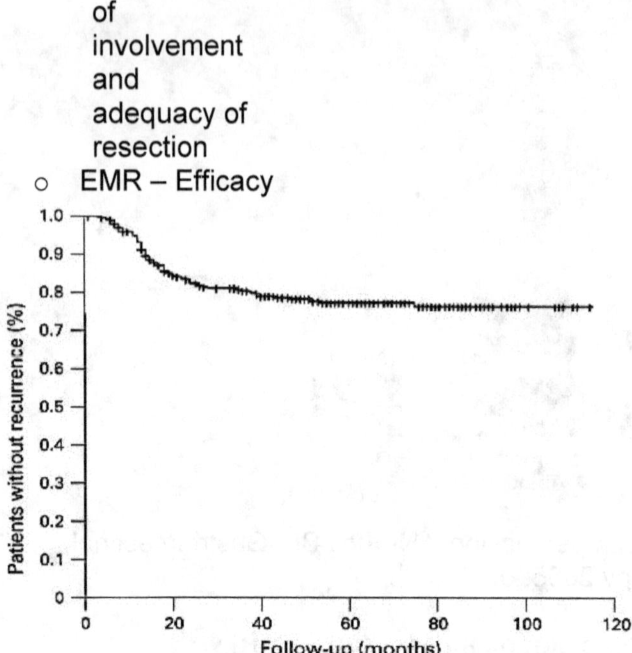

Kaplan–Meier plot for estimating the tumour freedom in 349 patients with high-grade intraepithelial neoplasia and early adenocarcinoma in Barrett's oesophagus treated with endoscopic therapy.

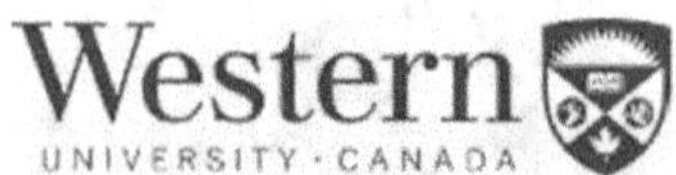

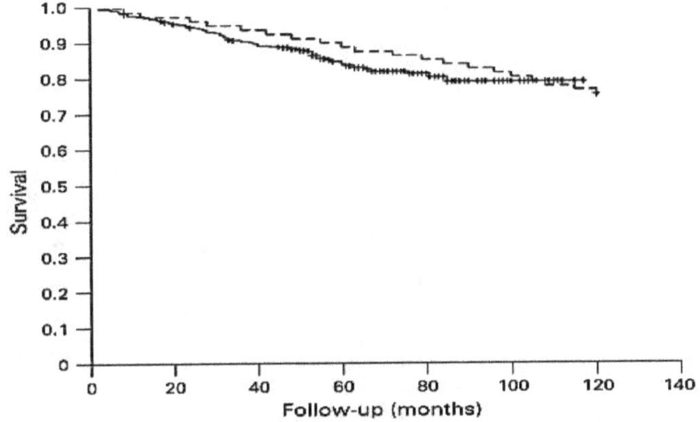

Kaplan–Meier plot for estimating the overall survival compared to the average German population with matched gender and age (dashed line) (p = not significant).

Printed with permission: Pech O et al. Gut 2008; 57:1200-6.

Conclusions on Endoscopic Therapies in BE

- Endoscopic therapy with PDT and RFA is superior to PPIs alone for preventing progression from HGD to cancer in BE
- RFA may have a better safety profile and is easier to administer than PDT
- Cohort studies have shown excellent long term survival rates for HGD treated with EMR

Esophagectomy

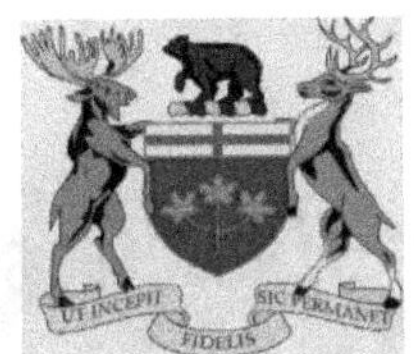

MANAGEMENT OF BARRETT ESOPHAGUS AND TREATMENT OF GERD

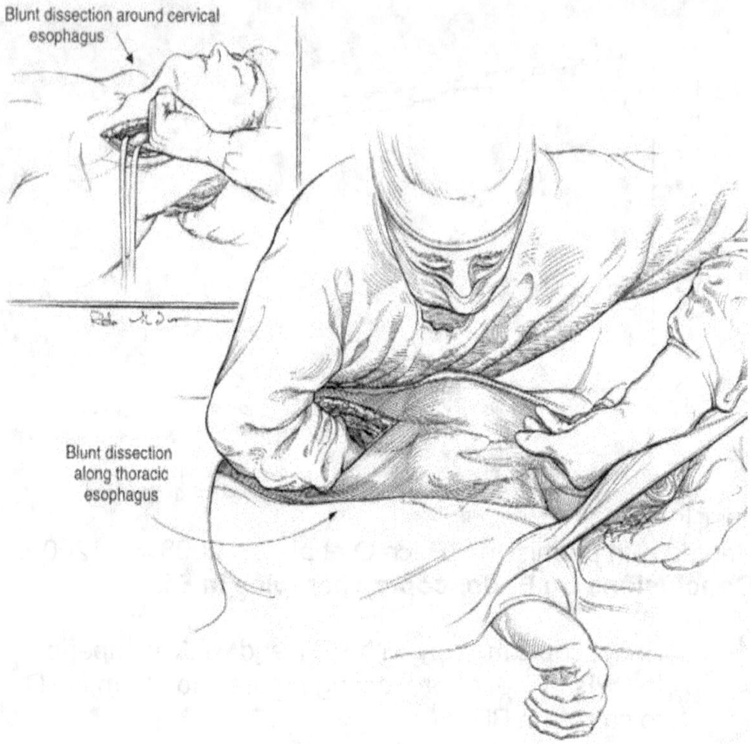

Blunt dissection around cervical esophagus

Blunt dissection along thoracic esophagus

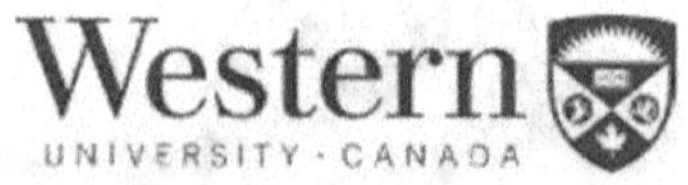

- PROS
  - Definitive removing all tissue at risk of malignancy
  - Provides a specimen for examination
  - Can assess local lymph nodes
  - Minimally invasive techniques being increasingly described
- CONS
  - High rate of morbidity & mortality
  - Long term complications include:
    - Dysphagia
    - Weight Loss
    - GERD
    - Dumping

➢ Factors Affecting Esophagectomy Mortality

	No. of hospitals	Patients	Actual mortality*
Cancer specialization			
National cancer institutions	12	310	13 (4.2%)
Community hospitals	13	30	4 (13.3%)
P value			0.05
Esophagectomy volume			
≥ 5 cases / y	5	266	8 (3.0%)
< 5 cases / y	20	74	9 (12.2%)
P value			0.004
Total operative volume			
≥ 3333 cases / y	10	263	12 (4.6%)
< 333 cases / y	15	77	5 (6.5%)
P value			NS
Hospital size			
≥ 600 beds	12	176	12 (6.8%)
< 600 beds	13	164	5 (3.0 %)
P value			NS

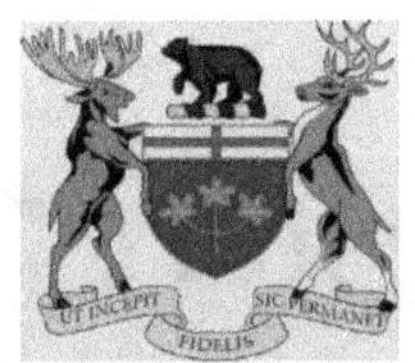

Printed with permission: Swisher SG et al. J Thorac Cardiovasc Surg 2000; 119:1126

Decision factors for esophagectomy vs. endoscopic management

	Favours Esophagectomy	Favours RFA/EMR
o Age	Younger	Older
o Life Expectancy	Longer	Shorter
o Extent of Metaplasia	Widespread	Limited
o Experience	Experienced surgeon	Experience endoscopist
o Risk Tolerance	Cancer Phobic	Surgery Phobic
o LN involvement	+	-

- Esophagectomy is a reasonable option for the treatment of BE-HGD but does carry high rate of morbidity if not performed in a high volume centre
- Endoscopic treatments for BE-HGD are effective, at least in the short term.

Should we treat LGD (Non Dysplastic BE)

Reasons to Treat	Reasons not to Treat
o Inability to predict who will progress to HGD/adenocarcinoma	- Low risk to actually progress to adenocarcinoma
o Inability to predict time course of progression	- No evidence treating LGD actually decreases long term mortality
o Risk of understaging due to inadequate sampling	- Risk of complications from treatment

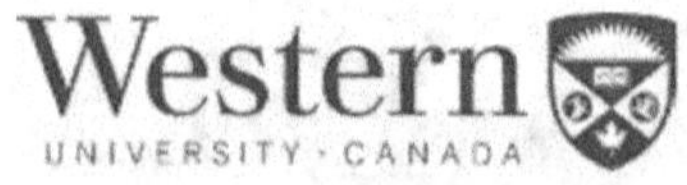

- Relieve patient anxiety of having a premalignant condition
  - May bury areas of Barrett under the ablated tissue

Treating LGD

- Ablative therapies can successfully eradicate BE / LGD
- It is not clear that this ablation reduces cancer risk and warrants the risks and substantial expense of ablative procedures.
- Thus, at present, there is limited evidence for ablating non dysplastic or LGD in BE
- ↑ risk with use of PPIs (or odds ratio)

	OR
– C.difficile infection	
▪ Incident	1.7
▪ Recurrent	2.5
– CAP / HCAP	1.27
– Fractures	
▪ Hip*	1.30
▪ Spine	1.56
▪ All sites	1.16

* Hazard ratio was higher in current and former smokers, 1.51.

Abbreviations: CAP, community acquired pneumonia; HCAP, healthcare associated pneumonia

- While there is an ↑ relative risk of metabolic bone disease in persons who used PPI > 2 years, the absolute ↑ risk was small:

Absolute risk of hip fractures per 1000 person-years

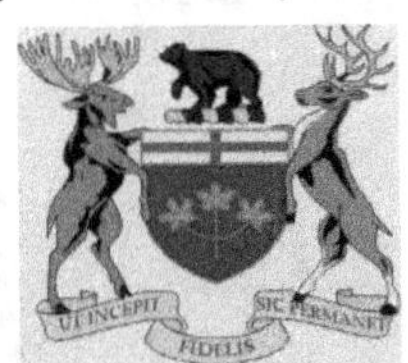

PPI non-users	Regular PPI users
1.51	2.02

- Give the influence of H. pylori infection on the PPI-associated risk of developing atrophic gastritis (gastric atrophy; atrophy of gastric glands) in the body of the stomach.

    - PPI user and annual incidence of atrophy of the mucosa of the gastric body

        - H. pylori
            - Negative 0.7
            - Positive 4.7

    Thus, practically (clinically speaking), the risk of gastric atrophy resulting from the long-term use of PPIs occurs mainly in persons who are H. pylori positive.

Risk of Longterm PPI

The malabsorption of iron and vitamin B12 in persons taking PPIs chronically may not necessarily be clinically significant. However, the malabsorption of calcium and reduction in osteoclastic activity with PPIS is associated with an ↑ risk of osteopenia and osteoporosis.

- Give the physiological explanation why some cardiac patients with congestive heart failure who are chronically taking PPIs require monitoring of their serum magnesium concentration.

    - PPIs lower the serum concentration, as also do diuretics and digoxin, placing persons consuming

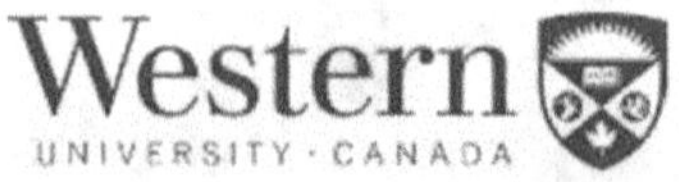

these medications at risk of the adverse effects of hypomagnesemia.

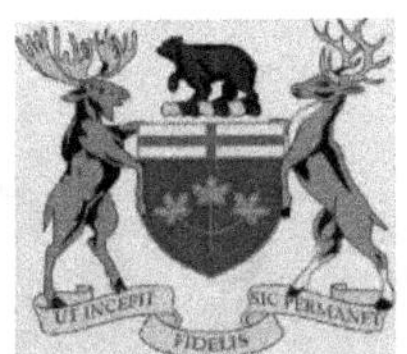

MANAGEMENT OF BARRETT ESOPHAGUS AND TREATMENT OF GERD

- Give 8 potential risks of long-term PPI therapy.

	Risk magnitude/possible consequence
➢ Associated with hypergastrinemia	
○ Hypergastrinemia-induced carcinoid tumours	- Not demonstrated in humans
○ Accelerated progression of atrophic gastritis/gastric cancer with concomitant *H. pylori* gastritis	- No documentation of an increase in atrophic gastritis and no basis to recommend testing or treatment for *H Pylori* before long-term PP use
○ Formation of gastric fundic gland polyps	- Odds ratio of 2.2 for developing Fundic gland polyps within 1-5 years, negligible, if any, risk of dysplasia - Some patients show decreased vitamin B_{12} levels after years of acid inhibition, case reports (2) of clear deficiency
➢ Malabsorption	
○ Vitamin B_{12} malabsorption	- Nested case-control study of UK patients older than 50 years; adjusted odds ration of 1.44 (95% confidence interval, 1.30-1.59) of hip fracture with PPI use longer than 1 year
○ Calcium Malabsorption	

	Risk magnitude/possible consequence
○ Iron malabsorption	– Poor response to oral iron supplement absorption in 2 iron-deficient individuals improved after cessation of Omeprazole; no clear clinical relevance
○ Increased risk of *C difficile* colitis	– PPI use is independent risk of *C difficile* diarrhea in antibiotic users, odds ratio of 2.1 (95% confidence interval, 1.2-3.5)
○ Increased risk of community-acquired or nosocomial pneumonia (presumably aspiration)	– Nested case-control analysis, adjusted odds ratio for pneumonia with PPI use of 1.73 (95% confidence interval, 1.33-2.25)

- ○ Drug-drug interactions; PPIs metabolized by cytochrome P450 and may induce or inhibit drug metabolism (phenytoin, warfarin, Plavix®)
- ○ Possible increased risk of gastric cancer theoretical consideration: Gastric colonization with bacteria that convert nitrates to carcinogenic *N*-nitroso compounds that then reflux

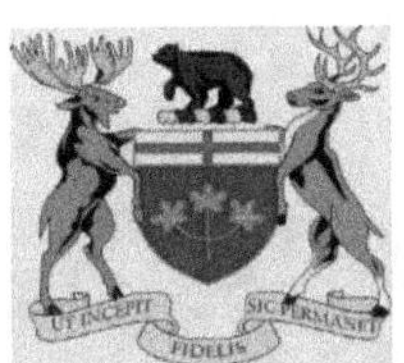

	Risk magnitude/possible consequence
o Cancer	– Data on PPI use and increased gastric *N*-nitrosamine remain uncertain and the risk of cancer is speculative
	– Based on 345 accidental exposures compared with 787 controls, no observed increased teratogenicity
o Safety in pregnancy (Omeprazole crosses placenta and is pregnancy safety category C; other PPIs are category B)	– Clinically significant PPI drug-drug interactions are rare (<1/million prescriptions); clinical significance of some PPIs reducing effectiveness of Plavix is uncertain
o Collagenous colitis	– Few case reports with lansoprazole
o Anaphylaxis	
o Acute interstitial nephritis	– 64 cases worldwide, partially reversible (one case requires dialysis, no deaths), estimated risk 1/12,500 patient-years of therapy)
o Pancreatitis	

Printed with permission: AGA Technical Review. *GE* 2008;135: pg. 1392-1413.

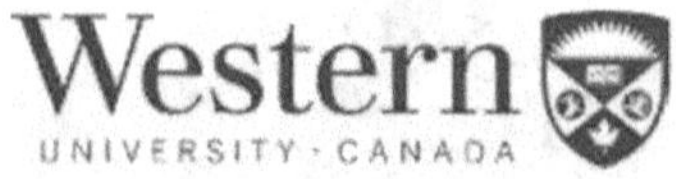

GERD Treatment in Pregnancy

- Give the FDA category for the safety of drugs used to treat GERD in pregnancy and recommendations for breast-feeding.

Drugs	FDA category	Recommendations for breast-feeding
➢ *Antacids*		
○ Aluminum-, calcium or magnesium-containing antacids	None	Most are safe for use during pregnancy and for aspiration prophylaxis during labour because of minimal absorption Avoid long-term, high-dose therapy in pregnancy
○ Magnesium trisilicates	None	Not safe for use in pregnancy as cause fluid overload and metabolic alkalosis
○ Sodium bicarbonates	None	No teratogenecity in animals. Generally regarded as acceptable for human use because of minimal absorption
➢ *Mucosal protectant*		
○ Sucralfate	B	A prospective, controlled study suggests acceptable for use in humans

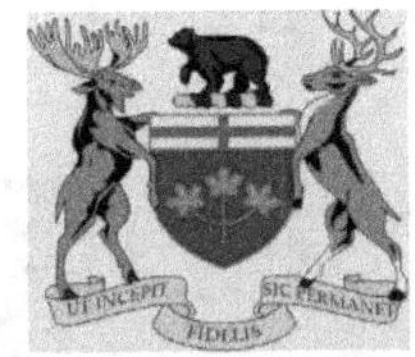

MANAGEMENT OF BARRETT ESOPHAGUS AND TREATMENT OF GERD

Drugs	FDA category	Recommendations for breast-feeding
➢ *Histamine2-receptor antagonists (H2RA)*		
○ Cimetidine	B	Same as above. Ranitidine is the only H2RA whose efficacy during pregnancy has been established
○ Ranitidine	B	Same as cimetidine, but paucity of safety data in humans
○ Famotidine	B	Not recommended during pregnancy. In animals, spontaneous abortion, congenital malformations, low birth weight and fewer live births have been reported. Little data in humans.
○ Nizatidine	B	
➢ *Promotility agents*		
○ Cisapride	C	Embryotoxic and fetotoxic in animals. Prospective controlled study in human suggest acceptable in pregnancy, but was removed because of cardiac arrhythmias

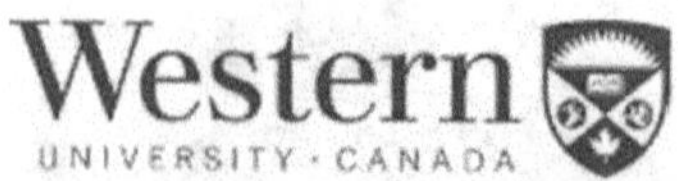

Drugs	FDA category	Recommendations for breast-feeding
○ Metoclopramide	B	No teratogenic effects in animals or humans reported Embryotoxic and fetotoxic in animals. Case reports in human suggest similar concerns. Possible cardiac damage.
➤ *Proton-pump inhibitors*		
○ Omeprazole	**C**	For all PPIs, no teratogenicity or harm, but only limited human pregnancy data
○ Lansoprazole	B	
○ Rabeprazole	B	
○ Pantoprazole	B	
○ Esomeprazole	B	

Printed with permission: Ali RAR, and Egan LJ. *Best Pract Res Clin Gastroenterol* 2007;21: 799-803.

- GER-related cough may be a diagnosis of exclusion. Name 6 conditions that must be excluded before considering the diagnosis of GER-related cough.
  - No exposure to environmental irritants
  - Not a present smoker
  - Not on an ACE inhibitor
  - Normal or stable chest radiograph
  - No symptomatic asthma (i.e. cough not improved on therapy, or negative methacholine inhalation challenge test)

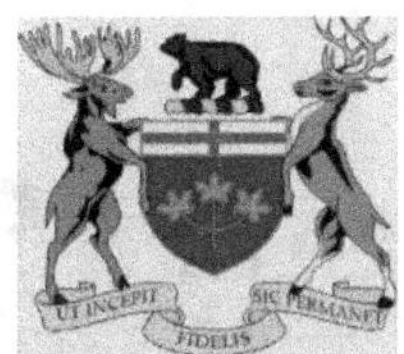

- No upper airway cough syndrome due to rhinosinus diseases ruled out (i.e. cough not improved by first generation H_1-receptor antagonists and 'silent' sinusitis ruled out)
- No non-asthmatic eosinophilic bronchitis (i.e. sputum studies negative or cough not improved by inhaled/systemic corticosteroids)

Abbreviations: ACE, angiotensin-converting enzyme; GER, gastroesophageal reflux

Printed with permission: Chandra KM and Harding SM. *Nat Clin Pract Gastroenterol Hepatol* November 2007;4(11): 606.

- Give the empiric medical trial for GER-related cough.

➢ Medications

- Twice daily PPIs 30-60 minutes before breakfast and dinner
- Consider adding a prokinetic agent initially if dysphagia is present or if cough does not improve with PPI
- Assess response to therapy within 1-3 months
- Lifestyle modifications (please see question 10, page 20)

➢ Further testing, as indicated by initial response

Abbreviations: GER, gastroesophageal reflux; PPI, proton pump inhibitor

Adapted from: Chandra KM and Harding SM. *Nat Clin Pract Gastroenterol Hepatol* 2007; 4(11): 606.

- Give 5 indications for open or laparoscopic surgical fundoplication in the patient with GERD.

- GERD symptoms responding to PPI, (penalty for failure of PPI as an indication)
- Intolerance to PPIs
- Cost of PPIs
- Patient preference, desire for a "cure"
- Persistent large volume regurgitation
- Large symptomatic hiatus hernia
- Respiratory complications from recurrent aspiration
- Recurrent peptic strictures in a young person

Abbreviations: GERD, gastroesophageal reflux disease; PPI, proton pump inhibitor

- Give 5 etiologies of benign, non-GERD related esophageal strictures.
  - Congenital—strictures, atresia
  - Drugs and chemicals—radiation, caustic, chemical, thermal, quinidine gluconate
  - Webs, rings
  - Sclerotherapy
  - Acid and non-acid causes of esophagitis
  - Surgery--complicated reflux strictures (NG tube, ZE syndrome), ischemia, anastomotic (staples)
  - Iatrogenic - EMR for BE, prolonged NG tube, therapy, PDT

Abbreviations: BE, Barrett epithelium; EMR, endoscopic mucosal resection; NG, nasogastric tube; PDT, photodynamic therapy; ZE, Zollinger-Ellison syndrome

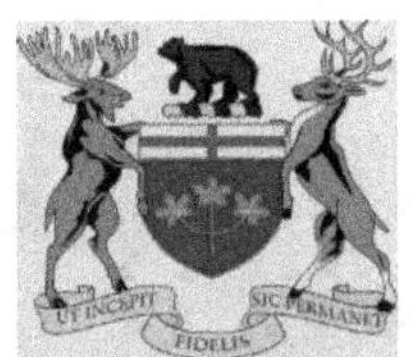

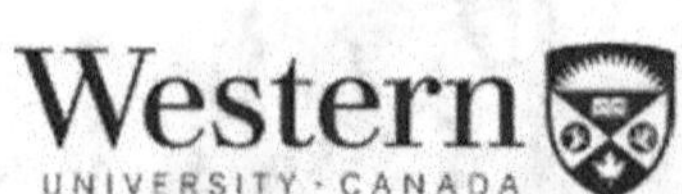

Doc , I Can't Swallow

Mohammed Aljawad

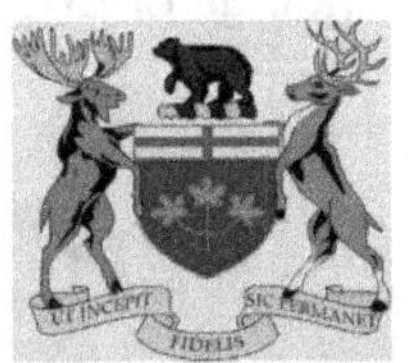

- Definition of EoE
  - Chronic, immune/antigen-mediated esophageal disease characterized
    - Clinically by symptoms related to esophageal dysfunction
    - Histologically by eosinophil-predominant inflammation

Source: Updated Consensus Recommendations; Liacouras CA, et al. J Allergy Clin Immunol. 2011; 128(1): 3-20.

- Demography
  - Incidence/prevelance of EoE – is it increase incidence or increase awareness
  - Esophgeal biopsies were reviewed in two periods to compare eosinophil infiltration
  - 1980-88 : 247 Bx from 188 subjects >> 62 subjects had esophageal disease
  - 2001-02 : 811 Bx from 322 subjects >> 132 subjects had esophageal disease
  - No change in number of esophageal eosinophils from 1980 until 2002, but steady increase from 2002 to the present, suggesting no change in EoE (> 15 Eo / hpf)
  - About 75% of persons with EoE are Caucasian

Abbreviation: hpf, high power field

Source: Lee JJ, et al. J Pediatr Gastroenterol Nutr. 2009; 48(1): 37-40.
2000 to 2007: Children and Adults

Bottom line: EoE is a New Disease

- ↑ barium swallows - No reports of characteristic barium swallow findings of EoE documented in old literature

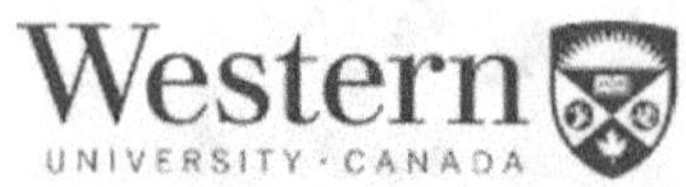

- ↑ EGDs and biopsies – No change in distribution of esophageal Eosinophils overtime
- Not likely ↑ awareness, but likely a true ↑ incidence of EoE
- Associated with ↑ incidence of other allergic conditions

➢ Diagnostic guideline (combination of clinical and pathological findings)

- Clinical
  - Symptoms of esophageal dysfunction
- Pathological
  - 15 eosinophils/hpf in the middle portion of the esophagus
- Exclude other causes of esophageal eosinophilia
- Response to treatment
  - No response to PPIs (persistence of eosinophils)
  - Dietary exclusion
  - Topical corticosteroids

Abbreviation: hpf, high power (microscopic) field

Source: Liacouras CA, et al. J Allergy Cin Immunol. 2011; 12891: 3-20.

- Give diseases associated with esophageal eosinophilia
  - Esophagus
    - GERD
    - EoE
    - Achalasia
  - Small bowel
    - Celiac disease
    - Crohn disease

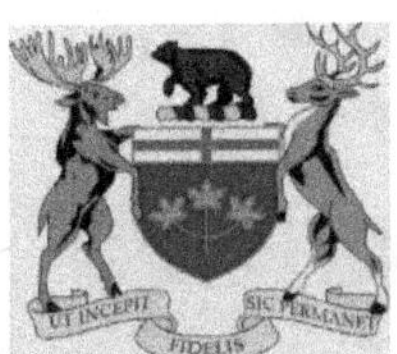

- Systemic disease
  - Eosinophilic gastrointestinal diseases
  - Hypereosinophilic syndrome
- MSK
  - Connective tissue disease
  - Graft-versus-host disease
- Drugs
  - Drug hypersensitivity
- Infection
- Skin
  - Vasculitis
  - Pemphigoid vegetans
- Although symptoms may be mistaken for GERD, and many patients respond to PPIs, EoE is a distinct entity

➤ Pathophysiology of EoE

- Eosinophils invade the epithelium of the esophagus
- Th2 cells release the cytokines interleukin 5, interleukin 13, and eotaxin-3.
- Eosinophils are recruited and invade the mucosa

➤ Clinical Manifestation

- Dysphagia
- Food impact heartburn
- Abdominal pain
- Nausea / vomiting
- Allergic disease or atopy in ~ 50%
- Inverse relationship with H.Pylori infection
- Possible association with Celiac Dx

Source: Dellon ES et al. Clin Gastroenterol Hepatol. 2009;7(12):1305-13.

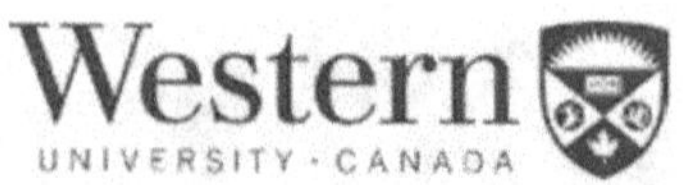

- Endoscopic Features
  - EoE is a biopsy diagnosis
  - Normal in 17%
    - If suspected clinically, then biopsy even if endoscopically normal
  - If the patient has esophageal symptoms, history of allergy / atopy, and abnormal EGD → biopsy (bx)
  - Take a minimum of 4-6 mucosal biopsies from middle and distal esophagus
  - Multiple circular rings
  - Inflammation in mid distal Esophagus
  - Mid Esophageal. tear
  - Food bolus
  - Meta analysis of endoscopic features
    - Esophageal rings
    - Linear furrows
    - Strictures
    - White plaques
    - Pallor / dec
    - Narrow caliber

Source: Kim HP, et al. Clin Gastroenterol Hepatol. 2012;10(9):988-96.

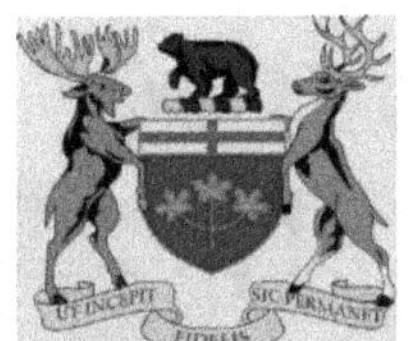

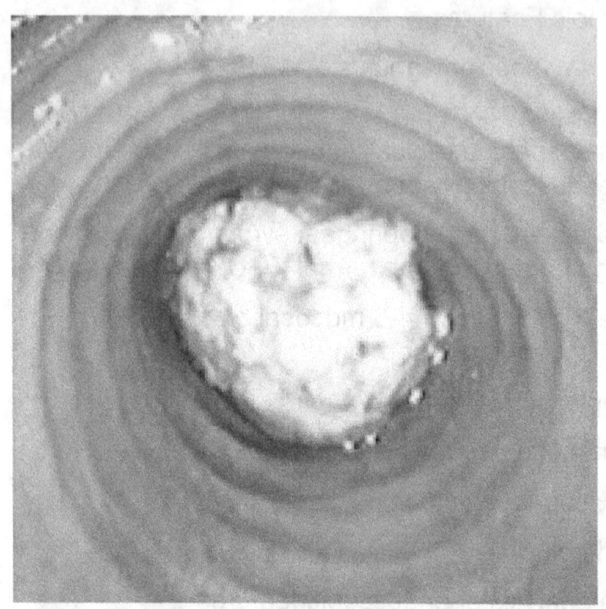

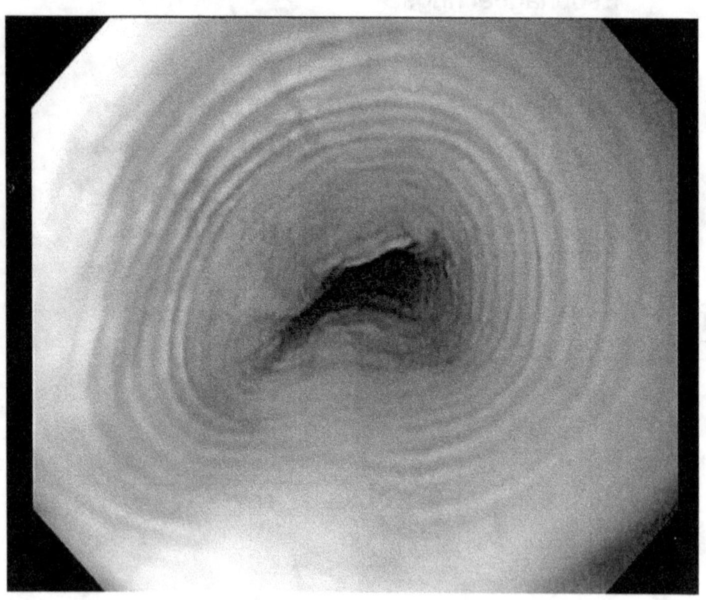

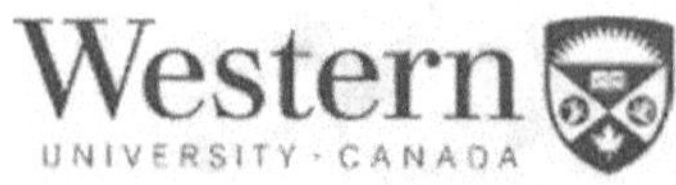
Western
UNIVERSITY · CANADA

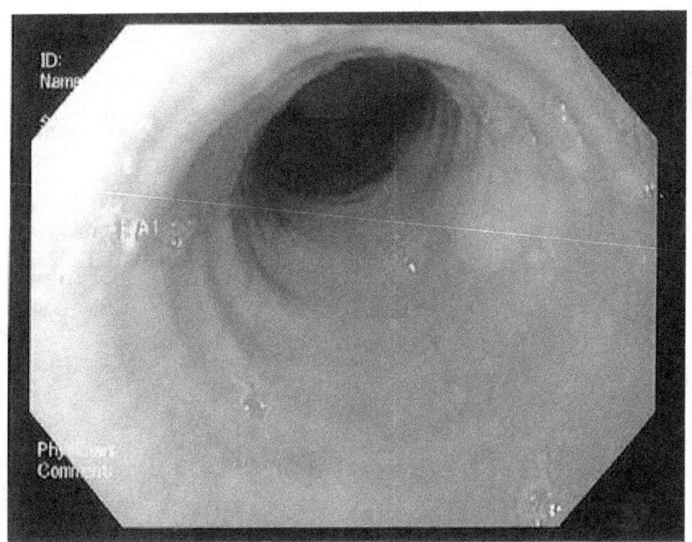

- Linear furrows
- White specks (micro-abscesses)

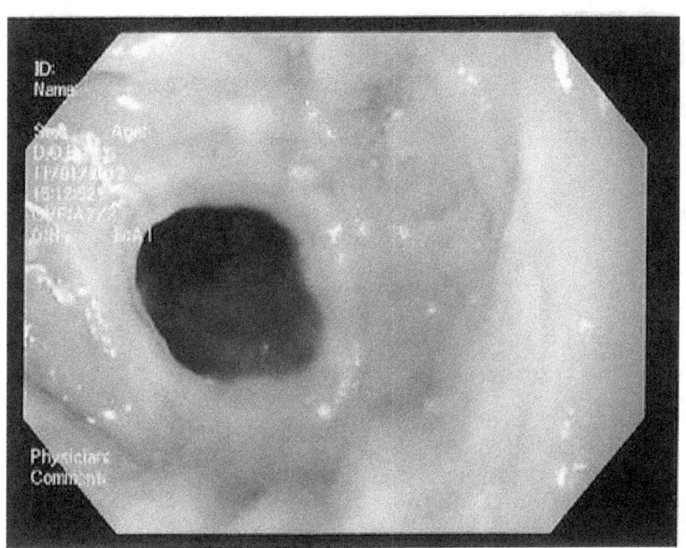

- Narrowing, suggestive of stricture or ring

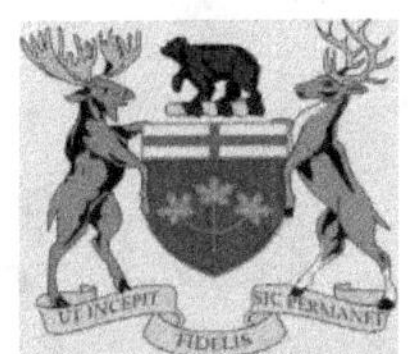

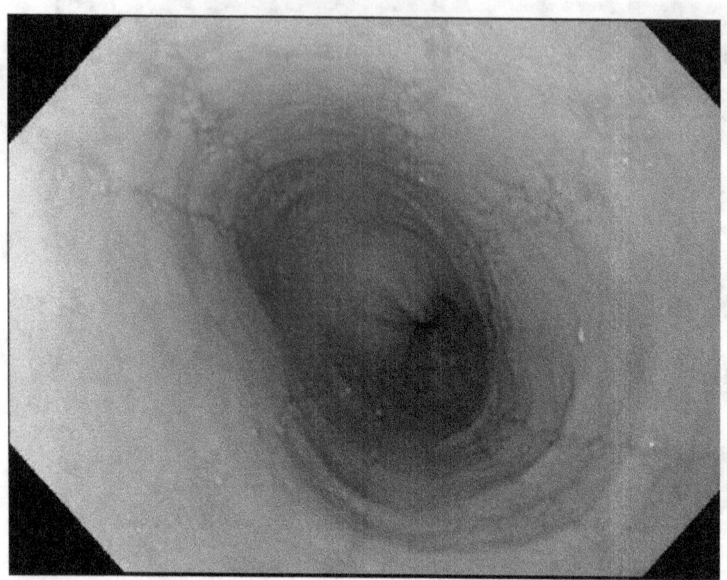

- Narrowing, suggestive of stricture or ring

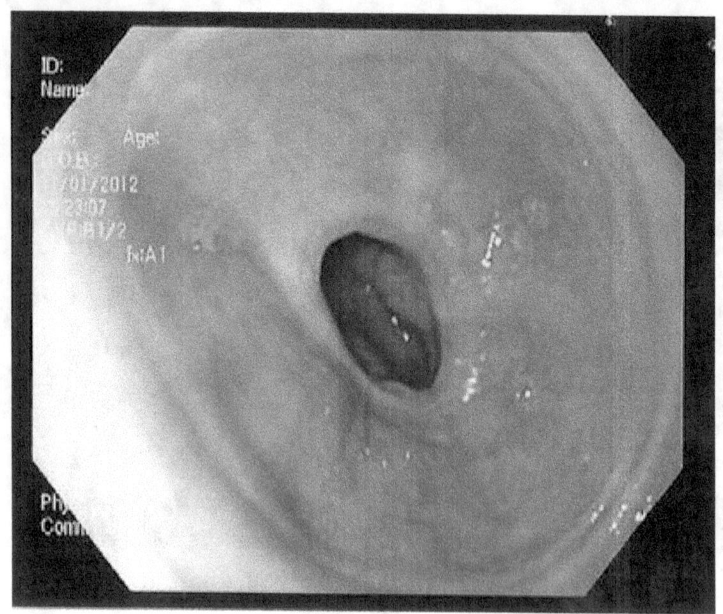

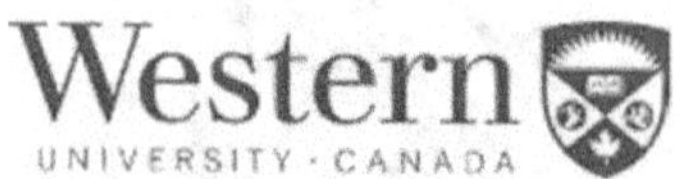

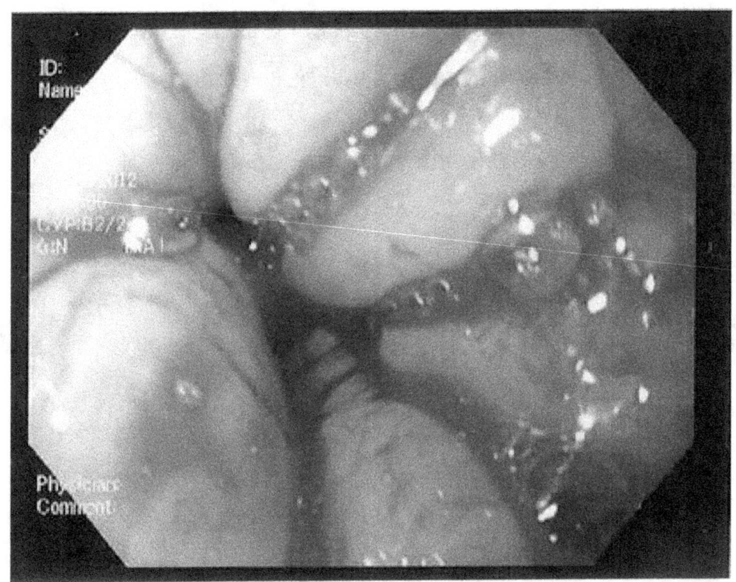

- Bleeding post dilation

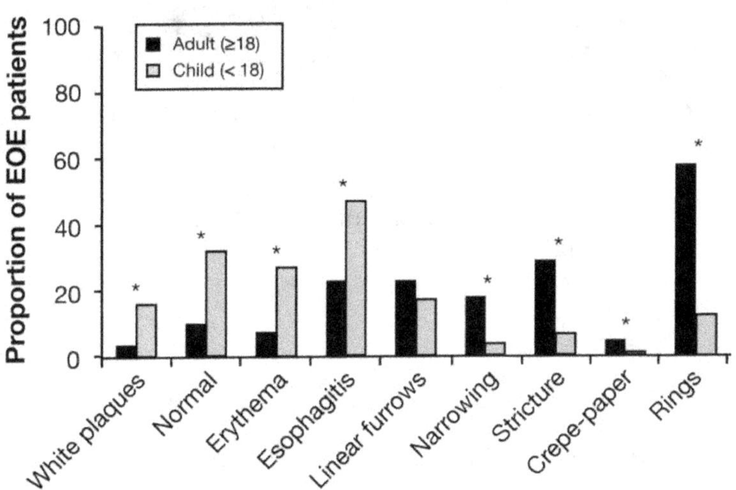

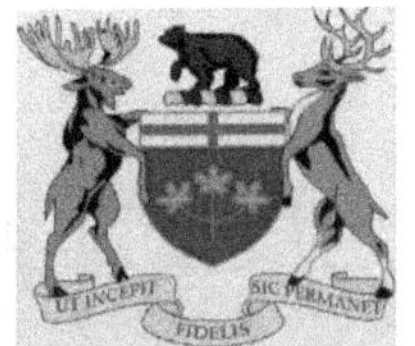

- Clinical features may suggest GERD
- > 90% of adult patients will have features suggestive of EoE
- If endoscopic features of EoE seen, then biopsy esophagus

Source: Dellon ES, et al. Clin Gastroenterol Hepatol. 2009;7(12):1305-13.

- Histopathology

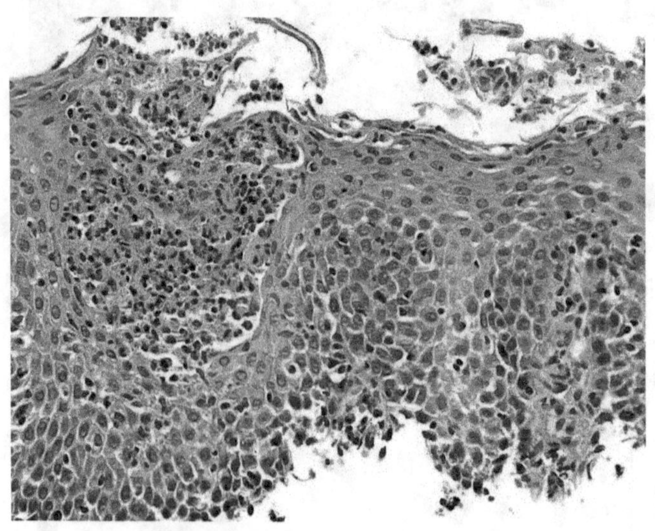

- Sensitivity, based on numbers of mucosal biopsies

  1: 73 %
  2: 84 %
  3: 97 %
  6: 100 %

Source: Shah A, et al. Am J Gastroenterol. 2009;104(3):716-21.

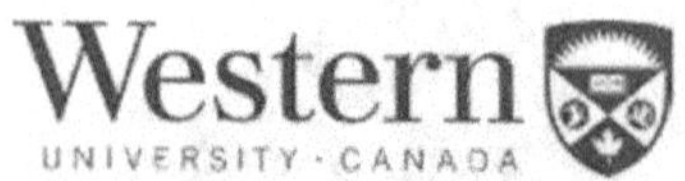

- Give the histopathology of EoE.
    - Eosinophils
        - Superficial layering
        - Sheets
        - Microabscesses
        - Extracellular eosinophil granules (degranulated cells)
    - Subepithelial and lamina propria fibrosis and inflammation
    - Basal cell hyperplasia (usually ≥ 50% of thickness of epithelial layer)
    - Papillary lengthening (may reach the upper 1/3 of the squamous epithelium
    - Dilated intercellular spaces
    - Dilated intercellular spaces
    - Vacuolation of keratinocytes
    - Increased numbers of mast cells, B cells, and IgE-bearing cells
    - Vacuolation of keratinocytes

- Give the histopathological features distinguishing EoE from GERD

	EoE	GERD
o Eosinophils		
– Diffuse intraepithelial distribution of eosinophils	Upper and lower half	Usually only to the lower half)
– Eosinophilic microabscesses	Frequent	Uncommon
– Degranulated eosinophils	Upper and lower half	Rare

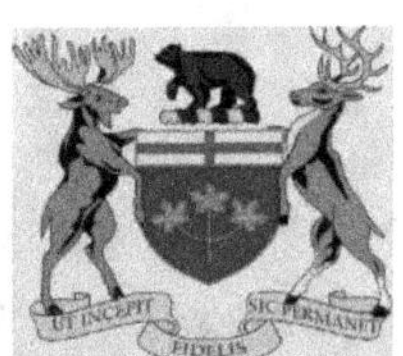

	EoE	GERD
o Basal cell hyperplasia (% of thickness of epithelium)	Usually ≥50%	Usually ≤25%
o Lamina propria fibrosis	Frequent	Rare

- Laboratory Finding in EoE
    - Peripheral eosinophilia ~ 50%
    - ↑ total IgE in some patients

- Treatment

- PPIs
    - 75% of all patients with Eo infiltration achieve clinicopathological remission with PPI
    - EoE-like profile patients: response rate 50 %
    - Esophageal pH monitoring poorly predicts PPI response

Source: Molina-Infante J et al.Clin Gastroenterol Hepatol 2011;9:110-7

- PPI Responsive Esophageal Eosinophilia :
    - Should be differentiated from EoE
    - A trial of PPI bid for 2 months followed by endoscopy and biopsy is recommended
- Improvement in dysphagia
    - Budesonide :72 %
    - Placebo: 22 %

Source: Straumann A et al. Gastroenterology. 2010;139(5):1526-37.

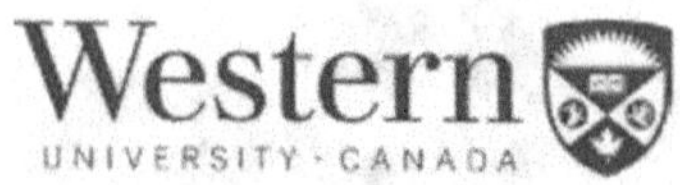

- Budesonide (Topical steroid) include
    - RCT, 18 patients for each arm
    - Oral Viscous Budesonide (OVB) : 1 mg twice daily for 15 days
    - Eosinophils (Eos) / hpf
        - Budesonide : 68.2 >>>> 5.5
        - Placebo : 62.3 >>> 56.5

- Maintenance of Remission

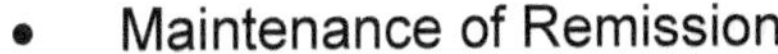

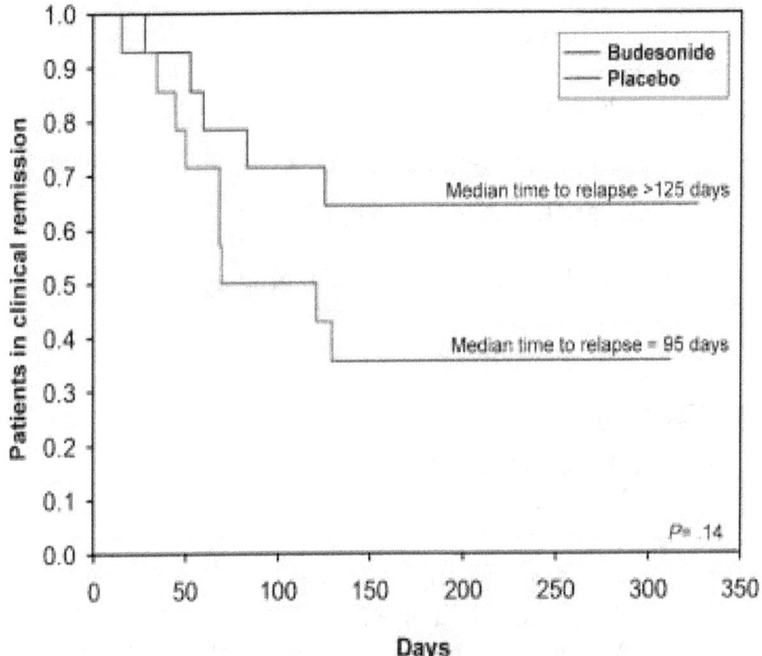

- Nebulized Budesonide (NEB) 0.25 mg bid for 50 weeks
- Therapeutic gain, ~30%

Source: Straumann A, et al. Clinical Gastroenterol Hepatol;2011;9(5):400-9; Dellon ES, et al. Gastroenterology 2012;143(2):321-4.

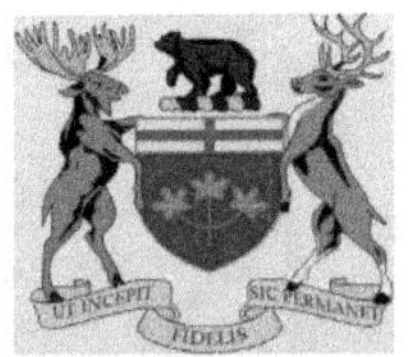

- Six Food Elimination Diet (SFED)
- Food triggers
  - Wheat 60 %
  - Milk 50 %
  - Soy 10 %
  - Nuts 10 %
  - Egg 5 %
  - Sea Food < 1%
- Skin test predictability only 13%
- Prospective clinical trial of SFED, 50 patients, 6 weeks
- > 75% ↓ Eos / hpf
- Symptom scores decreased 94%
- EGD appearance improved in 78 %

Source: Gonsalves N, et al.Gastroenterology 2012;142(7):1451-9.

➤ Esophageal Dilation

- Goal esophageal diameter
  - 15 to 18 mm
- Benefit
  - Relief of dysphagia, > 90 %
  - Patient satisfaction ~75%
  - Average duration of symptoms relief, 1- 2 yrs
- No effect on underlying inflammation
- Esophageal Dilation: Post-procedure

(Schoepfer AM et al.Am J Gastroenterol. 2010;105(5):1062-70)

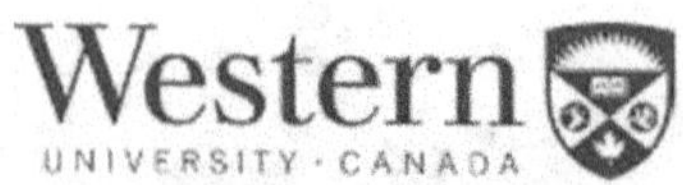

Safety of Esophageal Dilation in EoE

- 1 study
  - 293 dilations in 161 patients
  - 74 % balloon and 26 % Savory dilation
  - Deep mucosal tear - 9%
  - Immediate perforation -1.0%

Source: Jung KW et al. Gastro Endo. 2011;73(1):15-21.

- Meta analysis
  - Only one perforation in 671 dilations (0.15%) in 468 patients
  - Superficial esophageal tear was common, but not clinically important

Source: Jacobs JW et al. Dig Dis Sci. 2010;55(6):1512)

"Attitude is a little thing that makes a big difference."

Winston Churchill

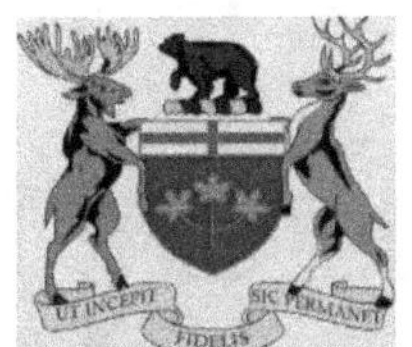

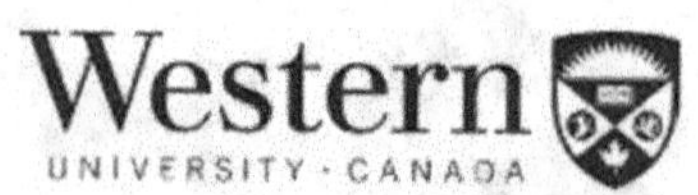
Western
UNIVERSITY · CANADA

Esophageal Motility Testing

Keith McIntosh

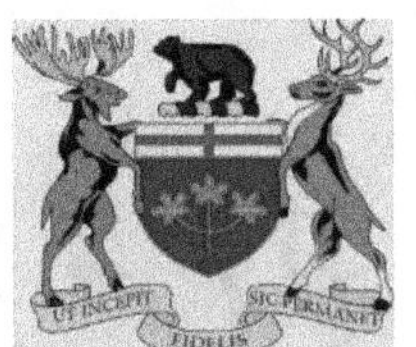

- Indications for Esophageal Manometry
  - Dysphagia – endoscopy negative
  - Chest pain – endoscopy & cardiac negative
  - Pre-24 hr pH testing
  - Pre-anti-reflux surgery
  - For definitive diagnosis of any suspected primary or secondary esophageal motility disorder

- Causes

- Primary

- Give a classification of primary esophageal manometry disorders.
  - Achalasia
    - Type I
    - Type II
    - Type III
  - EGJ Outflow Obstruction (Achalasia variant IV)
  - Diffuse Esophageal Spasm (DES)
  - Hypercontractile Esophagus
    - Jackhammer Esophagus
    - Nutcracker Esophagus
  - Primary Peristaltic Abnormailities
    - Absent Peristalsis
    - Frequent Failed Peristalsis
    - Weak Peristalsis with Large or Small Breaks
  - Non-specific Motor Disorder

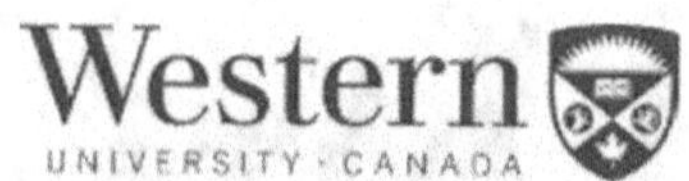

- Secondary
- Give 5 secondary causes of esophageal motility disorders.
  - Connective Tissue Disorders (scleroderma, MCTD)
  - Diabetes Mellitus
  - Alcohol Abuse
  - Amyloidosis
  - Neurologic Disorders (MS, Parkinson's)
  - Muscular Dystrophy
  - Radiation
  - Drugs (narcotics)

Abbreviations: MCTD, mixed connective tissue disorders; MS, multiple sclerosis

Conventional Esophageal Manometry

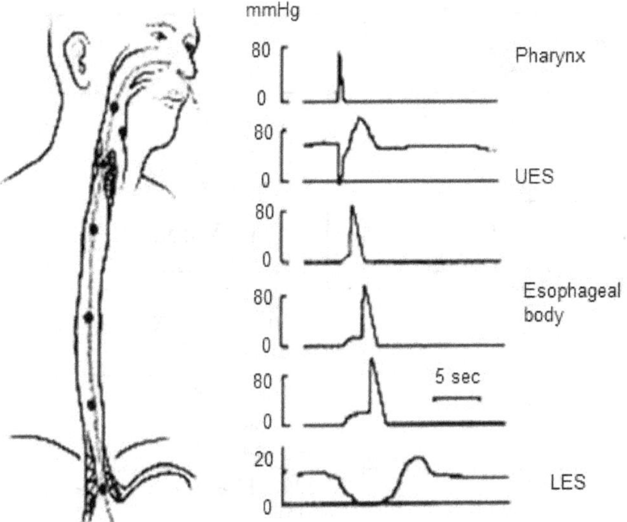

High Resolution Manometry Pressure Topography (Clouse) Plot

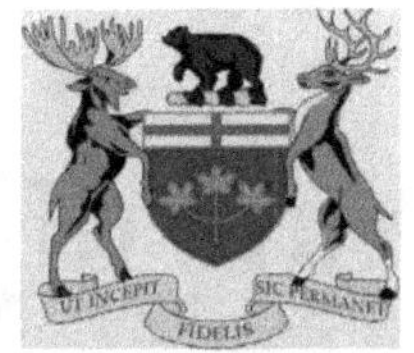

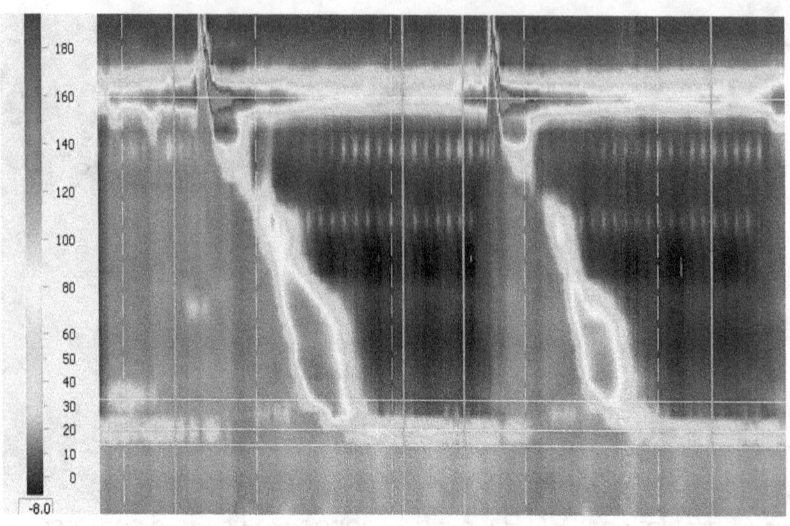

Normal Parameters of Conventional and High Resolution Manometry (HRM)

Convential			HRM	
LES Resting Pressure	15-45mm Hg			
LES Residual Pressure	<8 mm Hg		Integrated Relaxation Presssure (IRP)	< 15 mm Hg
Peristaltic Amplitude	30 – 180 mm Hg		Distal Contractile Integral (DCI)	500 – 5000 mmHg.cm.s
Peristaltic Velocity	<9 cm/s		Contractile Front Velocity (CFV)	< 9 cm/s
			Contractile Deceleration Point (CDP)	
			Distal Latency (DL)	> 4.5 s

Peristaltic Breaks

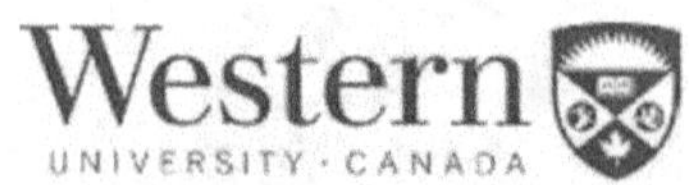

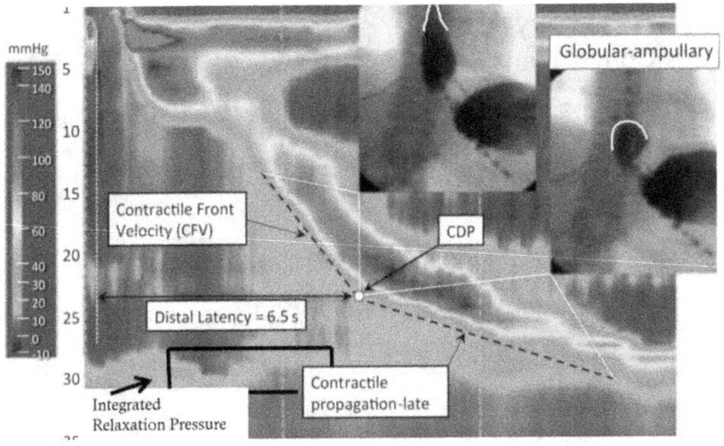

Achalasia

- Diagnostic imaging
  - Barium swallow

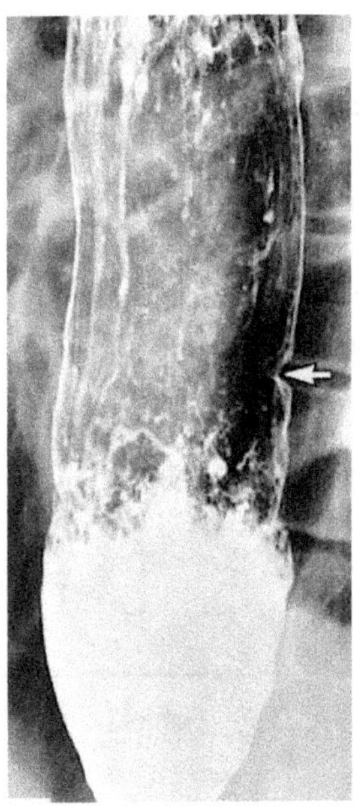

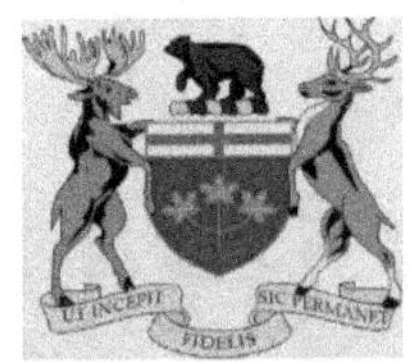

- Manometry
- Conventional
    - Impaired LES relaxation
    - +/-Elevated LES resting pressure
    - Aperistalsis
    - Elevated baseline intraesophageal pressure
    - Common cavity phenomenon

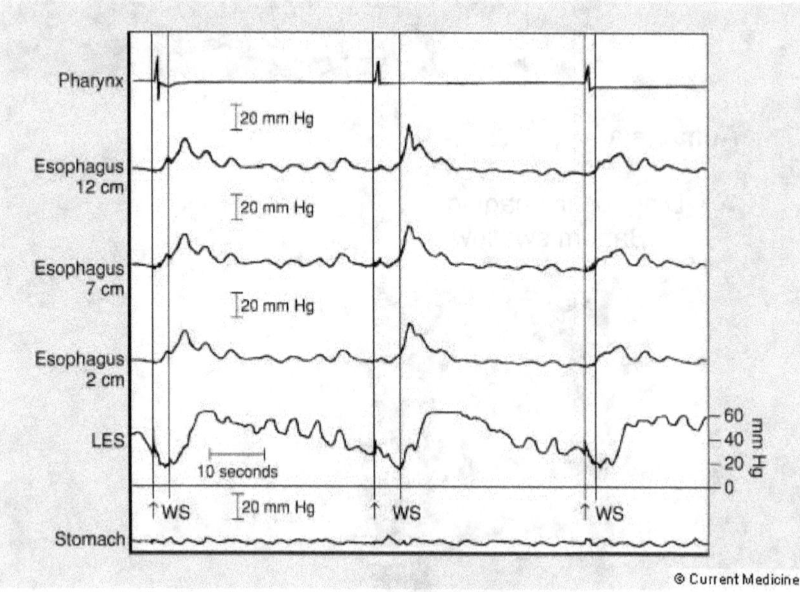

HRM

Subtype	
Type I	IRP > ULN, 100% Failed Peristalsis

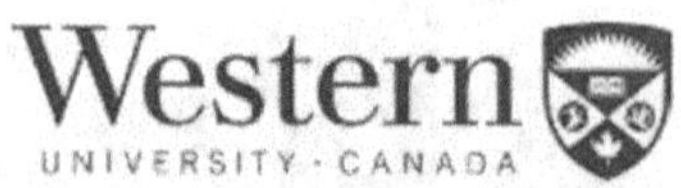

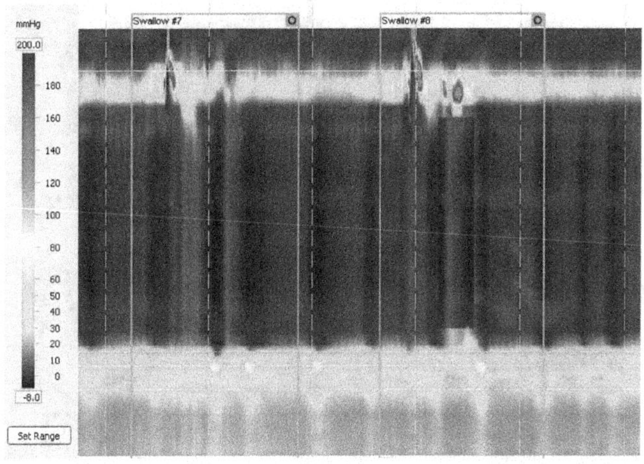

Subtype	
Type II	IRP > ULN, no normal peristalsis, Panesophageal pressurization >20%

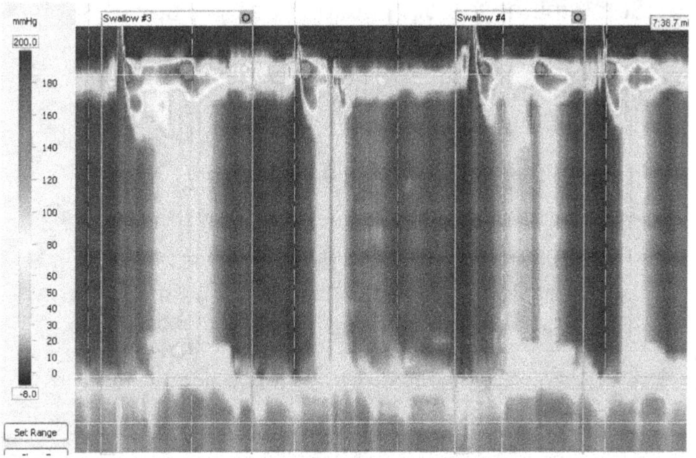

Type III	IRP > ULN, no normal peristalsis, premature contractions distal esophagus >20%

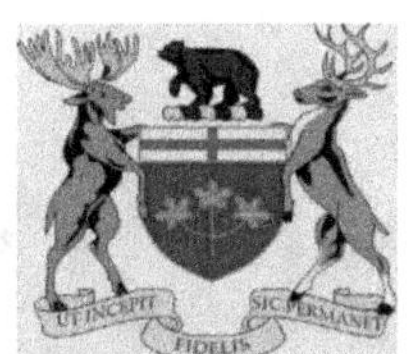

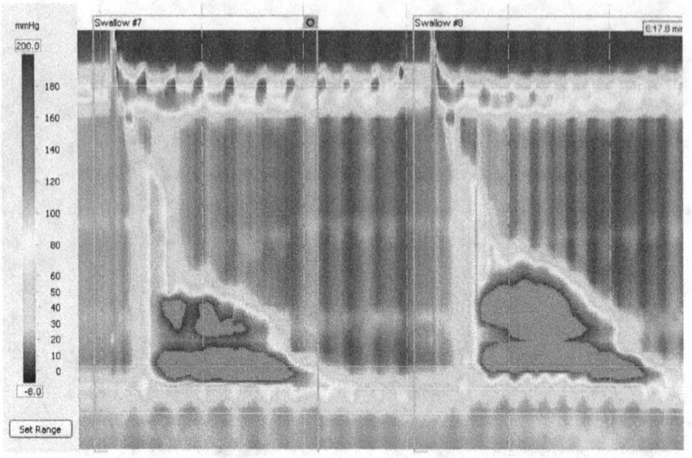

Type IV, achalasia variant

- EGJ Outflow Obstruction
- IRP > ULN
- Some instances of intact or weak peristalsis such that criteria for achalasia are not met
- Rule out mechanical obstruction

"To give pleasure to a single heart by a single act is better than a thousand heads bowing in prayer."

Mahatma Gandhi

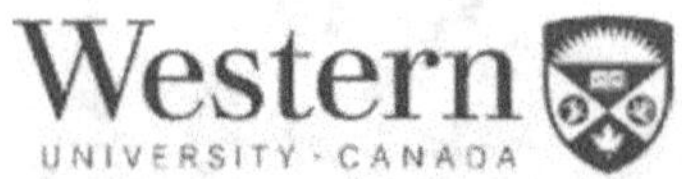

Diffuse Esophageal Spasm (DES)

- Now being referred to as distal esophageal spasm
- Intermittent dysphagia or atypical chest pain (aka NCCP, non-cardiac chest pain)

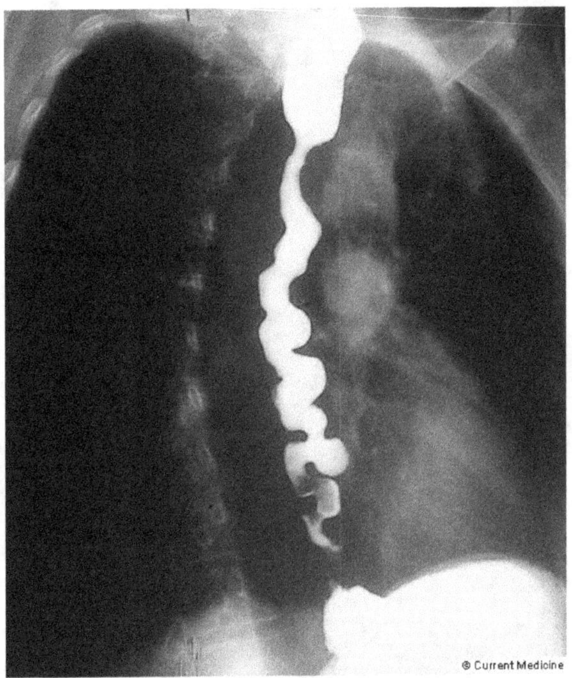

- Types

Conventional	HRM
- Normal LES relaxation - >20% Simulatenous contractions	- Normal IRP - DL < 4.5 sec with > 20% of contractions

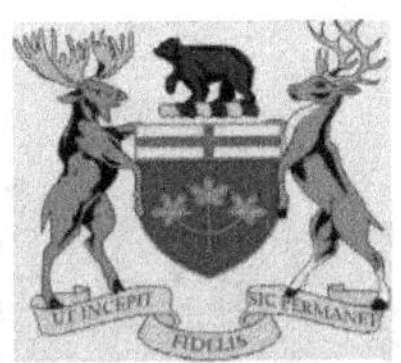

- Frequently high amplitude contractions

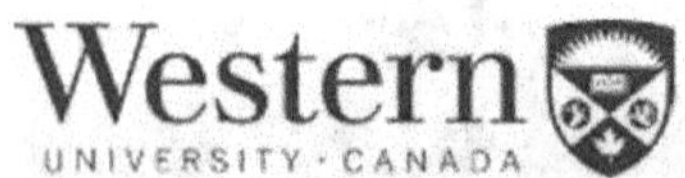

- Conventional Manometry

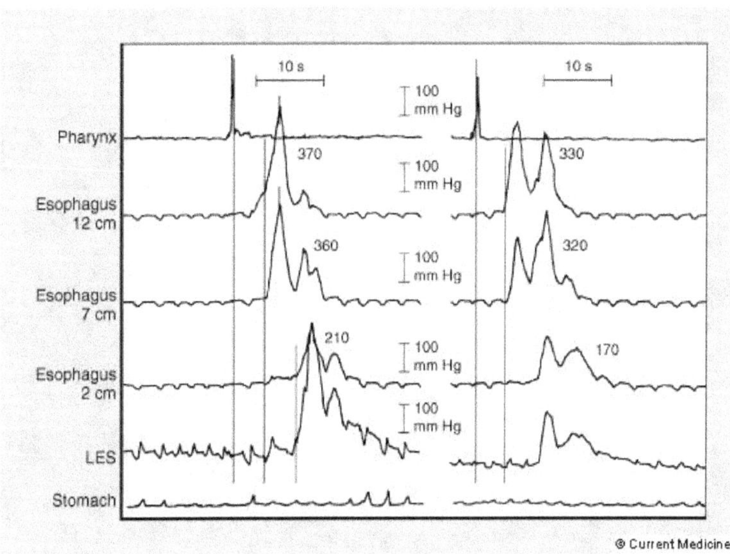

- High Resolution Manometry (HRM)

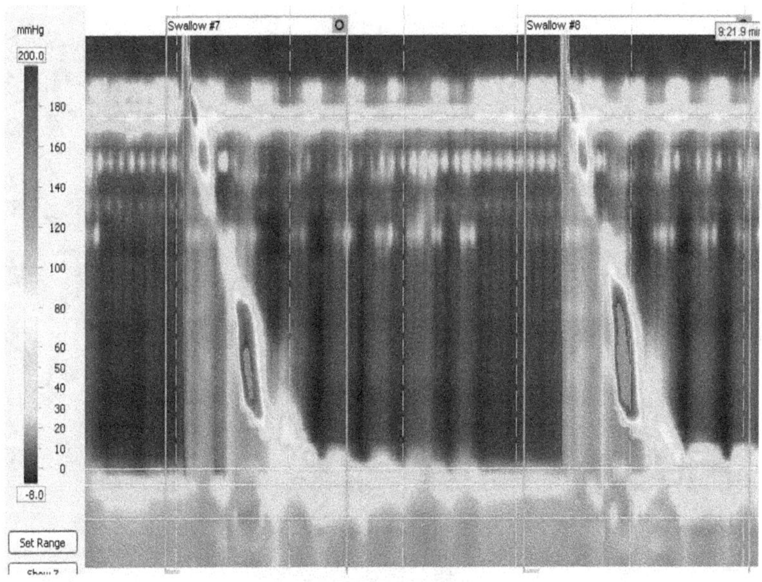

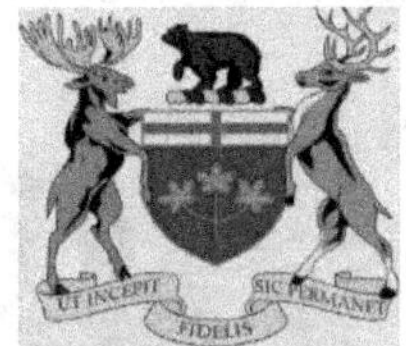

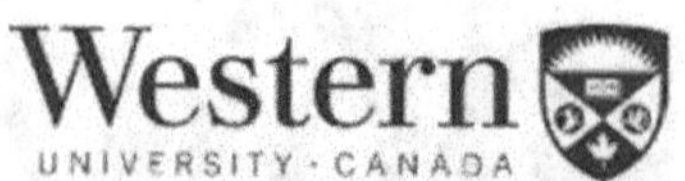
Western
UNIVERSITY · CANADA

Nutcracker Esophagia

➢ Manometry

- Conventional

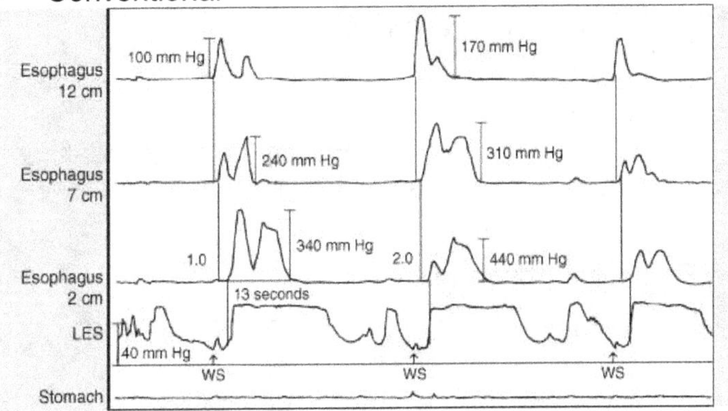

  - o Atypical chest pain plus odynophagia
  - o High amplitude, peristaltic contractions
  - o ↑ amplitude >180mmHg
  - o Any contraction >250mmHg

- HRM

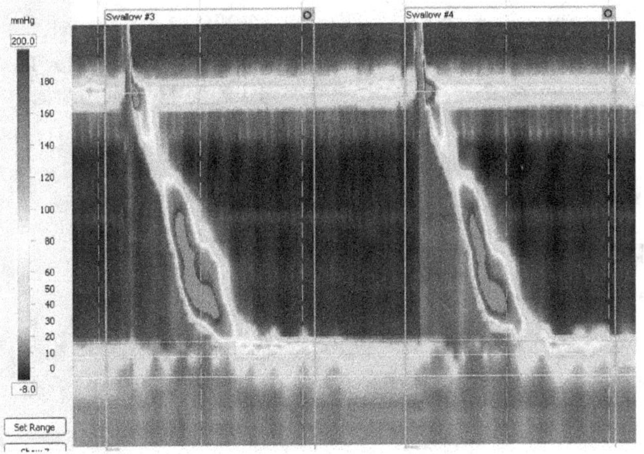

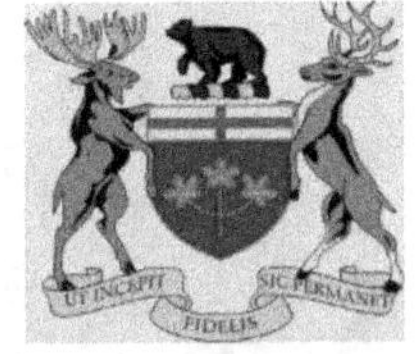

Hypercontractile Esophagus

- HRM
  - Jackhammer
    - At least one swallow with DCI > 8000 mm Hg.cm.s
  - Nutcracker
    - Mean DCI > 5000 mm Hg.cm.s but not meeting criteria for "Jackhammer"
  - Peristaltic Abnormalities
    - Absent Peristalsis – IRP N, 100% of swallows failed peristalsis
    - Frequent Failed Peristalsis – IRP N, >30% but <100% failed peristalsis
    - Weak Peristalsis with large breaks – >20% swallows with > 5 cm break in 30 mm Hg isobaric contour
    - Weak Peristalsis with small breaks – >20% of swallows with 2-5 cm break in 30 mm Hg isobaric contour

Scleroderma Esophagus

- Aperistalsis
- Hypotensive LES

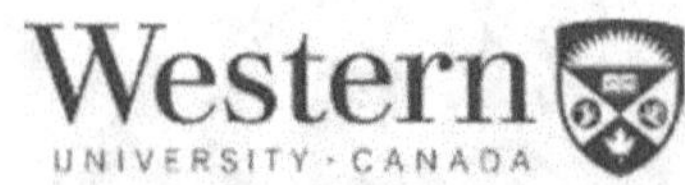

➢ Conventional Manometry

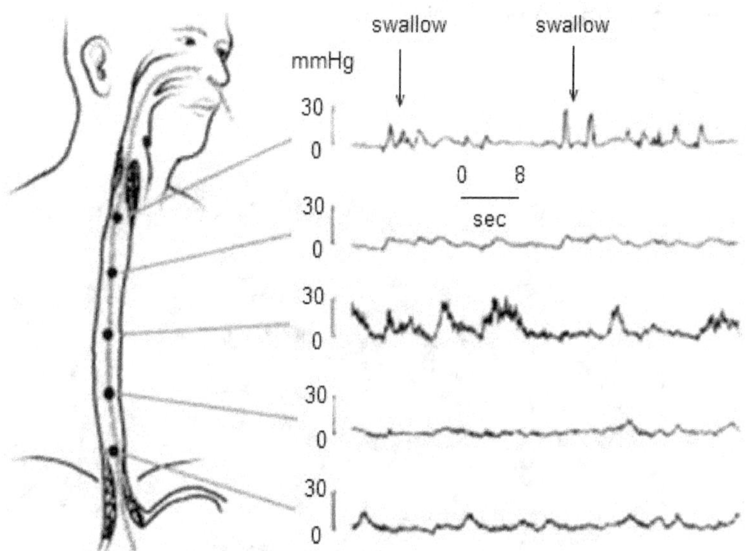

• HRM

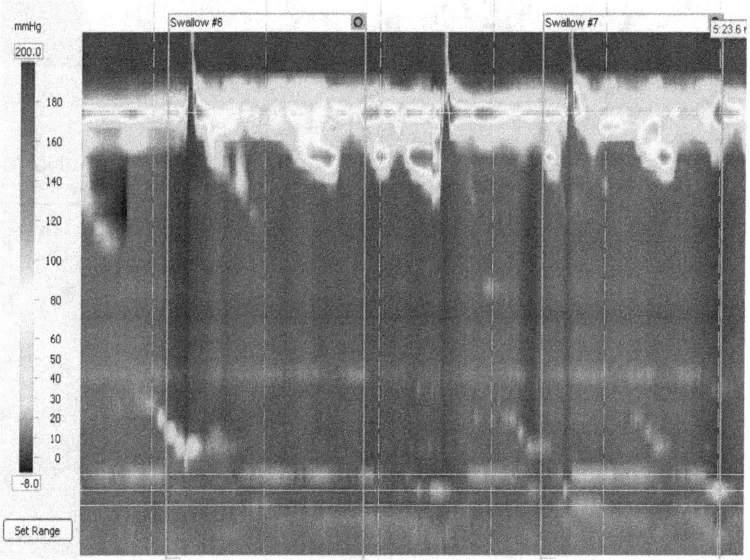

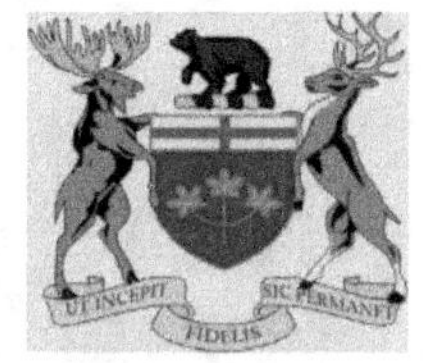

Cases: in the following 4 cases, comment on the HRM, including the EMS parameters, their meaning and the likely esophageal manometric diagnosis.

Case #1

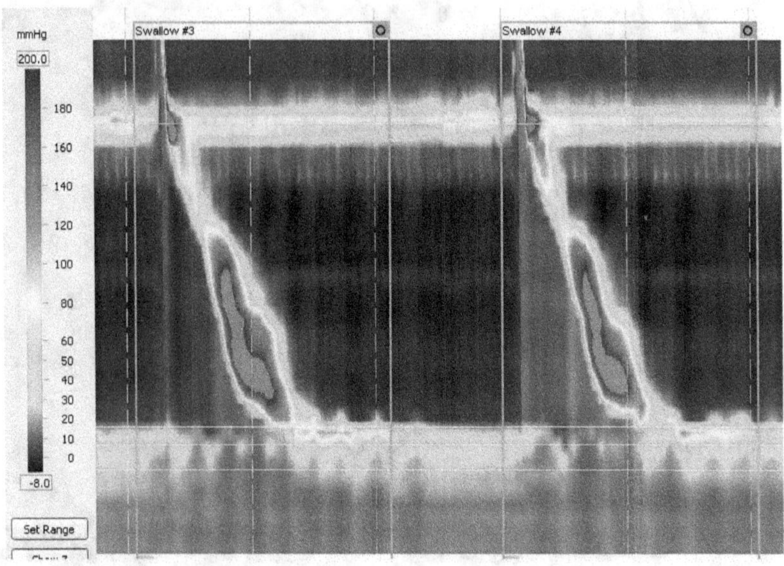

EMS Parameter	Mean	Normal
LES Resting Pressure (mm Hg)	26.9	13-43
IRP (mm Hg)	5.7	<15.0
Distal Wave Amplitude (mm Hg)	213.4	43-152
DCI (mmHg.cm.s)	5016	500-5000
CFV (cm/s)	3.3	< 9
Distal Latency (s)	6.0	>4.5
% Peristaltic	100%	

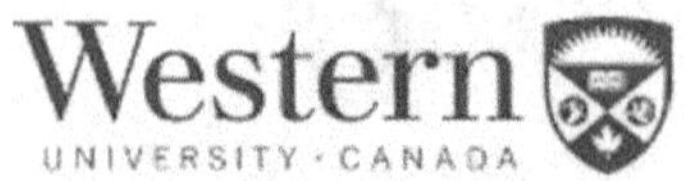

Case #2

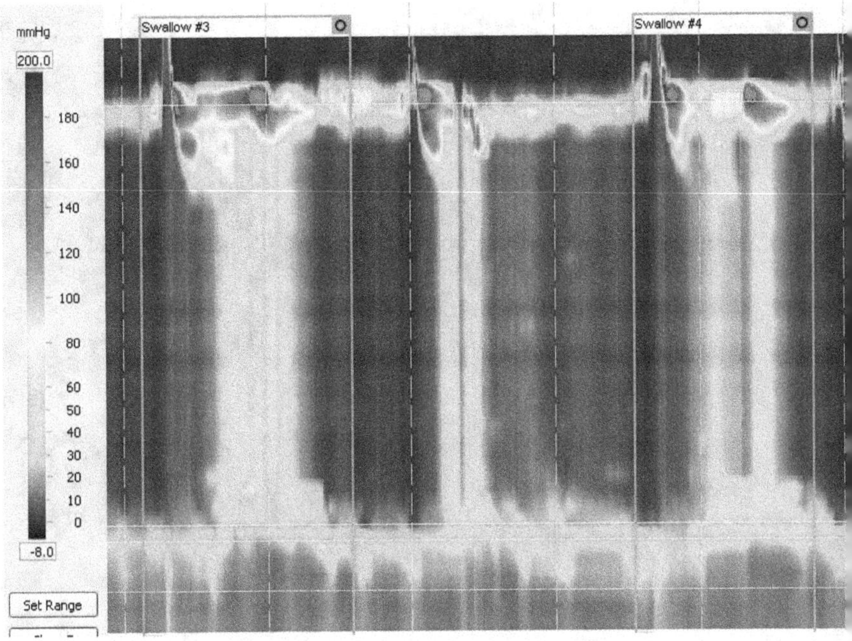

EMS Parameter	Mean	Normal
LES Resting Pressure (mm Hg)	24.7	13-43
IRP (mm Hg)	18.2	<15.0
Distal Wave Amplitude (mm Hg)	N/A	43-152
DCI (mmHg.cm.s)	N/A	500-5000
CFV (cm/s)	N/A	< 9
Distal Latency (s)	N/A	>4.5
% Simultaneous	100%	

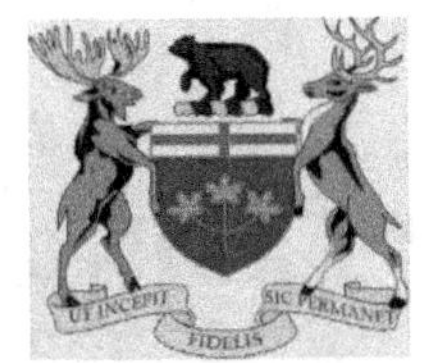

Case #3

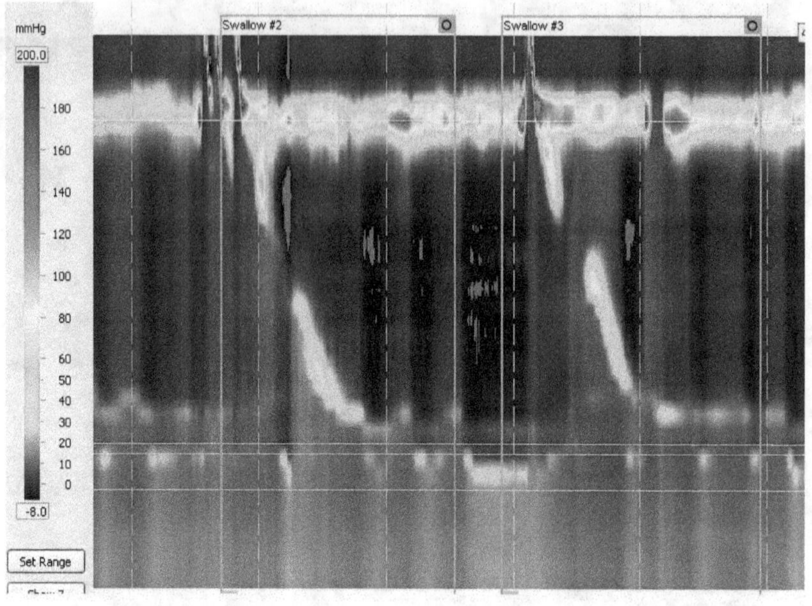

EMS Parameter	Mean	Normal
LES Resting Pressure (mm Hg)	10.7	13-43
IRP (mm Hg)	1.7	<15.0
Distal Wave Amplitude (mm Hg)	45.5	43-152
DCI (mmHg.cm.s)	453	500-5000
CFV (cm/s)	1.9	< 9
Distal Latency (s)	8.3	>4.5
% Peristaltic contractions	100%	

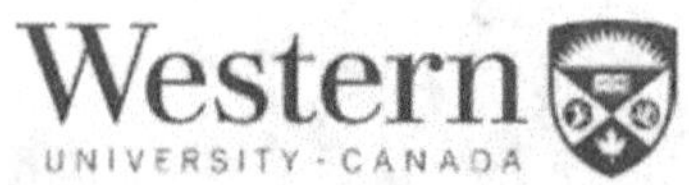

Case #4

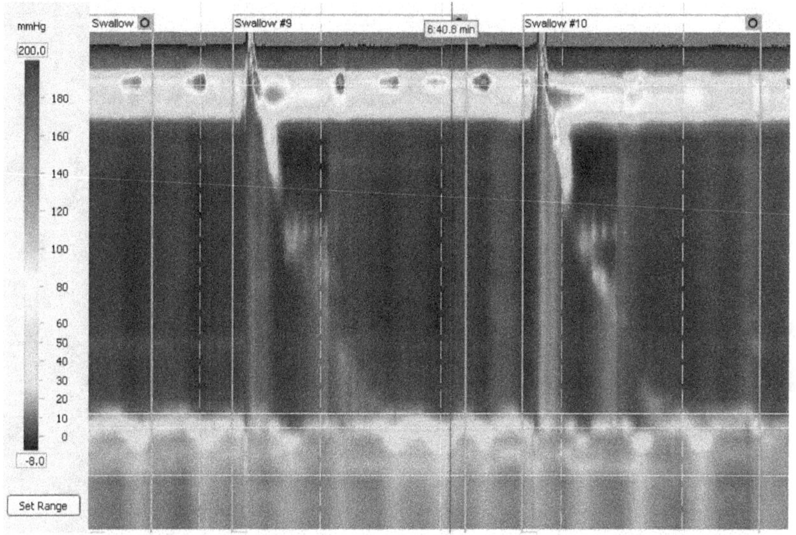

EMS Parameter	Mean	Normal
LES Resting Pressure (mm Hg)	21.1	13-43
IRP (mm Hg)	5.3	<15.0
Distal Wave Amplitude (mm Hg)	19.8	43-152
DCI (mmHg.cm.s)	173	500-5000
CFV (cm/s)	2.0	< 9
Distal Latency (s)	9.5	>4.5
% Peristaltic contractions	10%	

Answers

1. Nutcracker Esophagus
2. Achalasia (Type II – panesophageal pressurization)
3. Hypotensive LES, Weak Peristalsis with small breaks, (frequently seen in GERD), hiatal hernia
4. Frequent Failed Peristalsis

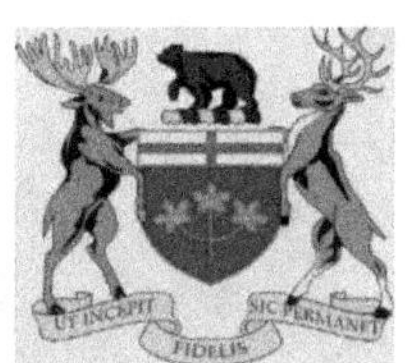

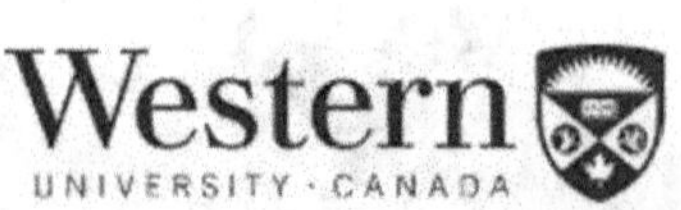

STOMACH

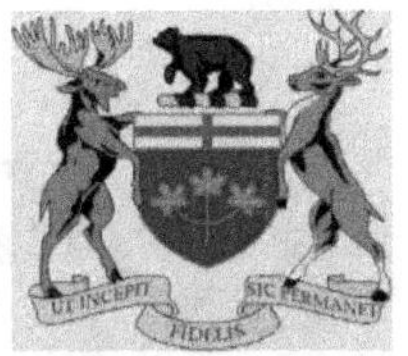

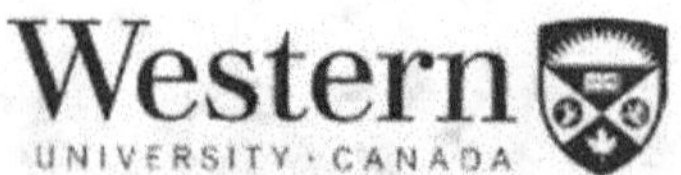

Dyspepsia

Nilesh Chande

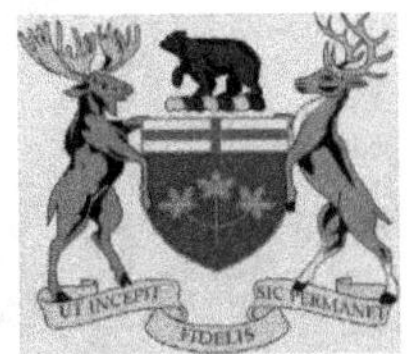

➢ Definition

- Canada:
  - Symptom complex of epigastric pain or discomfort thought to originate in the upper GI tract, in the absence of any organic, systemic, or metabolic disease that is likely to explain the symptoms
  - May include any of:
    - Heartburn
    - Acid regurgitation
    - Excessive burping/belching
    - Increased abdominal bloating
    - Nausea
    - Feeling of abnormal or slow digestion
    - Early satiety
  - A dyspepsia with "VBAD" alarm symptoms are not part of this definition of dyspepsia, and should lead to further investigation, including EGD.
    - VBAD
      - Vomiting
      - Bleeding – hematemesis, melena
      - Anemia
      - Dysphagia, odynophagia
    - FWLMS
      - Family history of upper GI cancer
      - Weight loss (non-intentional)
      - Liver disease jaundice, ascites
      - Mass in abdomen, or lymphadenopathy
      - Surgery on stomach in past

Note: the PPV (positive predictive value) of alarm symptoms is low, but the NPV (negative predictive value) is 99%; so, absence of "red flag" or "alarm" symptoms argues against upper GI malignancy being a cause.

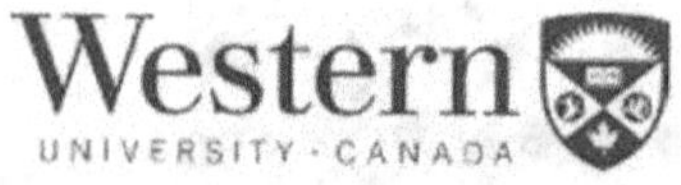

- There is so much overlap in symptoms that it is not possible to confidently distinguish between the usual causes of dyspepsia (i.e. poor specificity)
  - GERD (gastroesophageal reflux disease)
  - PUD (peptic ulcer disease, comprised of DU [duodenal ulcer] and GU gastric ulcer])
    - DU classically
      - On an empty stomach
      - 2 to 3 hours pc, hen buffering acid of food has been lost, and HCl
      - Secretion is no longer high between 11 pm to 2 am
  - NERD (normal endoscopy reflux disease) and NUD (non-ulcer dyspepsia) describe the same condition of reflux-like dyspepsia and non-ulcer dyspepsia, in which the patient suffers from dyspepsia, but the EGD is normal (thus NERD and NUD are forms of "investigated dyspepsia" since an EGD has been performed).

- Warning: exceptions – although the absence of VBAD FWLML alarm symptoms is reassuring (NPV, 99%) in the dyspeptic person, the presence of upper GI tract malignancy must be excluded by EGD in several circumstances:
  - Age over a cut-off (guidelines vary from 45 to 55 years of age; suggestion – use age 50, or earlier if one of the following is present)
  - Family or personal history of cancer of esophagus or stomach
  - Personal origin from an ARGD of the world with a high incidence of GCa; e.g. Japan, South America
  - Personal origin from an area or group of persons with a high prevalence of H. pylori infection (because H. pylori infection may be a factor causing GCa)

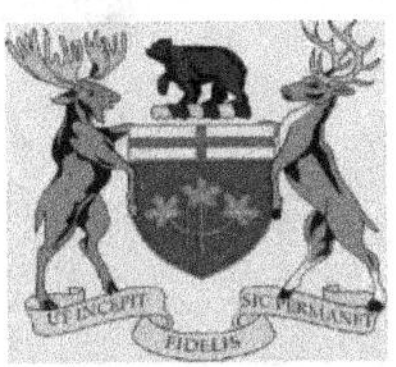

- The age cut-off is determined by the point at which the incidence of ECa / GCa begins to rise; e.g. 1% at age < 50 in N. Europe, USA, Canada
- Middle aged Caucasian male with > 10 year history of moderately severe GERD occurring ≥ 3 times per week (risk of Barrett esophagus and ECa)

- Also call: the odds ratio of gallstones in a dyspeptic is low or 2.0 and even if the patient is shown to have gallstones on abdominal ultrasound, that is not sufficient proof that the dyspepsia is not caused by GERD, PUD, NERD / NUD), or ECA / GCa.
- Overlap with IBS
  - Dyspepsia in persons with IBS, 14%
  - Reflux-like dyspepsia in IBS, 32%
  - IBS in persons with dyspepsia, 37%
- Most important difference from Rome III criteria is inclusion of heartburn in definition
  - Allows distinction of 3 subtypes:
    - Reflux-like
    - Ulcer-like
    - Dysmotility-like
- Uninvestigated dyspepsia
  - Dyspepsia for which no cause has yet been sought (in reality, an EGD has not been performed EGD is normal)
- Functional dyspepsia
  - Dyspepsia for which investigation has shown no cause
  - Would also include nonulcer dyspepsia

- Rome III
  - Dyspepsia is pain or discomfort in the upper abdomen which may be associated with symptoms described as heartburn, indigestion, nausea,

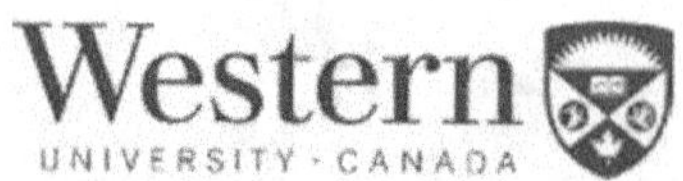

fullness, poor digestion some described as heartburn, e.g. Rome III

Functional Gastrointestinal Disorders
o Functional dyspepsia - Postprandial distress syndrome
o Belching disorders - Aerophagia - Unspecified excessive belching
o Nausea and vomiting disorders - Chronic idiopathic nausea - Functional vomiting
o Rumination syndrome in adults

Diagnostic Criteria* for Functional Dyspepsia

- One or more of:
  - Bothersome postprnadrial fullness
  - Early satiation
  - Epigastric pain
  - Epigastric burning

plus

- No evidence of structural disease (including at upper endoscopy) that is likely to explain the dyspeptic symptoms

** Criteria fulfilled for the last months with symptom onset at least 6 month before diagnosis*

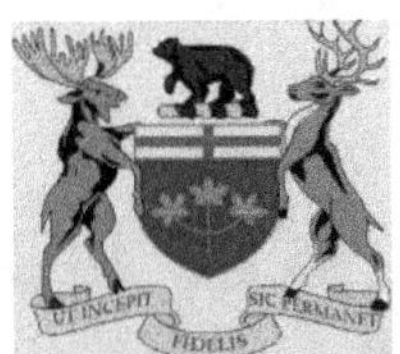

- Types
    - Epigastric pain syndrome (EPS)
    - Postprandial distress syndrome
    - Early satiation
        - A feeling that the stomach is overfilled soon after starting to eat, out of proportion to the size of the meal being eaten, so that the meal cannot be finished.
        - Previously, the term "early satiety" was used, but satiation is the correct term for the disappearance of the sensation of appetite during food ingestion

o Epigastric pain	- Epigastric pain to the region between the umbilicus and lower end of the sternum, and marked by the midclavicular lines. - Pain refers to a subjective, unpleasant sensation; some patients may feel that tissue damage is occurring. - Other symptoms may be extremely bothersome without being interpreted by the patient as pain
o Epigastric burning	- Epigastric refers to the region between the umbilicus and lower end of the sternum, and marked by the midclavicular lines. - Burning refers to an unpleasant subjective sensation of heat.

Printed with permission: Drossman DA. The functional gastrointestinal disorders and the Rome III process. Gastroenterology. 2006; 130(5):1377-90.

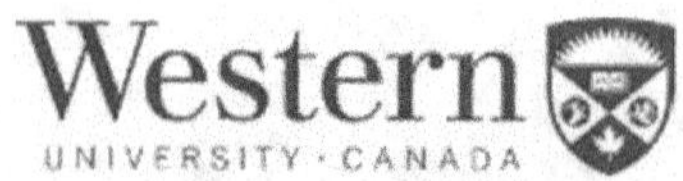

- **Epigastric Pain Syndrome (EPS)**

The diagnosis of EPS must include *all* of the following:

- Pain or burning localized to the epigastrium of at least moderate severity at least once perweek
- The pain is intermittent
- Not generalized or localized to other abdominal or chest regions
- Not relieved by defecation or passage of flatus
- Not fulfill criteria for gallbladder and spincter of Oddi disorders

** Criteria fulfilled for the last 3 months with symptoms onset at least 6 months before diagnosis*

- The pain may be of a burning quality but without a retrosternal component
- The pain of commonly induced or relieved by ingestion of a meal but may occur while fasting
- Postprandial distress syndrome may co-exist

➢ Diagnostic Criteria* for Postprandial Distress Syndrome

Must include *one or both* of the following:

- Bothersome postprandial fullness, occurring after ordinary sized meals, at least several meals.
- Early satiation that prevents finishing a regular meals, at least several times per week

*Criteria fulfilled for the last 3 months with symptoms onset at least 6 months before diagnosis

- Upper abdominal bloating or postprandial nausea or excessive belching can be present
- EPS may co-exist
- Excludes heartburn (unlike Canadian definition of dyspepsia)

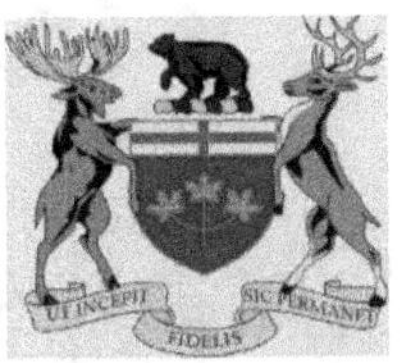

Rome III

- GERD may overlap with and IBS
  - Presence of GERD or IBS does not exclude dyspepsia
  - Presence of typical reflux symptoms should lead to a provisional diagnosis of GERD
  - Presence of heartburn does not exclude PDS or EPS if dyspepsia persists despite an adequate PPI trial
  - Overlap of IBS with PDS or EPS is common
    - May share similar pathophysiological mechanisms
- EPS: Epigastric pain or burning (termed "epigastric pain syndrome")
- PPD: Postprandial fullness (termed "postprandial distress syndrome")
- **Early satiation** (meaning "inability to finish a normal sized meal or postprandial fullness)

➢ Demography

- General prevalence in Western populations of dyspepsia – 25-50%
- Natural history – persisting/recurring symptoms
- Lower quality of life in dyspepsia patients compared to healthy controls and compared to those with PUD

➢ Causes / associations

- 1040 with uninvestigated dyspepsia
- Prompt endoscopy within 7-10 days after presenting to family MD
- No therapy given before endoscopy

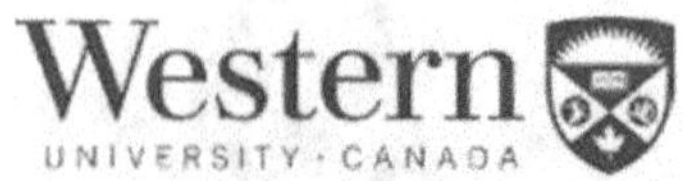

- Subgroups of symptoms:
  - Ulcer-like – 45%
  - Reflux-like – 38%
  - Dysmotility-like – 18%
  - Alarm symptoms in 2.8%

CADET-PE study (Aliment Pharm Ther 2003)

Prevalence of clinically significant findings by age

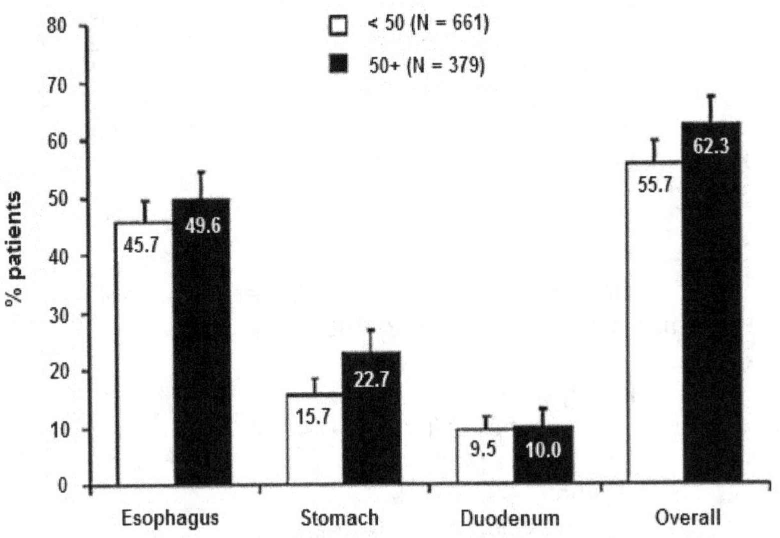

Printed with permission: Thomson AB, et al. Aliment Pharmacol Ther. 2003;17(12):1481-91.

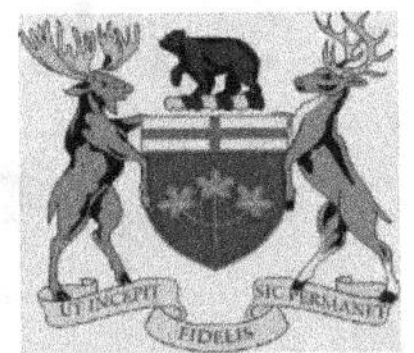

Most severe dyspeptic symptom at baseline

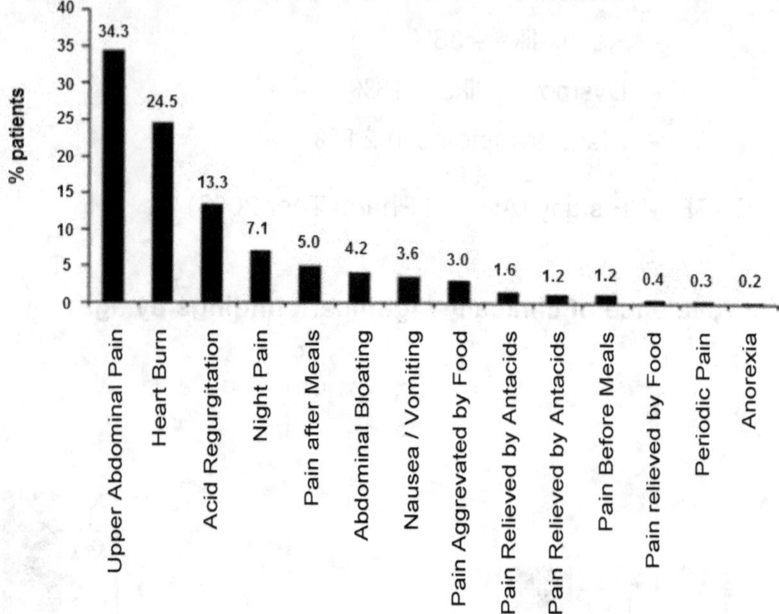

Printed with permission: Thomson AB, et al. Aliment Pharmacol Ther. 2003;17(12):1481-91.

- Findings at endoscopy
  - No significant findings – 42%
  - Clinically significant findings – 58%
  - Esophagitis – 43%
    - 55% of those with reflux-like dyspepsia
    - 36% of those without reflux-like dyspepsia
  - PUD – 5.3%
    - Duodenal ulcer (DU) – 2.8% (69% HP-positive)
    - Gastric ulcer (GU) – 3% (55% H. pylori - positive)
  - Barrett – 2.4% (4.1% with reflux-like dyspepsia)
  - H. pylori positivity – 30%

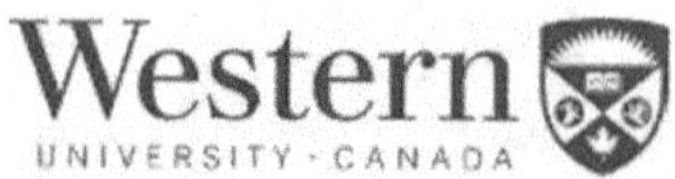

Other than slight increase in esophagitis in GERD-like symptoms, could not predict endoscopic findings by symptoms

- Give the approach to the patient with dyspepsia.
  - Uninvestigated
  - Associated with use of NSAIDs
  - H. pylori-ssociated
  - Non H. pylori-associated

Prevalence (95% CI) of clinically significant findings by dyspepsia sub-group (based on most bothersome symptom reported)

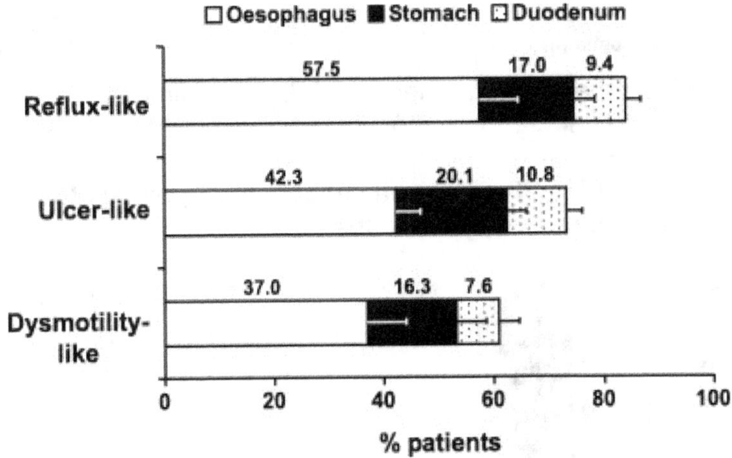

Printed with permission: Thomson AB, et al. Aliment Pharmacol Ther. 2003;17(12):1481-91.

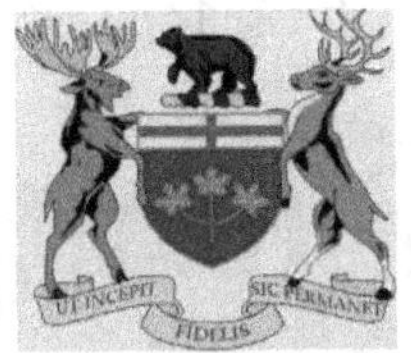

Most prevalent (95% CI) clinically significant findings by ASA/NSAID use

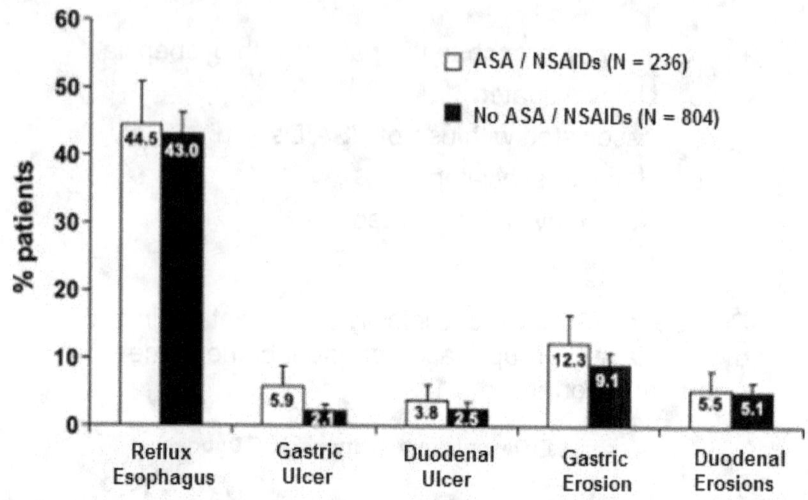

Printed with permission: Thomson AB, et al. Aliment Pharmacol Ther. 2003;17(12):1481-91.

Prevalence (95% CI) of erosive oesophagitis, gastric ulcer and duodenal ulcer by *H. pylori* status

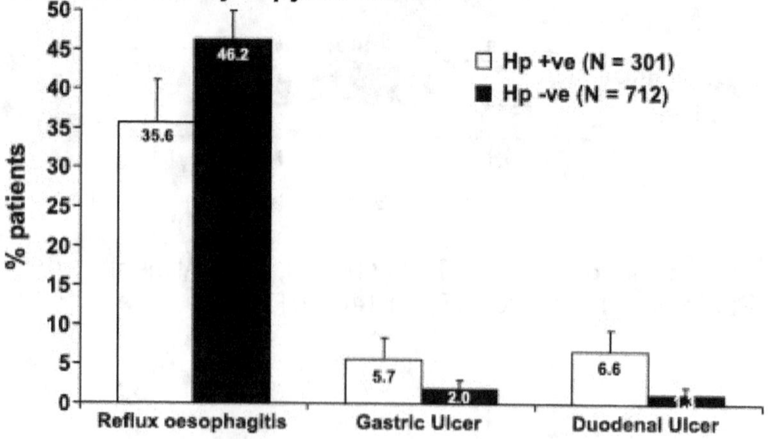

Printed with permission: Thomson AB, et al. Aliment Pharmacol Ther. 2003;17(12):1481-91.

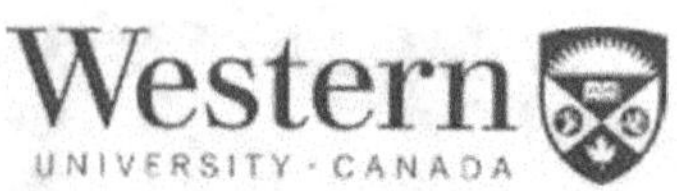

CADET-PE

- Alarm symptoms
  - No correlation between alarm symptoms and presence of clinically significant findings
- Malignancies
  - 2/1040 patients (0.2%) were found to have malignancy
    - Neither had alarm symptoms
  - 1 patient - esophageal carcinoma in situ
  - 1 patient - MALT lymphoma
- Conclusions
  - Clinically significant findings are common in dyspeptic patients
    - More common in older than younger patients
  - Types of presenting symptoms do not predict endoscopic findings
  - Most common findings are esophagitis and HP-related PUD
    - Can manage these patients with PPI or test-and-treat HP strategy (without endoscopy)
  - Malignancy is rare

➢ **Suggested clinical approach (CanDys Guidelines)**

- Age < 50 years, not in an "exception" group, no alarm symptoms → empiric anti-secretory, or
- T & T ("test and treat" for H. pylori) if in a high prevalence H. pylori area
- Age > 50 years, in an "exception" group, or with alarm symptom(s) → EGD
- There are pro's and con's for each approach
- If patient is in a low H. pylori risk area or group, then T&T is not the preferred approach

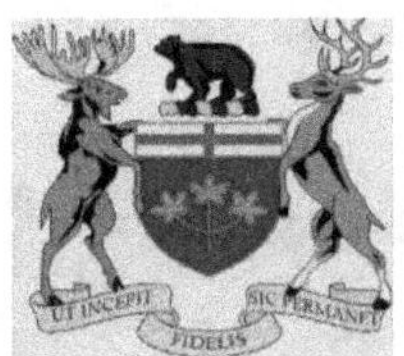

CanDys guidelines

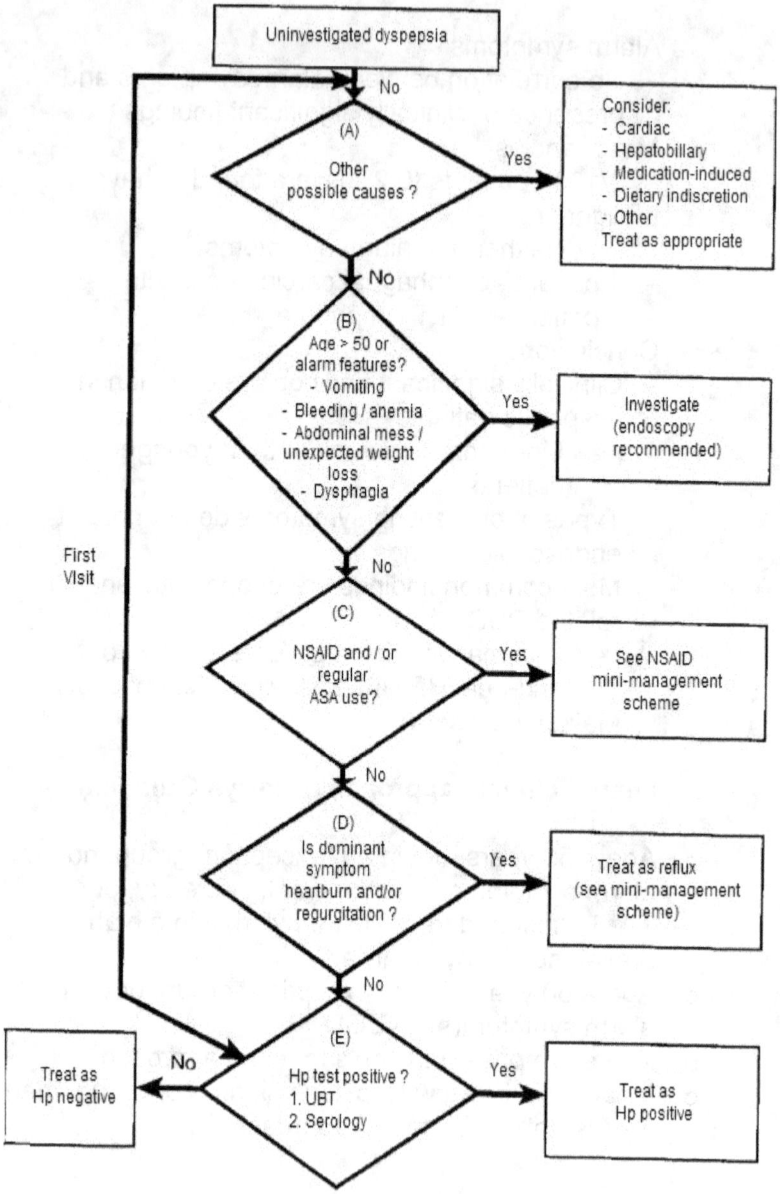

Uninvestigated dyspepsia

(A) Other possible causes ? — Yes → Consider:
- Cardiac
- Hepatobillary
- Medication-induced
- Dietary indiscretion
- Other

Treat as appropriate

No ↓

(B) Age > 50 or alarm features?
- Vomiting
- Bleeding / anemia
- Abdominal mess / unexpected weight loss
- Dysphagia

Yes → Investigate (endoscopy recommended)

No ↓

(C) NSAID and / or regular ASA use? — Yes → See NSAID mini-management scheme

No ↓

(D) Is dominant symptom heartburn and/or regurgitation ? — Yes → Treat as reflux (see mini-management scheme)

No ↓

First Visit → (E)

(E) Hp test positive ?
1. UBT
2. Serology

No → Treat as Hp negative

Yes → Treat as Hp positive

Printed with permission: Veldhuyzen van Zanten SJO, et al. Can J Gastroenterol 2005; 19(5): 285-303.

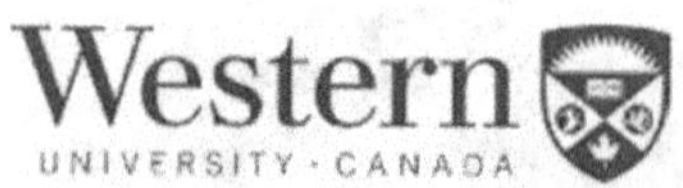

- CMAJ 2000:
  - "An evidence-based approach to the management of uninvestigated dyspepsia in the era of *Helicobacter pylori*"
- Can J Gastroenterol 2005:
  - "Evidence-based recommendations for short- and long-term management of uninvestigated dyspepsia in primary care: An update of the Canadian Dyspepsia Working Group (CanDys) clinical management tool"

- Why EGD > age 50?
  - This recommendation is based on "expert opinion", and some experts suggest that the age cut-off should be 55-yr
  - Incidences of gastric and esophageal cancers starts to rise at age 50
  - Recommended EGD > 45 years, ACG, AGA, BSG > 55 yrs
  - With frequent reflux-like symptoms, especially ≥ times per week, > 5-10 yr duration and moderately severe, Caucasian males, reasonable to perform EGD once-in-a-lifetime to look for Barrett esophagus.

- Why concern about "alarm" symptoms?
  - Most UGI malignancies present with alarm symptoms
  - Presence of any alarm symptom is an indication for EGD
    - Vomiting
    - Bleeding/anemia
    - Abdominal mass
    - Unexplained weight loss

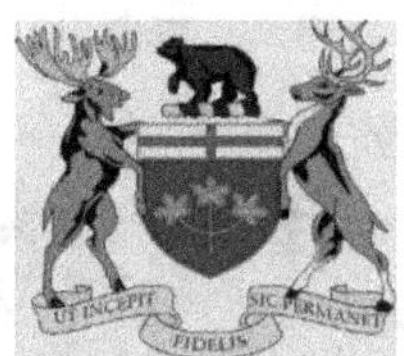

- Dysphagia

➢ Treatment

- Empiric therapy
    - Empiric anti-secretory approach with OTC (over-the-c) ounterantacids, H2RA (H2 receptor antagonists), and half-dose PPIs.
    - PPIs may already have been by the patient before consulting a physician
    - In guidelines, by "anti-secretory trial of therapy" is usually meant to be a standard dose of any PI, given po od ½ hour before breakfast, given for 4 to 8 weeks.

- Test-and-treat (for H. pylori)
    - Prevalence of H. pylori in Northern Europe / Canada is about ~25% (~10% amongst locally born children)
    - Distinguish between H. pylori infection and H. pylori disease, e.g. prevalence of H. pylori in Canadian adults, ~25% prevalence of GU / DU, ~5% (by EGD)
    - Empiric treatment of H. pylori infection in investigated dyspeptics is higher, in part because DU and GU associated disease is being treated, rather than just H. pylori-associated gastritis, the associated symptoms from which generally respond poorly to the eradication of H. pylori.
    - If using a biopsy-based test for H. pylori
        - Stop PI for at least 1 week before taking EGD biopsy
        - Take 2 EGD biopsies from gastric antrum, 2 from body, and 1 from angularis
    - Positive serology for H. pylori only indicates previous exposure; a negative serology test excludes H. pylori-associated disease

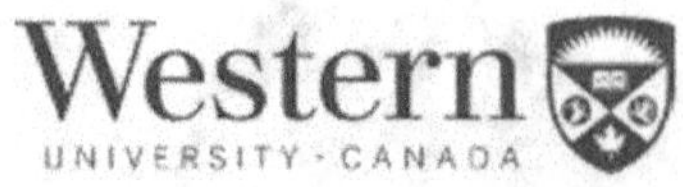

- Specificity is even lower with increasing age and in cirrhosis; determine presence of active infection with UBT or stool antigen test.

- Give the benefits and limitations associated with 5 interventional/ diagnostic approaches to the patient with dyspepsia who is under 50 years of age and who has no alarm symptoms.

Diagnostic approach	Benefits	Limitations
○ "Watchful waiting" only	– Patients with mild and transient symptoms are not prescribed medication or investigated	▪ No clinical studies
○ Empirical Antisecretory therapy (PPI or H2RA)	– Addresses symptoms immediately – Documented effect on reflux symptoms and ulcer-related symptoms	▪ Recurrence after therapy is the rule. EGD is often only postponed, and may be false negative.
○ Treat based on clinical diagnosis	– Clinically meaningful. Low costs	▪ Unreliable
○ Treat based on subgrouping and computer-based algorithms	– Clinically attractive. Low costs	▪ Does not reliably predict EGD diagnosis or response to therapy

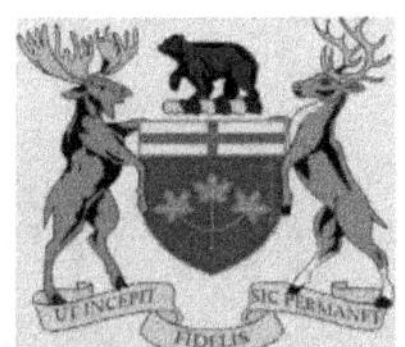

Diagnostic approach	Benefits	Limitations
○ H.*pylori* test-and-treat	– Infected patients with ulcer disease will have symptomatic benefits. Reduces endoscopy rates. Safe and cost-effective compared with endoscopy. Possible reduced risk of later ulcer development.	▪ Low benefit in those without peptic ulcer disease will not benefit. Continuing or recurrent symptoms may frustrate patients and clinician
○ H.*pylori* test-and-scope	– Potential to reduce upper EGD rates in H. pylori low-prevalence areas	▪ Only meaningful if a decision about eradication therapy in infected patients is influenced by endoscopy result. Increases endoscopy demands. Not applicable in H. pylori-high prevalence areas
○ Early endoscopy	– Diagnostic "gold standard". Might lead to reduced medication in patients with normal findings. Increased patient satisfaction in some trials.	▪ Invasive. Costly. About half of EGDs will be normal. Long waiting lists may lead to false negative results. Not the preferred option for many patients. Does not diagnose non-erosive reflux disease (NERD).

Abbreviations: EGD, esophagogastroduodenoscopy; H2RA, H2 receptor antagonist; NERD, non-erosive reflux disease; PPI, proton pump inhibitor.

Adapted from: Bytzer P. *Best Pract Res Clin Gastroenterol* 2004; 18(4): pg.683

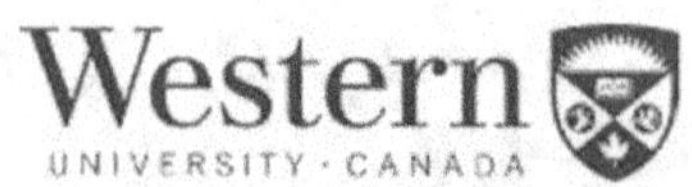

NSAID Mini-Management Scheme

Can the NSAID, ASA or COXIB treatment be stopped ?
- Yes → Is the patient improved ? → Yes → End
- No → Does the patient have a prior history of gastric or duodenal ulcer ?
  - Yes →
    1) Consider a non-invasive test for H. pylori infection and treat with eradication therapy if positive.
    2) I ulcer was related to ASA therapy, NSAID propylaxis may no longer be required if H. pylori eradication is confirmed.
    3) If ulcer was related to conventional NSAID therapy, NSAID prophylaxis is required, despite H. pylori status
  - No →
    1) If taking a conentional NSAID, consider switching to a COXIB or cotherapy with a PPI or misoprostol
    2) I taking ASA, consider cotherapy with PPI
    3) I taking a COXIB, consider switching to another COXIB or cotherapy with PPI

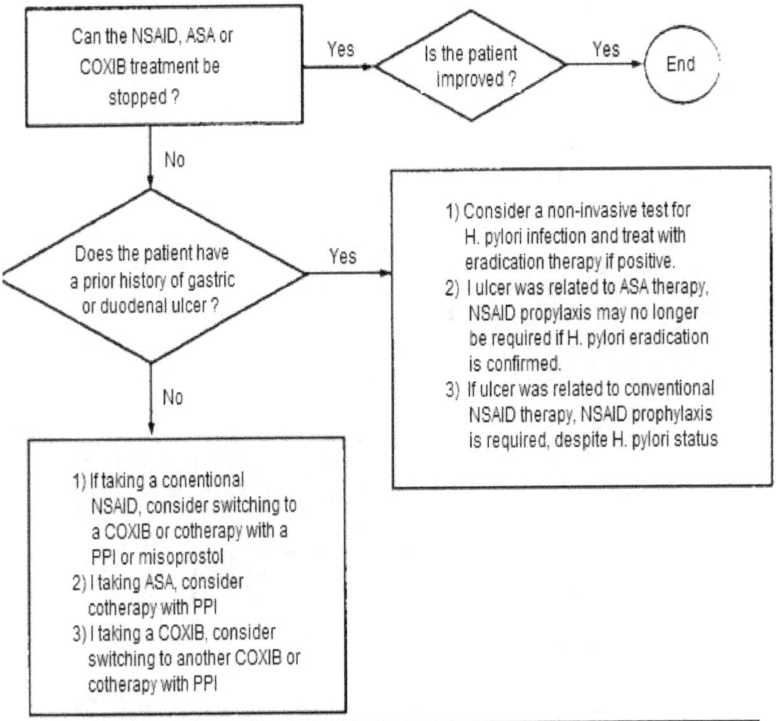

Testing for H. pylori infection in patients taking NSAIDs / ASA
Patient has a history of (bleeding ulcer or dyspepsia?Yes
Patient is intiating NSAID or ASA therapy Yes
Patient has taken NSAID or ASA for more than 6 months? No

Non-steroidal anti-inflammatory drug (NSAID) mini-management scheme; ASA, acetylsalicylic acid; COXIB, cyclooxygenase-2-selective inhibitor; PPI, proton pump inhibitor

Printed with permission: Veldhuyzen van Zanten SJO, et al. Can J Gastroenterol 2005; 19(5): 285-303.

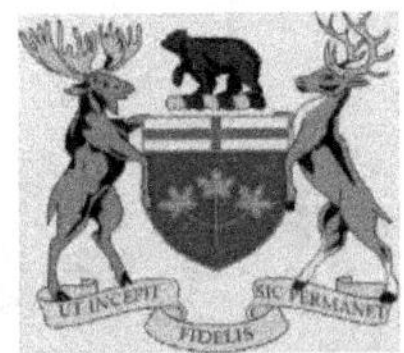

Algorithm for Treatment of GERD-like Dyspepsia

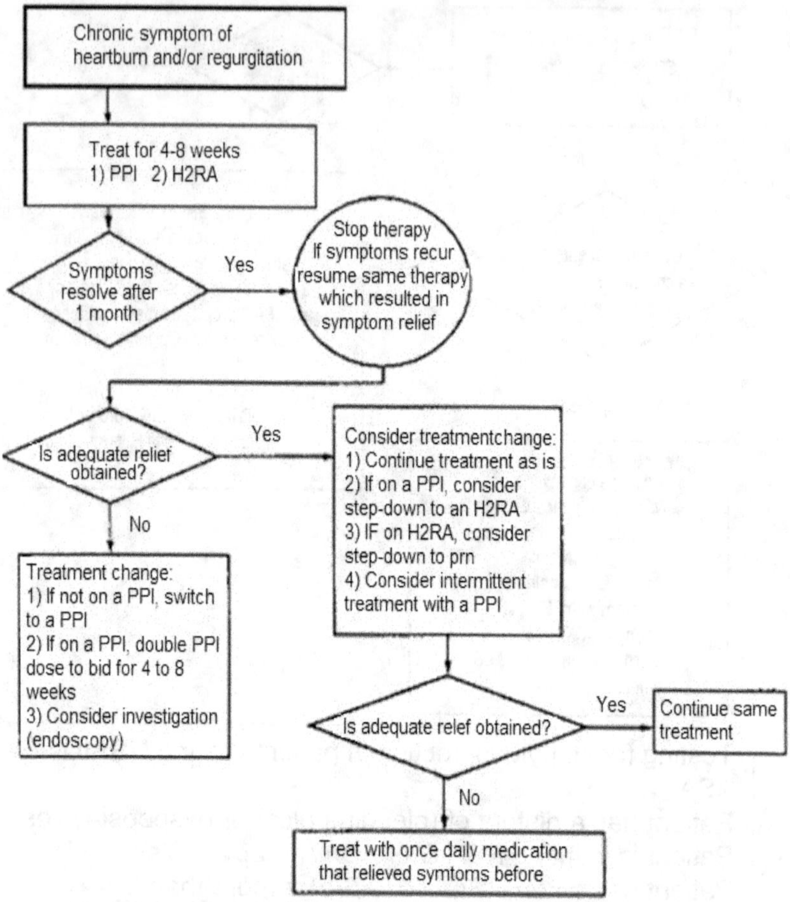

Chronic symptom of heartburn and/or regurgitation

↓

Treat for 4-8 weeks
1) PPI 2) H2RA

↓

Symptoms resolve after 1 month — Yes → Stop therapy. If symptoms recur resume same therapy which resulted in symptom relief

↓

Is adequate relief obtained?

Yes → Consider treatmentchange:
1) Continue treatment as is
2) If on a PPI, consider step-down to an H2RA
3) IF on H2RA, consider step-down to prn
4) Consider intermittent treatment with a PPI

↓

Is adequate relef obtained?

Yes → Continue same treatment

No → Treat with once daily medication that relieved symtoms before

No → Treatment change:
1) If not on a PPI, switch to a PPI
2) If on a PPI, double PPI dose to bid for 4 to 8 weeks
3) Consider investigation (endoscopy)

** Adequate symptom control is the goal regarding any treatment strategy

Consider endoscopy for the detection of Barrett's esophagus if chronic symptom of GERD have been present of more than 5-10 years
1) If no Barrett's mucosa is detected ------> no follow on endoscopy is required
2) If Barrett's mucosa is found --------> offer patient participation in a surveillance program

bid, twice daily; GERD, gastroesophageal reflux disease; H2RA, H2-receptor antagonist; prn, as needed; PPI, proton pump inhibitor

Printed with permission: Veldhuyzen van Zanten SJO, et al. Can J Gastroenterol 2005; 19(5): 285-303.

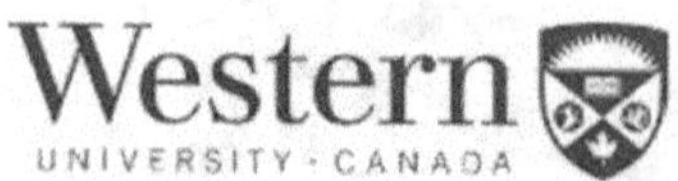

CLINICAL SCENARIO

An MCQ is directed at the issue of the recommended follow-up of a dyspeptic < 55 years whose UBT is positive and they are given successful triple therapy for H. pylori. You are tempted to answer that the correct follow-up is to repeat the UBT to determine if the infection has been eradicated.

Wrong. Successful triple therapy for H. pylori in this setting means the patient has lost her / his dyspepsia. The only circumstances were the UBT must be repeated is

- Persistent dyspepsia
- The patient with complicated H. pylori-associated peptic ulcer (e.g. hemorrhage) must be proven by repeat testing that the anti-H. pylori treatment has effectively eradicated the bug (expected cure rate for triple therapy is only 80%)

Uninvestigated Dyspepsia and H. pylori

- 294 patients with dyspepsia and +HP breath test
- OMC vs. PPI + placebo antibiotics x 7 days
- Results:
  - 50% improvement in treated group vs. 36% in control
  - ARR 14%, NNT 7
  - Reduction in mean annual health care cost by $53 in treated group
- Conclusion: HP test-and-treat strategy appropriate for dyspepsia without alarm symptoms

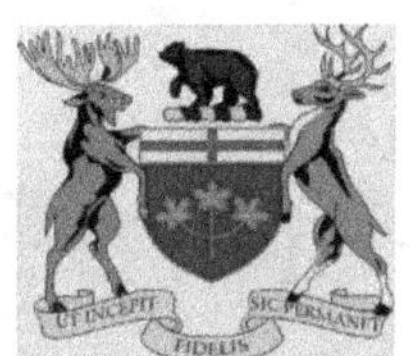

Abbreviations: ARR, absolute risk reduction; HP, H. pylori; OMC, omeprazole metronidazole clarithromycin; NNT, number needed to treat; PPI, proton pump inhibitor

CADET-HP (BMJ 2002)

Non-Ulcer Dyspepsia and H. pylori

- RRR 8%
- NNT 18 to cure dyspepsia
- Placebo rate 30% - thus NNT 3 in practice

Abbreviations: NNT, number needed to treat; RRR, relative risk reduction

Moayyedi (Cochrane Library)

Dyspepsia and pregnancy

- Upper GI symptoms are common in pregnant women, and when EGD has been performed the findings are esophagitis (34%) and gastritis (25%).
- Predictors of heartburn during pregnancy include young age of the mother, her parity, increasing gestational age, and the presence of heartburn before pregnancy (which occurs in 14% of mothers) (Marrero JM, et al. *Br J Obstet Gynaecol* 1992:731-4).
- Only calcium-containing antacids should be used for GERD symptoms, since
  - Aluminum-containing antacids may cause fetal neurotoxicity,
  - Alginic acid (Gaviscon, sucralfate) may cause fetal distress
  - Magnesium-containing antacids may cause renal stones, respiratory distress and cardiovascular impairment, and hypotemia.

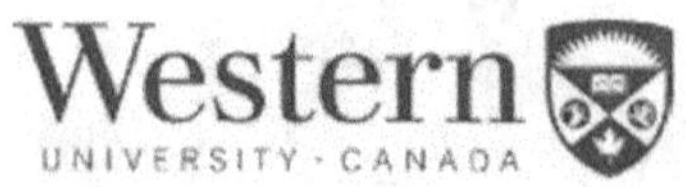

- Nizatidine is not recommended for lactating mothers (FDA C, due to report of growth retardation of rodent pups)

- Give 6 factors to consider when performing endoscopy in pregnant women.
  - A strong indication is always needed, particularly in high-risk pregnancies
  - Whenever possible, endoscopy should be deferred until the second trimester
  - The lowest possible dose of sedative medication should be used (wherever possible FDA category A or B drugs)
  - Procedure time should be short
  - To avoid inferior venal cava or aortic compression, the patient should be positioned in the left pelvic tilt or left lateral position
  - Presence of fetal heart sounds should be confirmed before sedation and after the procedure
  - Obstetric support should be immediately available
  - No endoscopy should be performed in patients with obstetric complications (placental rupture, imminent delivery, ruptured membranes, or pre-eclampsia)

Printed with permission: Keller J, et al. *Nat Clin Pract Gastroenterol Hepatol* 2008; 5(8): 435.

Pediatrics

- Give a differential diagnosis of vomiting in a newborn.
  - Gastroenteritis, gastroesophageal reflux, overfeeding, food allergy, milk protein intolerance, congenital duodenal atresia, pyloric stenosis, volvulus, meconium ileus, Hirschsprung's disease

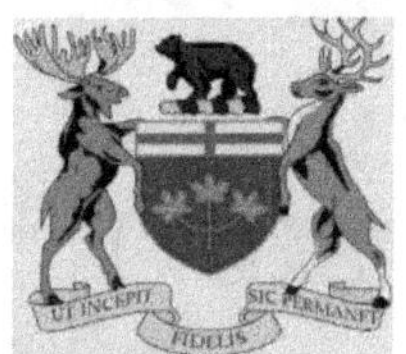

Helicobacter Pylori Positive Mini-Management Scheme

Patient *Hp* positive

↓

Eradicate Hp
a. PPI + AC or MC or
b. RBC + AC + or MC (bid x 7 days)
c. PPI +BMT (bid x 14 days)
(advise patient to return 4 weeks after treatment if symptoms recur or persist

↓

Symptoms resolved at follow-up ?

- Yes → No further therapy or investigation
- No ↓

Confirm Hp eradication by UBT or histology (not serology)

↓

Hp eradicated ?

- Yes → Treat as Hp negative (see mini-management scheme)
- No ↓

Switch regimen and retreat* or refer for investigation

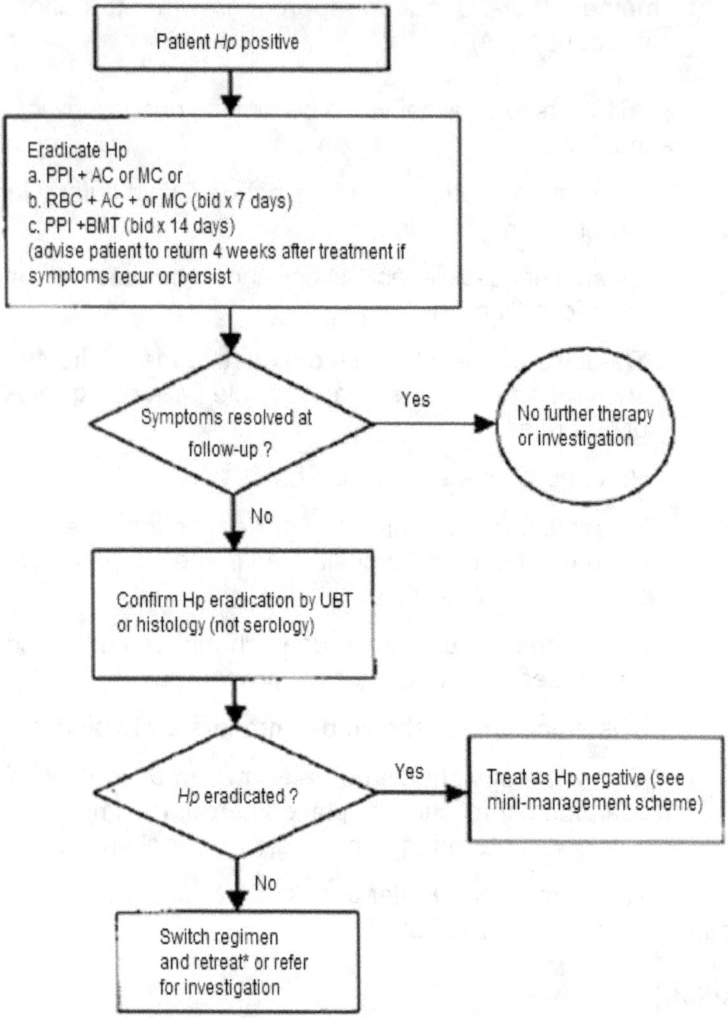

A = amoxicillin 1000 mg; B = bismuth subsalicylate (2 tablets); C = clarithromycin 250 or 500 mg (500 mg if treatment failure); M = metronidazole 500 mg (250 mg in BMT [bismuth-metronidazole-tetracycline] combimation therapy; PPI = lansoprazole 30 mg, omeprazole 20 mg or pantoprazole 40 mg; RBC = ranitidine bismuth citrate 400 mg; T = tetracycline 500 mg

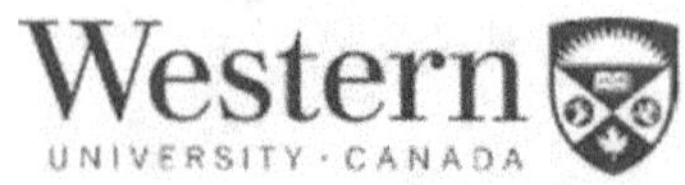

If PPI or RBC + MC (metronidazole + clarithromycin) was used, switch to PPI or RBC + AC (amoxicillin + clarithromycin) or vice versa, or switch to a 14-day course of PPI +BMT

Printed with permission: Veldhuyzen van Zanten SJO, et al. An evidence-based approach to the management of uninvestigated dyspepsia in the era of Helicobacter pylori. CMAJ 2000; 62 (12) suppl S3-S23.

Helicobacter Pylori Negative Mini-Management Schemes

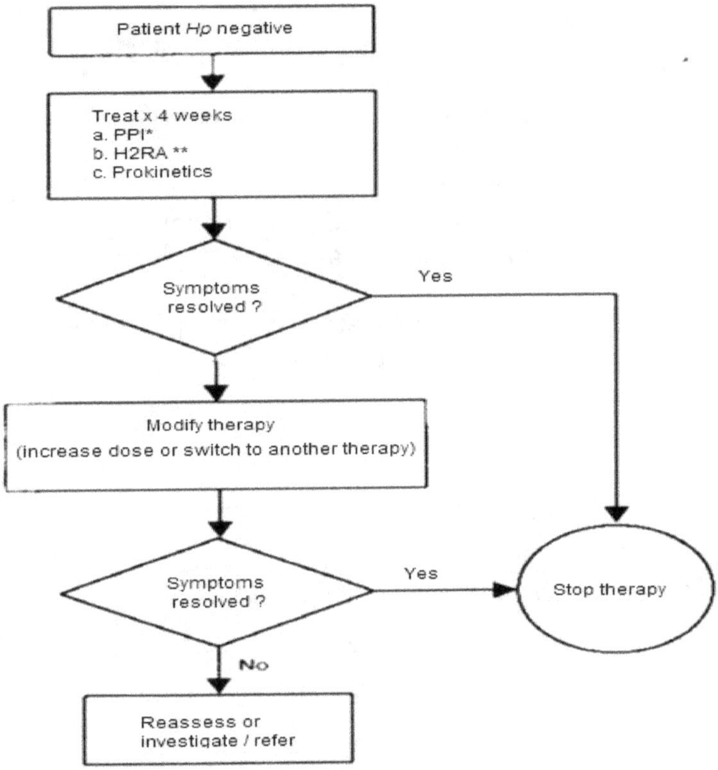

Patient *Hp* negative

↓

Treat x 4 weeks
a. PPI*
b. H2RA **
c. Prokinetics

↓

Symptoms resolved ? — Yes → Stop therapy

↓

Modify therapy
(increase dose or switch to another therapy)

↓

Symptoms resolved ? — Yes → Stop therapy

↓ No

Reassess or investigate / refer

* Most of the data available are for omeprazole (20 mg once daily), some for lansoprzole (20 mg once daily), some for lansoprazole (30 mg once daily)
** Most of the data are for ranitidine

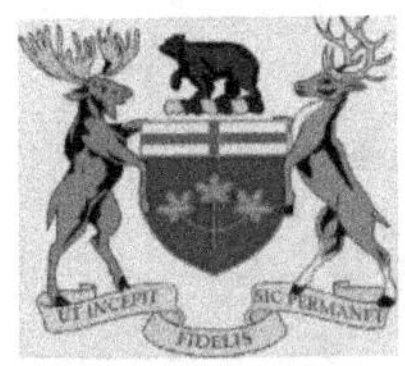

Printed with permission: Veldhuyzen van Zanten SJO, et al. An evidence-based approach to the management of uninvestigated dyspepsia in the era of Helicobacter pylori. CMAJ 2000; 62 (12) suppl S3-S23.

- Dyspepsia is common
- Use an algorithmic approach (such asto maximize treatment benefits but minimize costs
- CanDys guidelines
- Not everybody needs EGD
- Rome III Management Recommendations
  - Similar to CanDys
  - Recommend endoscopy for all "patients over a threshold age (45-55 years, depending on health care access and incidence of malignant disease)"
  - Suggest that "endoscopy first might be more cost-effective in older patients"

"Hard work and good intentions are admirable, but for the successes of life, you have to put the puck in the net."
Grandad

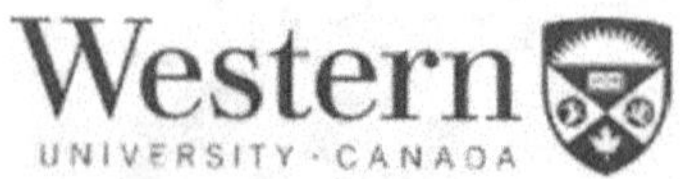

H. Pylori Infection and Associated Diseases

Aze Wilson

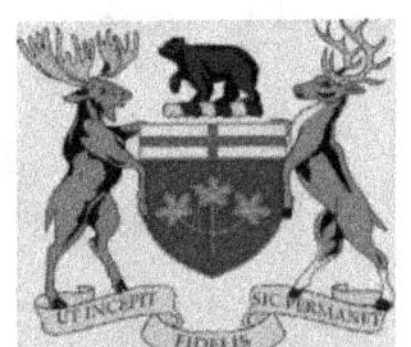

Helicobacter pylori

- A gram-negative bacterium
  - Selectively colonizes human gastric epithelium, causing a spectrum of pathological conditions ranging from gastritis to peptic ulcer disease to gastric cancer

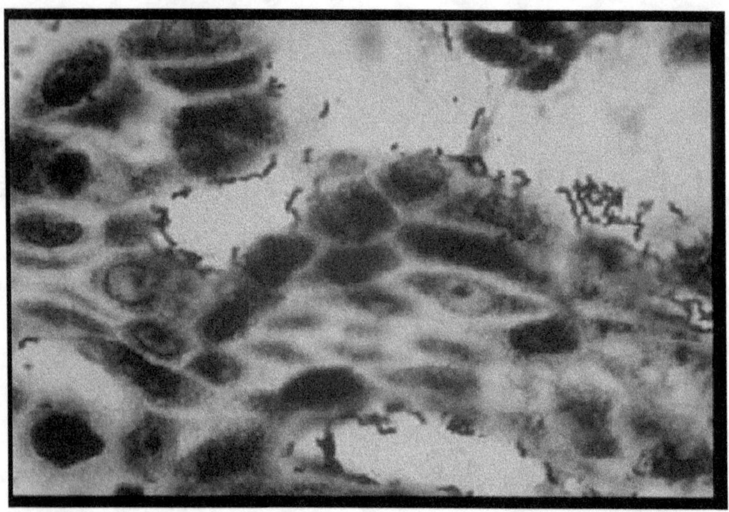

A silver stain (Warthin Starry) of HP on gastric mucus-secreting epithelial cells

Marshall BJ and Warren JR. Lancet. 1984;1(8390):1311-5.

- Linked to multiple GIT diseases (Peek RM Jr and Crabtree JE. J Pathol. 2006;208:233-48)
  - Gastric/duodenal ulcers (10%)
  - Gastric adenocarcinoma (1-3%); listed as class 1 carcinogen by WHO
  - MALT lymphoma (0.7%)
  - Gastric non-Hodgekins lymphoma

Abbreviations: MALT, mucosa associated lymphoid tissue; WHO, World Health Organization

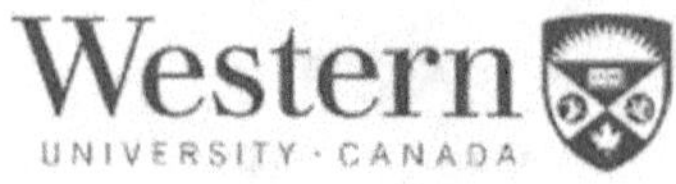

- Genetic studies suggest idea that humans have
  - Co-evolved with H.pylori, and
  - Have been colonized for > 58,000 years

Linz B et al. Nature. 2007;445(7130):915-8.

- Prevalence of HP by Region
  - A low of~30% in Canada and the United Kingdom, to a high of 80% to 90% in Africa and parts of China
  - Prevalence may vary within a country, for example, in Canada
    - Children < 10 yr born in Canada,~10%
    - Adults 20-40 yr old born in Canada~30%
    - First Nations Canadians~70-80%

- Transmission and Sources of Infection:
  - Mechanism of acquisition is unknown (Kusters JG et al. Clin Microbiol Rev. 2006;19:449-90)
  - Human-to-human (po-po or fecal-po)
  - No conclusive evidence for zoonotic transmission
  - Detected in saliva, vomitus, feces, gastric refluxate (Allaker RP, et al. J Med Microbiol. 2002;51:312-7;
  - No increased risk in: dentists, GIs, RNs or partners of HP+ individuals[3]
  - No conclusive evidence for predominant transmission via any of these products. Acquisition most likely occurs in childhood from close family members

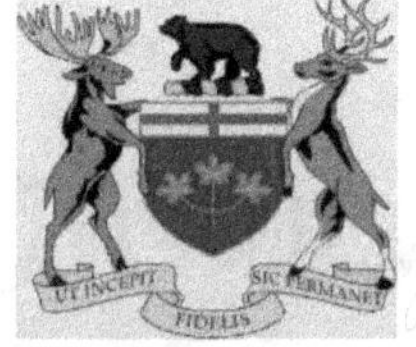

- Risk Factors for Infection (Patel P, et al. Lancet. 1994;344(8921):511-2)
  - Age (older)
    - Usually acquired by year 10
  - Socioeconomic status during childhood
    - As the levels of household hygiene increased the preavlence of HP in the younger generations has declined in industrialized regions, but remains fairly constant in developing nations
    - Childhood crowding
    - Sharing a bed
    - Absence of fixed hot water supply
  - Country of origin (Graham DY, et al. Dig Dis Sci. 1991;36(8):1084-8)
  - Genetic factors (Malaty HM, et al. Ann Intern Med 1994;120(12):982-6)
    - MZ twins near/far>DZ twins

Abbreviations: DZ, dizygote; MZ, monozygote

HP Strategy to Survive in the Stomach

- Multiple polar flagellae propel the bacterium through the stomach's mucus and unstirred water (UWL) layer
- The H. pylorum survives in the alkaline microenvironment of the UWL, partially created with the urease optimum of pH 6.2, and creating a non-acidic microzone that proects the bacteria.
- Use of adherence factors (adhesions) to avoid being shed during cell turnover to enable HP to bind specifically to gastric-type epithelium to avoid being shed during cell and mucous turnover.

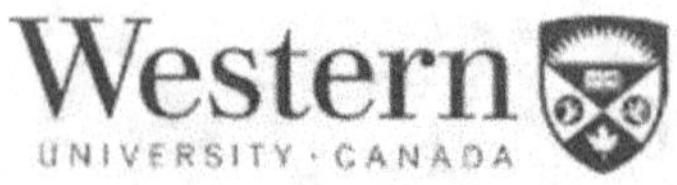

Method of Colonization

- Antibody to H. pylori is detected
- Reason for poor IS immune response
- HP is able to avoid host immune surveillance via molecular mimicry.
  - HP is lined by Lewis (Le) Ag – identical to components of human blood
  - Disguise is imperfect and results in a reduced immune response contributing to injury of the gastric mucosa (gastritis)
- Avoidance of detection via genetic variability
  - HP chromosome analysis = high degree of variability

➢ Factors mediating tissue injury:

- Lipopolysaccharides
  - Glycolipids found in the cell envelope of gram-negative bacteria (endotoxins)
  - Endotoxins are proteins which induce inflammatory reactions by binding to the bacterial membrane
  - Stimulate the release of cytokines (Th1 response)
  - Interfere with the gastric epithelium-laminin interaction
    - Loss of mucosal integrity,
    - Decreased mucin synthesis
    - Stimulation of pepsinogen secretion
  - Endotoxins are less potent than LPP of E. Coli
  - This may account for its adaptation for LT residence

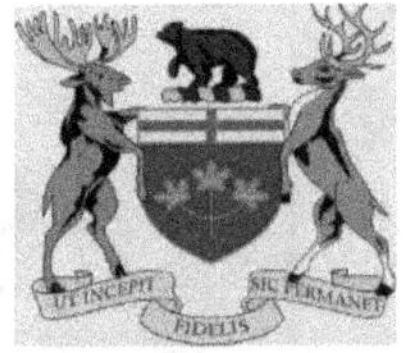

- Other leukocyte recruitment and activating factors[1]
  - LPS-independent soluble surface protein recruitment of PMNs and monocytes to the lamina propria
    - H. pylori PMN-activating protein (napA gene) (Evans DJ Jr et al. Infect Immun. 1995;63:2213-20)
    - Immunologically active porins (Tufano MA et al. Infect Immun. 1994;62:1392-9)

Abbreviations: LPS, lipopolysaccharides; PMN, polymorphonucleal neutrophils

- Vacuolating cytotoxin (VacA)[1]
  - Induces vacuole formation in eukaryotic cells
  - Increases IC permeability allowing more nutrients to be available to H. pylori
- Outer membrane inflammatory protein(OipA)[1]
  - Enhances inflammatory response within the mucosal lining
    - Synergistic with CagA (cytotoxin associated antigen)
- Heat shock proteins
  - HspA and HspB (unclear role in pathogenesis of infection)
- Cytotoxin associated antigen (CagA)
  - Associated with pathogenicity island" = CagA
  - Virulence factor associated with increased inflammatory response
  - Pathogenicity island is a sequence of genes associated with the development of a certain outcome (eg. GU, DU)

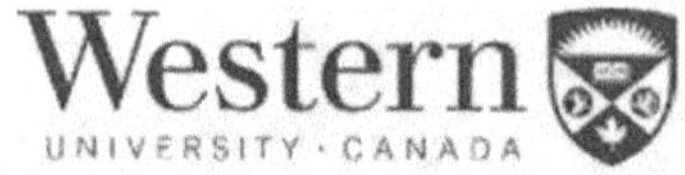

- Pathogenesis of Inflammation:
  - HP stimulates the release of a variety of inflammatory mediators:
    - **Direct**: bacterial products of the CagA pathogenicity island and OipA
    - **Indirect**: interaction with gastric mucosa
      - Release of IL-8 (recruits PMNs)
      - Production of reactive O_2 metabolites
      - Upregulation of PMN expression of CD11b/CD18 (↑ PMN adherence via CAM-1)
      - PMN adhesion ↑ microvascular pemeability and mast cell degranulation.

Chronic H. pylori Infection:

- All infected individuals in industrialized countries have a chronic active, non-atrophic superficial gastritis[1]
  - Marked lymphoplasmacytic inflammation and PMNs
  - Inflammation is concentrated in the luminal aspect of the bx
  - Pititis
  - Foveolar hyperplasia
  - Prominent lymphoid aggregates/follicles
  - HP occur as "seagull wing" shaped rods

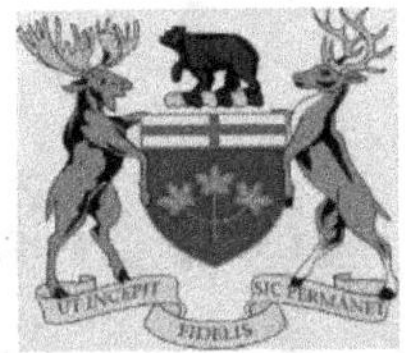

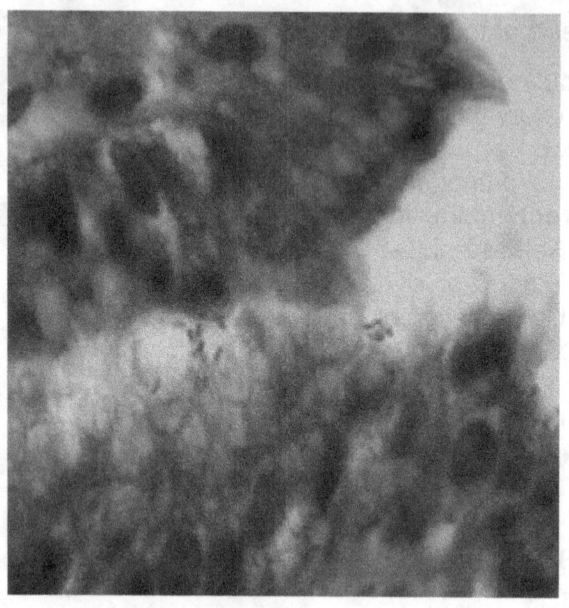

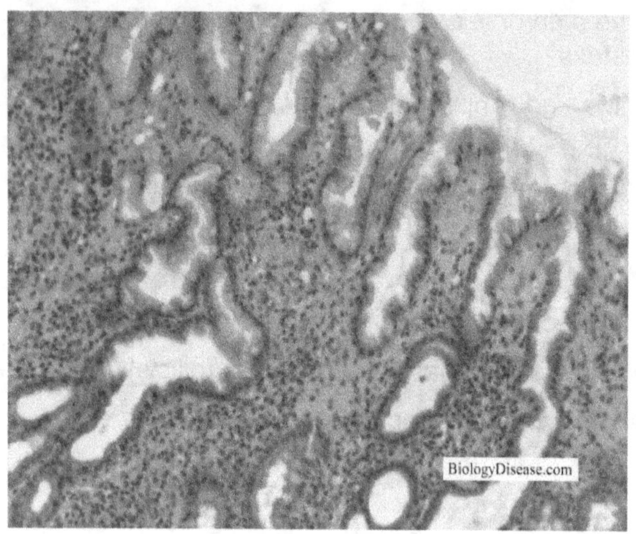
BiologyDisease.com

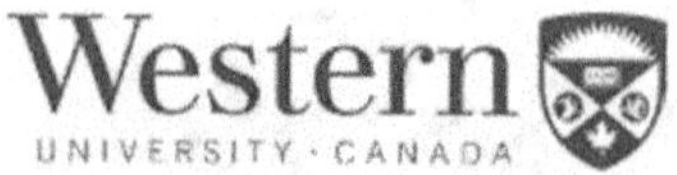
Western
UNIVERSITY · CANADA

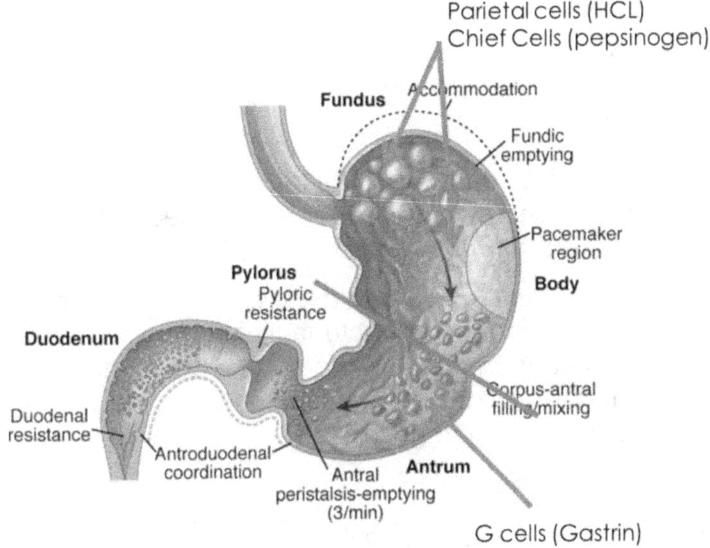

- Level of acid secretion correlates with distribution of inflammatory response effect on acid secretion (gastritis)
- Risk for different symptomatology is predicted by the pattern of gastritis:
- Antral-predominant gastritis = DU (increased delivery of unbuffered acid to the duodenal bulb.
- Chronic atrophic pan-gastritis = GU, gastric adenoca, gastric lymphoma

- Chronic atrophic pan-gastritis (CAPG)
  - In low acid states
    - Inflammatory infiltrate influences parietal cell function
    - Release of acid inhibitory cytokines, IL-1
    - HP colonization of the corpus > antrum

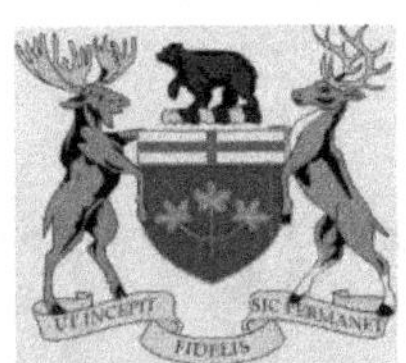

- CAPG
  - GU
  - GCa
  - GL
- Intact acid secretion: HP colonizes the gastric antrum where there are fewer acid secreting parietal cells (antrum predominant gastritis
- Impaired acid secretion (PPI, etc) have a more even distribution of bacteria in antrum and corpus and bacteria in the corpus are in closer contact with the mucosa leading to a corpus predominant pan gastritis

- Progression to gastric atrophy
  - Chronic active gastritis can progress to atrophic gastritis
    - Loss of glandular tissue from repeated mucosal injury
    - Replacement with fibrous tissue
    - Pathway to gastric adenoCa

➢ DU pathogenesis:
- HP stimulates release of gastrin (by unknown mechanism) → ↑ HCl secretion
- ↑ HCl in D1 (first part of duodenum) can cause gastric metaplasia (defense mechanism)
  - Spread of HP to DI
  - Acute/chronic inflammation and frank ulceration in some

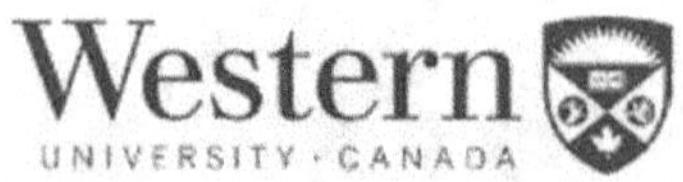

H. pylori Infection vs. H. pylori-asssociated disease

- Disease outcome is the result of the intricate, ongoing interplay between environmental, bacterial, and host factors.
  - Strain-to-strain genetic variability in bacterial virulence factors *affects the ability of the organism* to colonize and cause disease
- On the host side, variations in the host immune response to the chronic presence of *H. pylori directly impact H. pylori-associated gastric* disease and affect gastric acid output and thereby the density and location of *H. pylori cells.*

"Mediocrity is metric modulation, bringing people back (regression) to the mean."

Grandad

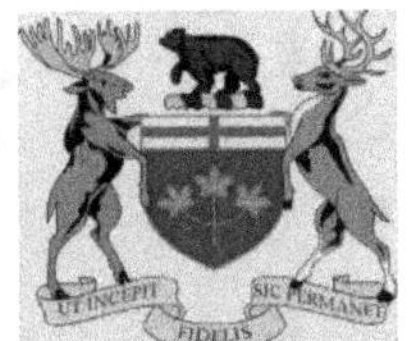

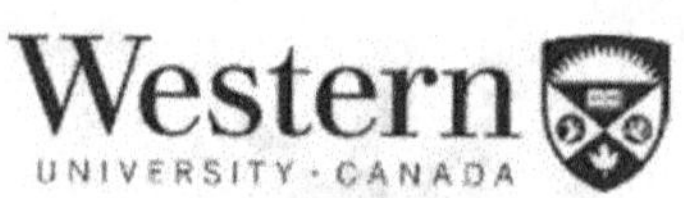
Western
UNIVERSITY · CANADA

MINI UPDATE

SMALL BOWEL

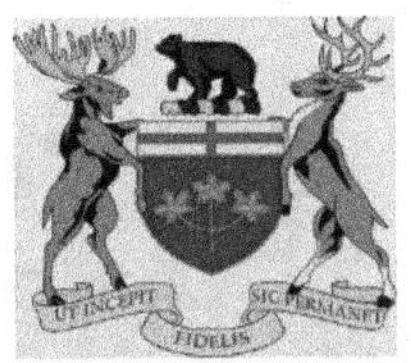

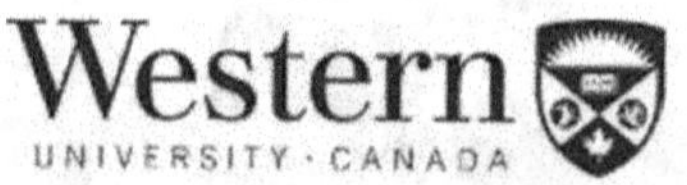

Celiac Disease

Melanie Beaton

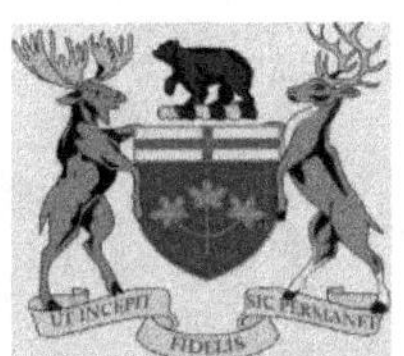

- Demography
  - Age
    - Mean age presentation; 45yr
    - 25% > 60yr
    - Teen years often a time of spontaneous remission, unusual to manifest in adolescence
    - May or may not have history consistent with unrecognized CD in childhood
    - Many develop CD for 1st time in adulthood.

- Clinical

- GI
  - Diarrhea
    - Episodic > Continuous, steatorrhea
    - Osmotic (malabsorption), Secretory (bacterial action creates hydroxy fatty acids)
  - Highly Variable and Non Specific
    - Some CD patients even present with constipation
    - Prevalence of CD in IBS is ↑4-fold, ACG recommendations for evaluation of
    - IBS-D include screening for CD (Source: Spiegel et al, Gastroenterol 2004; Ford et al. AIM 2009)
    - Bloating, Dyspepsia, Heartburn, Flatulence, Apthous ulcers
  - Weight loss

- Extraintestinal Manifestations
  - Cutaneous
    - Bruising
    - Edema
    - Dermatitis Herpetiformis
    - Follicular hyperkeratosis
    - Dermatitis
    - Acute stomatits

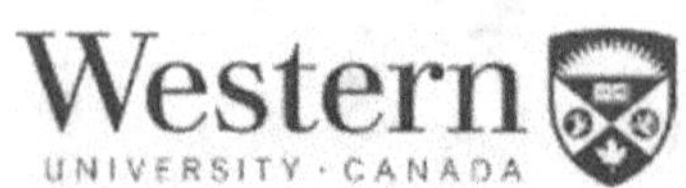

- Endocrine
  - DM Type 1
    - 5% DM 1 have CD & 5% CD have DM 1
  - Thyroid
    - Hypo > Hypertheriod
  - Secondary Hyperparathyroidism
  - Osteopenia (#1 complication, 70% of untreated celiac due to $\downarrow Ca^{2+}$ & Vit D absorption)
  - Osteoporosis (25%)
  - Short stature
  - Impotence
- Hematologic
  - IgA Deficiency
    - 2% w/CD (20 fold higher than general population)
  - Anemia (iron, folate > B12)
  - Hemorrhage (vitamin K)
  - Thrombocytosis
  - Howell-Jolly bodies (hyposplenism)
- Hepatic
  - ↑ transaminases
  - Association with PBC, PSC
- Musculoskeletal
  - Atrophy
  - Tetany
  - Weakness
  - Sjogren syndrome
  - Rheumatoid arthritis
  - Systemic Lupu Erythromatosus
  - Polymyositis
- OB/Gyn
  - Amenorrhea
  - Delayed Menarche
  - Early Menopause
  - Infertility
  - Slightly higher risk of post-partum hemorrhage

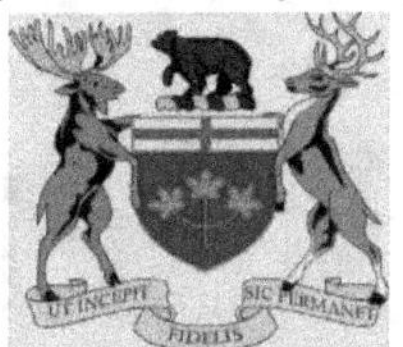

- Neurologic
  - Chronic fatigue
  - Depression (10%)
  - Peripheral neuropathy
  - Gluten Ataxia (thought to be from immunological damage to cerebellum
  - Spinal cord & peripheral nerves)
  - Demyelination
  - Seizures
  - Night blindness (Vitamin A deficiency)
  - Peripheral. Neuropathy & Ataxia usually do not respond to gluten withdrawl*
  - Possible neurological associations: Autism, ADHD, Cognitive deficits
- Gastrointestinal
  - IBD (Crohn Disease and ulcerative colitis)
  - Microscopic Colitis
  - Primary Sclerosing Cholangitis
  - Primary Biliary Cirrhosis
  - Collagenous sprue
- Collagenous colitis
- Lymphocytic colitis
- Lung
  - Interstitial lung disease
  - Idiopathic pulmonary hemosiderosis
- Kidney
- Miscellaneous
  - Down and Turner syndrome
  - IgA deficiency and nephropathy

Dermatitis Herpetiformis (DH)

- Skin Changes
  - Multiple grouped (herpetiform) papules & vesicles
  - Intensely pruritic

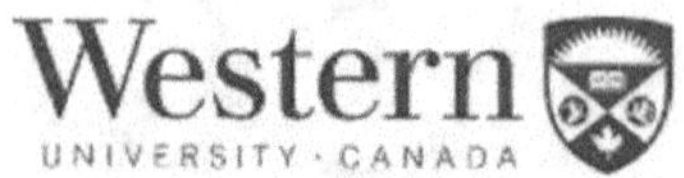

- Normally on elbows, dorsal forearms, knees, scalp & back
- 10-25% of CD patients have DH
- Up to 85% DH have CD (often asymptomatic)

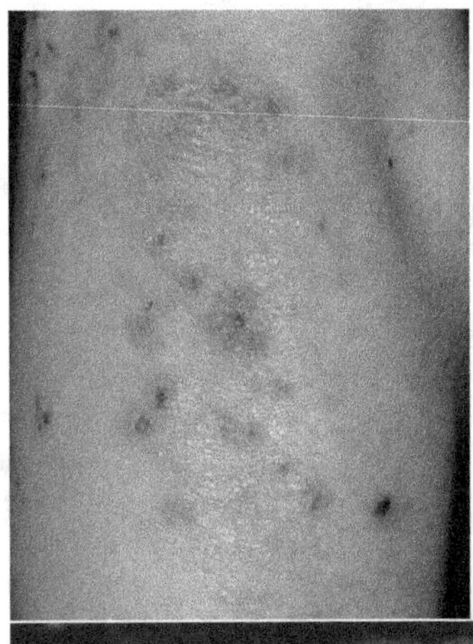

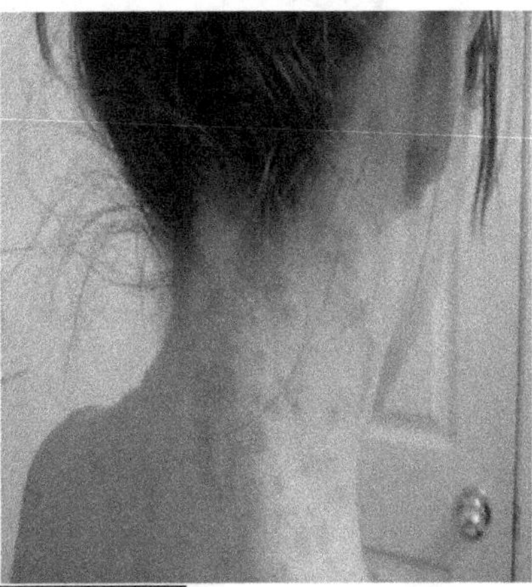

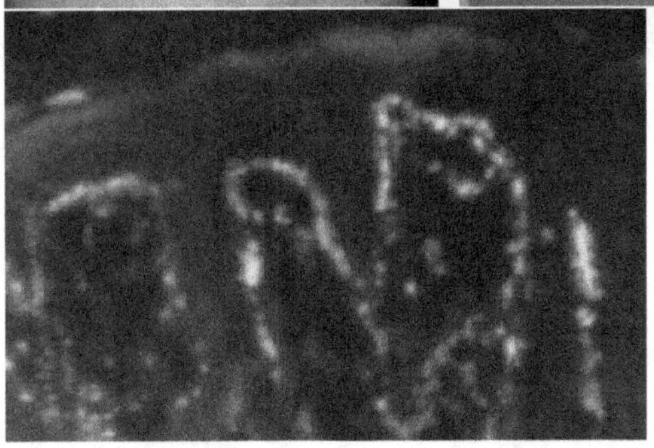

- Skin biopsy
  - Granular IgA deposits along basement membrane
- ↑Serum anti-TTG
- Diagnostically abnormal small bowel mucosal biopsy
  - Dapsone – quickly improves DH skin changes (no affect on bowel)
  - Gluten free diet (GFD) plus dapsone →Rapid gi improvement

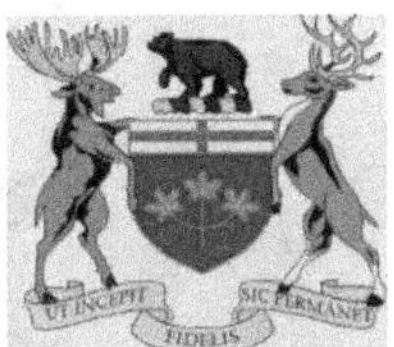

- Pathogenesis

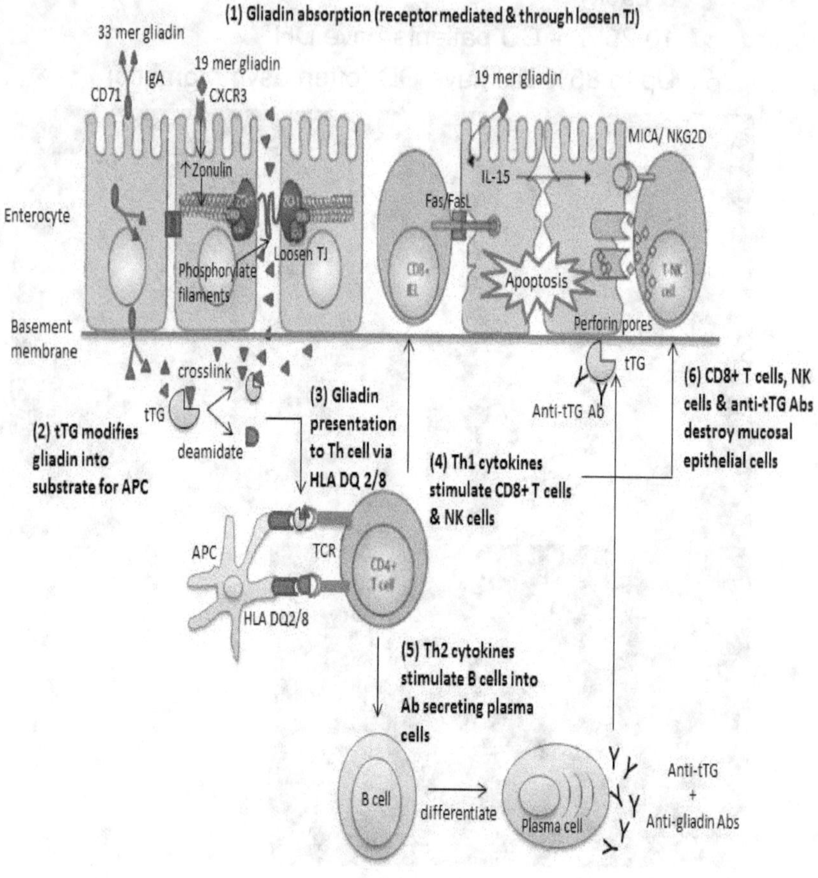

(1) Gliadin absorption (receptor mediated & through loosen TJ)
33 mer gliadin
IgA
CD71
19 mer gliadin
CXCR3
↑Zonulin
19 mer gliadin
MICA/ NKG2D
IL-15
Fas/FasL
Enterocyte
Loosen TJ
Phosphorylate filaments
CD8+ IEL
Apoptosis
T-NK cell
Perforin pores
Basement membrane
crosslink
tTG
deamidate
(2) tTG modifies gliadin into substrate for APC
(3) Gliadin presentation to Th cell via HLA DQ 2/8
tTG
Anti-tTG Ab
(4) Th1 cytokines stimulate CD8+ T cells & NK cells
(6) CD8+ T cells, NK cells & anti-tTG Abs destroy mucosal epithelial cells
APC
TCR
CD4+ T cell
HLA DQ2/8
(5) Th2 cytokines stimulate B cells into Ab secreting plasma cells
B cell
differentiate
Plasma cell
Anti-tTG + Anti-gliadin Abs

Printed with permission: Gujral N, et al. World J Gastroenterol. 2012;18(42):6036-59.

- Gliadin peptides cross the epithelium by paracellular tight junctions (TJ) as a consequence of ↑release of zonulin leading to ↓ mucosal integrity upon 19 mer gliadin binding to CXCR3 receptor, or via transcytosis, or retrotranscytosis of secretory IgA through transferrin receptor CD71.

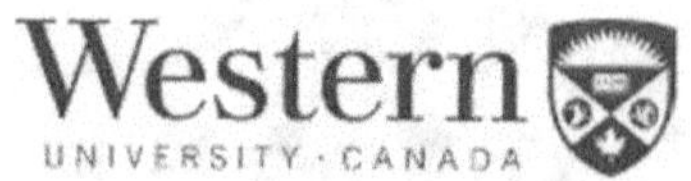

- Tissue transglutaminase (tTG) deamidates or crosslinks 33 mer gliadin, which is then recognized by HLA-DQ2 or -DQ8 molecules of antigen presenting cell (APC).
- APC presents the toxic peptide to CD4+ T (αβ) cells.
- Activated gluten-reactive CD4+ T-cells produce high levels of pro-inflammatory cytokines.
- Th1 cytokines promote increased cytotoxicity of intraepithelial lymphocytes (IELs; γδ T cells) and natural killer (NK) T cells which cause apoptotic death of enterocytes by the Fas/Fas ligand (FasL) system, or interleukin 15 (IL-15)-induced perforin/granzyme and NKG2D–MICA signaling pathways.
- The production of Th2 cytokines activate and induce clonal expansion of B cells, which differentiate into anti-gliadin and anti-tTG antibody secreting plasma cells.
- Interaction between with the extracellular tTG (mtTG) and anti-tTG-autoantibody may induce epithelial damage.

➢ Serology

- IgA tTG & EMA – both based on tTG as target antigen vs. AGAs where gliadin is target antigen
- Performance characteristics

Serologic Test	Sensitivity (%)	Specificity (%)	PPV (%)	NPV (%)
tTG IgA	95-100	97-100	80-95	100
IgA	85-98	97-100	98-100	80-95

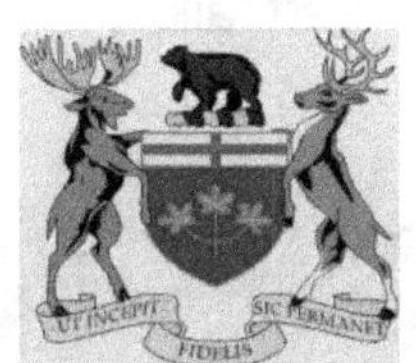

Serologic Test	Sensitivity (%)	Specificity (%)	PPV (%)	NPV (%)
tTG IgG	Sens - 40% (but higher in IgA deficiency) Spec - 98%			
AGA	75-95	82-95	28-100	65-100
AGA	69-85	73-90	20-95	41-88

Abbreviations: AGA, antigliadin antibody; EMA, antiendomysial antibody; NPV, negative predictive value; PV, positive predictive value; SENS', sensitivity; TTG, transglutaminase antibody

- Uses
  - Evaluate patients with suspected CD
  - Monitor adherence to GFD (gluten free diet)
    - IgA-tTG Antibody half-life is approximately 6-8wk
    - Often normalizes in 3-12mon
- Causes of **false negative** IgA-TTG serology
  - < 2 yr of age
  - IgA deficiency
  - Mild CD
  - Treated CD
    - GFD (gluten free diet)
    - TPN (total parenteral nutrition)
    - immunosuppression
- Causes of **false positive** IgA-TTG serology
  - Autoimmune conditions associated with CD, e.g.,
    - DM I, type 1 diabetes
    - Thyroid disease
    - IBD, inflammatory bowel disease
    - Some chronic liver diseases e.g., PBC
  - Severe HF (heart failure)

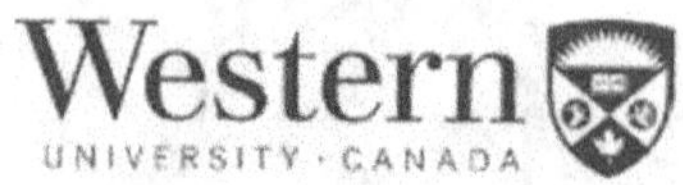

- Deamidated gliadin peptide (DGP) antibodies
  - More sensitive & specific than IgA & IgG AGA
  - May be slightly less sensitive than tTG

- Endoscopy
  - Features
    - Scalloping
    - Loss of duodenal folds
    - Fissures
    - Mosiac-appearance
  - 5-8 endoscopic mucosal biopsies (1-2 from cap of duodenum and 4-6 from distal duodenum)
    - Cap may have architectural distortion due to other causes, e.g.,
      - Brunner glands
      - peptic duodenitis

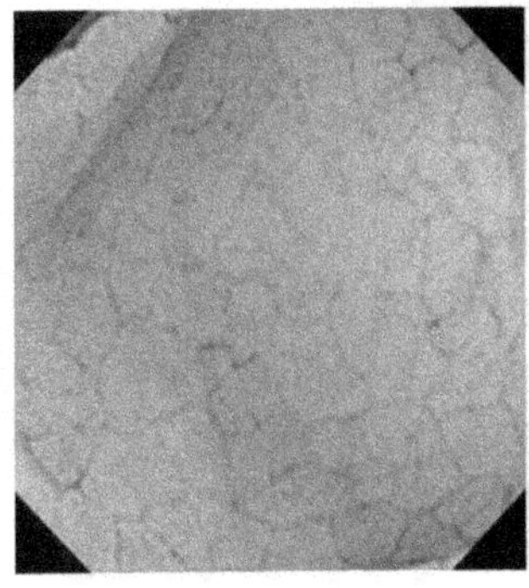
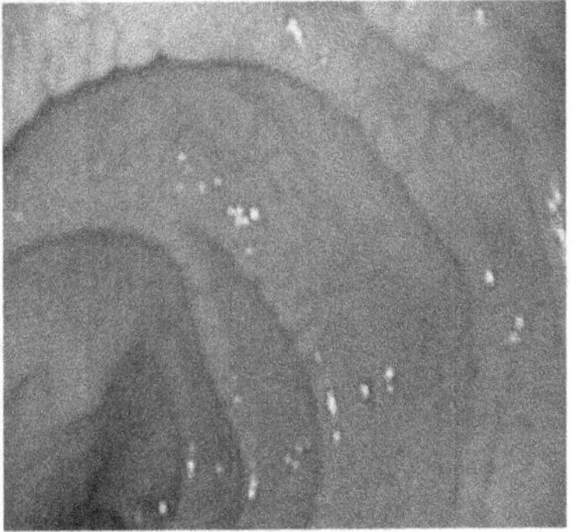

- Pathology
  - ↑ intraepithelial lymphocytes and change in types of T cells
  - Crypt hyperplasia
  - Villous shortening
  - The biopsy is "compatible" with diagnosis of CD, but other conditions may cause ↑IELs +/- villous shortening

Source: Lebwohl, GIE 2011

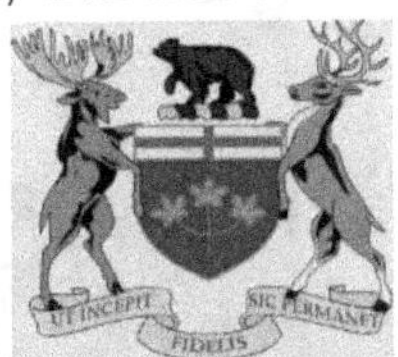

- Does everyone need a scope for Biopsy Confirmation of Diagnosis of CD?
  - "Four out of five" criteria proposed:
    - Typical CD symptoms
    - High titer autoantibodies (tTG/DGP IgA)
    - HLA DQ2 &/or DQ8 genotypes
    - Celiac enteropathy on biopsy
    - Response to GFD
  - Controversial whether biopsy for CD is a "must"

Source: Sapone, BMC Med 2012; Catassi, AJM 2010

Gluten Challenge Test (usually done only in a reseach setting)

- Consider a GCT (gluten challenge test) if person has already initiated GFD without serology and biopsy
- HLA-DQ2/8 is required ("permissive") to develop CD, so do genotyping to exclude CD prior to initiating GCT
- Start gluten 3g/d (1-1.5 bread slice) & double q2-3d until equivalent of ≥4 slices/d (10g), and continue for 6-8wk
  - Histological changes of CD can be seen by 2wk, even if patient can tolerate only 3g/d of gluten
  - Repeat serology after 6-8wk & if still negative, repeat again after longer gluten
  - If TTG and small bowel biopsy still negative
    - Monitor symptoms on normal (gluten-containing) diet
    - Consider repeat testing in 6mon

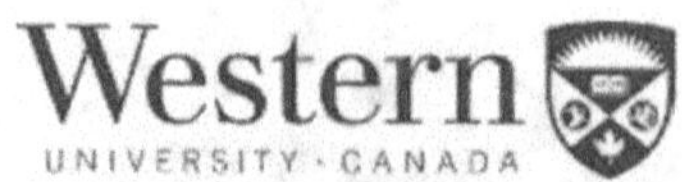

➢ Treatment

Key elements in management of CD

C – Consultation with Dietician
E – Education about disease
L – Lifelong adherence to GFD; "read the label" (of food products)
I – Identify & Treat nutritional deficiencies
A – Attend advocacy group meetings
C – Continue long-term f/u with medical team

- Gluten-Free Diet (GFD)
  - Avoid all wheat, rye & barley
  - Initially avoid all oats
  - Avoid malt unless clearly derived from corn
  - Avoid beer, lager, ale, stouts
  - Carefully read all labels for ingredients
  - Beware:
    - Medications / Food Supplements
    - Food Additives
    - Emulsifiers or Stabilizers
  - Initially limit milk products (often maybe lactose intolerant before GFD begins to heal CD mucosa)

- Response to GFD
  - Many have significant symptom improvement within 48 hr!
  - Usually wks to months for full clinical remission
  - Serology and histology abnormalities may lag behind clinical response
    - Improvement in villous architecture in 2-3 mon to 12 mon

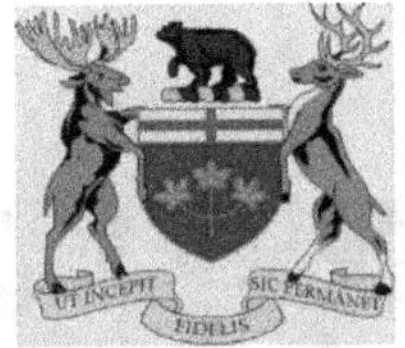

- Can be up to 2yr for complete resolution
  - Children usually fully resolve
  - Adults show only 'partial resolution' in 50%

NONRESPONSIVE CELIAC DISEASE (NRCD)

- Definition: *"Persistence of symptoms, signs or laboratory abnormalities typical of celiac disease despite adherence to a GFD for 6-12 months"*
- Affects ~1% of CD patients
- ↑TTG is common
- Common causes continued gluten ingestion
  - Associated lactose/fructose intolerance

Refractory Celiac Disease (RCD)

- *"Symptomatic, severe small intestinal villous atrophy that mimics celiac disease but does not respond to at least 6 months of strict GFD and is not accounted for by other causes of villous atrophy or overt intestinal lymphoma"*
- Very uncommon
- Sometimes a diagnosis of exclusion

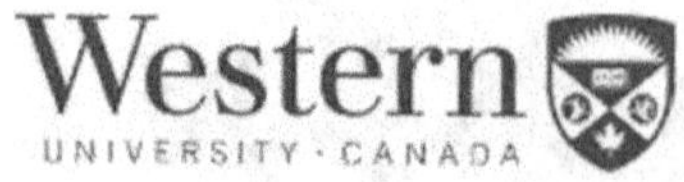

➢ Approach to Non Responsive Refractory Celiac Disease

Non-responsive celiac disease[1]

↓

Confirm accuracy of celiac disease diagnosis ⇐

Supporitng evidence:
- Confirmation of small-bowel histolgy findings consistent with celiac disease
- Positive EMA, tTGA, or DGP serology at some time during the clinical course
- Presence of HLA-DQ2 or HLA-DQ8
- Biopsy-proven dermatitis herpetiformis
- Clinical and/or histological response to GFD
- Strong family history of celiac disease
- Presence of associated auto-immune disorders

Yes / No

No ⇒ Evaluated for other causes of villous atrophy[2] and /or other condition with celiac-like clinical presentations[3]

Yes ↓

Celiac serologies[4] & expert dietician evaluation: gluten ingestion and/or other food intolerances identified?

Yes → Adjust diet & monitor progress

No → Small-bowel biopsy (with colonic biopsies if persisting diarrhea)

↓

Enteritis with villous atrophy?

Yes → Reconsider and exclude other etiologies for villous atrophy[2]

No → Consider alternative etiologies for ongoing symptoms[3]

↓

Refractory celiac disease (RCD)[5]

↓

Abnormal or clonal intestinal T lymphocytes?[6]

Yes → Type II RCD

No → Type I RCD

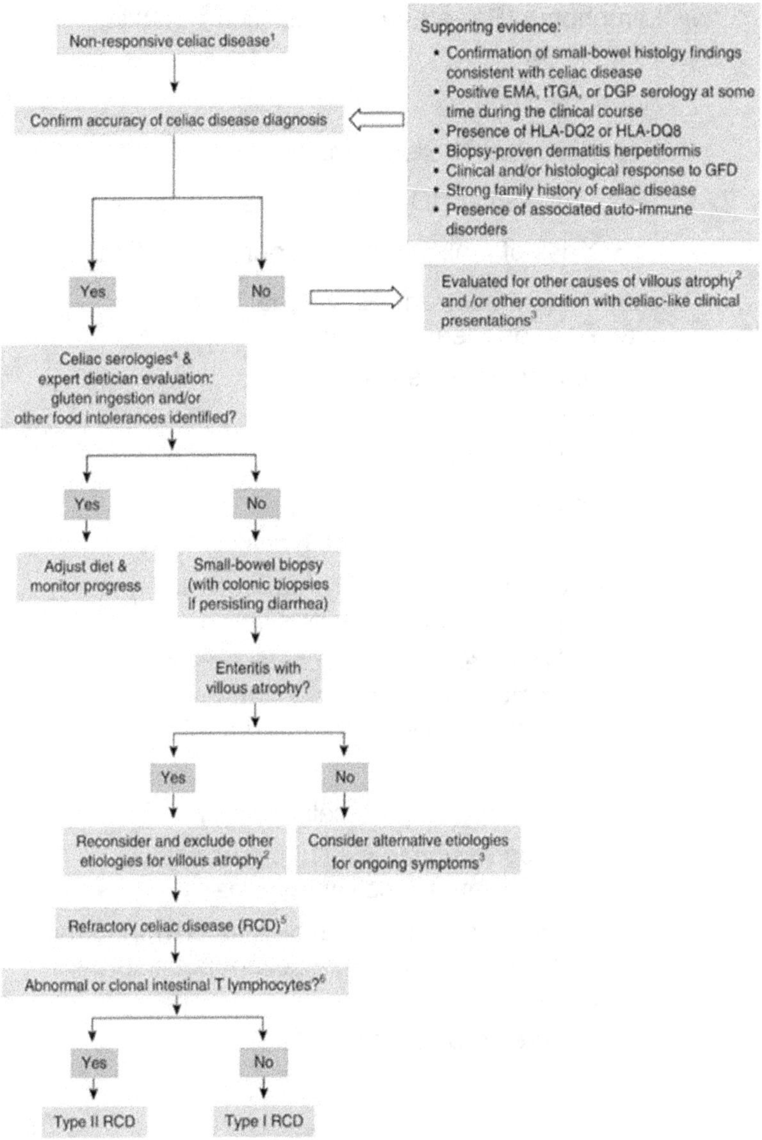

Printed with permission: Rubio-Tapia A, et al. Am J Gastroenterol 2013; 108:656.

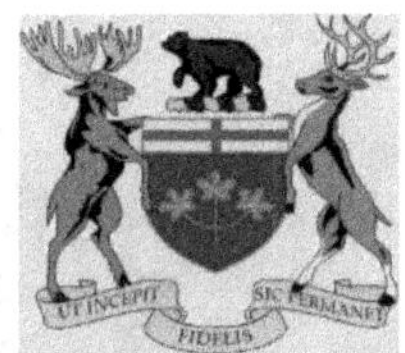

Celiac Disease & Malignancy

- Lymphoma (B- and T-cell NHL (non Hodgkin lymphoma)
- Adenocarcinoma
- Possibly ↓ risk of breast cancer
- ↑Risk 2-6-fold in CD, but absolute risk low
- Lower risk of malignancy with duration of GFD!
- Determine if aberrant IELs/clonal T-cells are present in duodenal biopsy by
  - Immunohistochemistry,
  - Flow cytometry, or
  - DNA for PCR:
  - Type I
    - No aberrant IELs or T-cell clonality
    - Low probability of lymphoma, ulcerative jejunitis or collagenous sprue
    - Treatment with corticosteroids, or immunosuppressive (Azathioprine, Cyclosporine, MTX, Infliximab)
  - Type II
    - Aberrant IELs, T-cell clonality
    - Progression to EATL (enteropathy-associated T-cell lymphoma)
    - High probability of evolution to lymphoma, ulcerative jejunitis or collagenous sprue
    - Poor prognosis may need TPN (total parenteral nutrition)

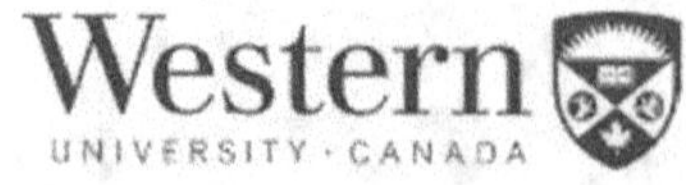

Ulcerative Jejunitis

- Rare, serious complication of CD
- Ulceration & hemorrhage
  - Strictures cause small bowel obstruction
- Many are ultimately diagnosed with lymphoma
- Suspect if abdominal pain & diarrhea not responsive to GFD weight loss
- Diagnosis: small bowel
  - Diagnosis imaging
  - Endoscopy
  - Surgery

Enteropathy-Associated T-cell Lymphoma (EATL)

- Transformation from Type II RCD
- Clues
  - Insidious
  - Ulcers
  - Unresponsive to GFD
  - Obstruction
  - Anemia
  - Adenopathy
  - Hypoalbunemia
- Commonly fatal

Possible Future Nondietary (gluten-free) Treatments for CD

- Genetically modified wheat
  - "Detox" peptides, difficult d/t large # peptides capable of triggering immune response in CD

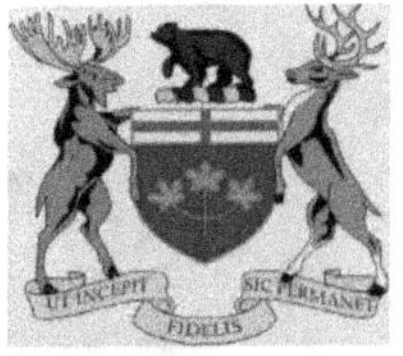

- Oral Glutaminases
  - Cleave gluten in stomach and jejunam into inactive fragments
- Inhibitors of paracellular permeability
  - Increased intestinal permeability feature of celiac & can facilitate gluten passage & uptake by T-cells
- Oral IgY binding to gluten
- Vaccination
  - 3 Dominant HLA DQ2 epitopes identified which may protect against other peptides ("Nexvax2" being trialed)
  - ↑Risk of immunogenicity by ↓ immune tolerance
- tTG Inhibitors
  - Prevent conversion to more potent form (but as tTG deamidates other biological processes, may have unwanted effects)

List of abbreviations:

CD, Celiac Disease;

IBS, Irritable Bowel Syndrome;

IBS D, Diarrhea predominant IBS;

IBD, Inflammatory Bowel Disease;

DM; Diabetes mellitus;

GFD; Gluten Free Diet

IEL, Intraepithelial Lymphocytes

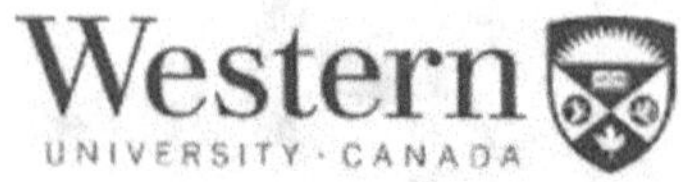

COLON

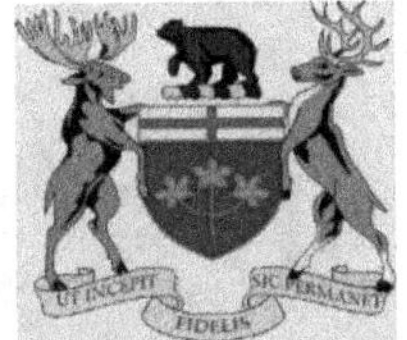

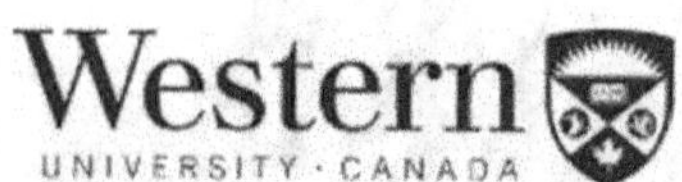
Western
UNIVERSITY · CANADA

MINI UPDATE

Defecation Disorders and Constipation

Mohammed Aljawad

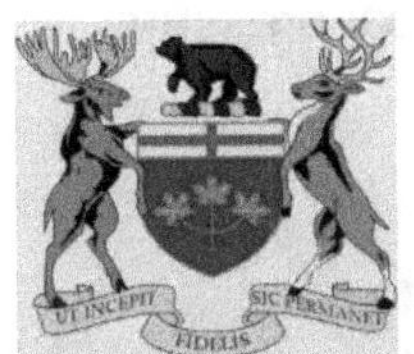

DEFECATION DISORDERS AND CONSTIPATION

Disorders of Defecation

- Defecation

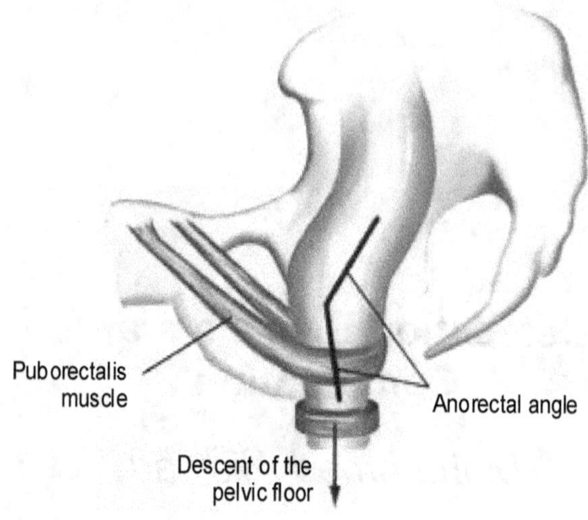

- Demography
    - Starts in childhood
    - Learned behaviour to reduce discomfort associated with the passage of large hard stools
    - Common in asymptomatic healthy women

- Pathophysiology
    - Inability to coordinate the abdominal, rectoanal and pelvic floor muscles

- Clinical
    - Constipation
    - Fecal incontinence
    - Inability to complete fecal evacuation
    - Perineal pain
    - Sensation of local pressure

- Appearance of a bulge at the vaginal opening on straining
- Need to use thumb or fingers to support the posterior vaginal wall to complete defecation
- Need to use a finger to evacuate the rectum digitally
- Rarely associated with structural abnormalities:
  - Rectal intussusception
  - Obstructing rectocele
  - Megarectum
  - Excessive perineal descent

➢ Types
- Rome III criteria for **functional defecation disorders**
  - The patient must satisfy diagnostic criteria for functional constipation
  - During repeated attempts to defecate, the patient must have at least two of the following:
    - Evidence of impaired evacuation, based on balloon expulsion test or imaging
    - Inappropriate contraction of pelvic floor muscles (i.e., anal sphincter or puborectalis) or less than 20% relaxation of basal resting sphincter pressure by manometry, imaging, or EMG
    - Inadequate propulsive forces assessed by manometry or imaging

➢ Disorders of the **anorectum and pelvic floor**
- Descending perineum syndrome
- Diminished rectal sensation
- Functional fecal retention (FFR)

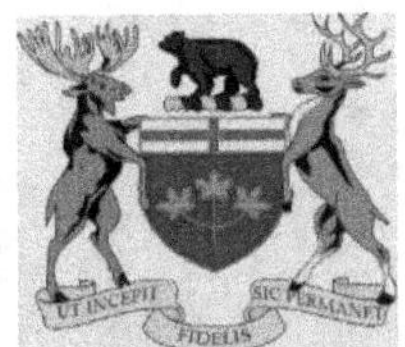

- Rectal prolapse
- Rectocele
- Solitary rectal ulcer syndrome

- **Descending perineum syndrome**
  - Pelvic floor muscle weakness
  - Pelvic floor descends to a greater extent than normal (1 to 4 cm) when the patient strains
  - Anorectal angle is widened and the rectum is more vertical
  - Rectal expulsion is difficult
  - Electrophysiologic studies
    - Partial denervation of the striated muscle and evidence of pudendal nerve damage

- **Rectal prolapse**
  - Pelvic floor muscle weakness
  - Asymptomatic in 33% of patients
  - History
    - Prolonged straining in response to a constant desire to defecate
    - Sense of incomplete evacuation
    - Infrequent passage of small hard stools
    - Abdominal pain and distention
  - DRE - > 4 cm descent of perineum when asking the patient to strain, as if to defecate
  - Treatment
    - Symptomatic
    - Surgery

- Give the pathophysiology of disorders of the anorectum and pelvic floor, which contribute disordered defecation.

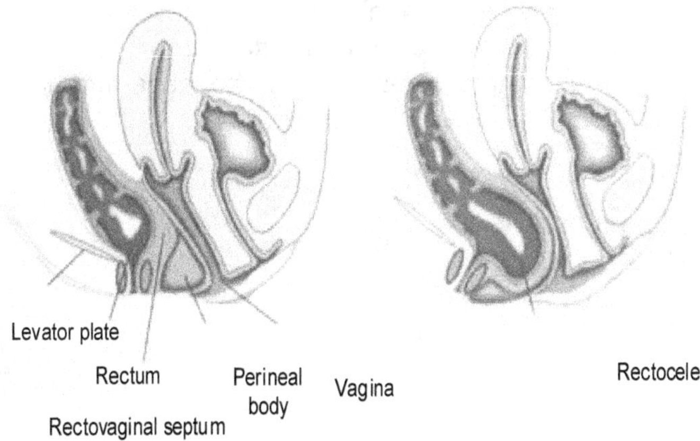

- **Solitary rectal ulcer syndrome**
  - Due to chronic straining
  - Varying degrees of rectal prolapse exist
  - Paradoxical contraction of the puborectalis muscle
  - Mucus and blood per rectum
  - Endoscopic finding
    - Erythema
    - Hyperemia
    - Mucosal ulceration
    - Polypoid lesions
    - Commonly of the anterior rectal wall
  - Treatment
    - Biofeedback
    - Symptomatic – bulk laxatives and dietary fiber
    - Surgery

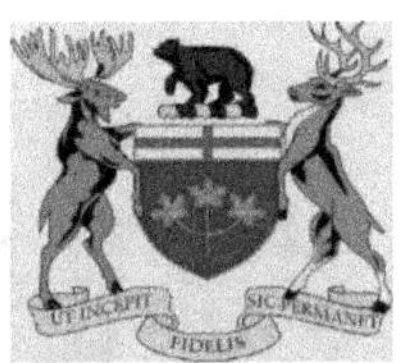

- **Functional fecal retention (FFR)**
  - Most common defecatory disorder in children
  - The most common cause of encopresis (fecal incontinence) because of leakage of liquid stool around a fecal impaction
  - A learned behaviour that results from withholding defecation, often because of fear of a painful bowel movement

- Diagnosis
  - Algorithm
  - Blood tests
    - TSH, Ca^{2+}, blood sugar
  - Exclude structural disorders
    - Barium enema
    - SBFT
    - colonoscopy
  - Measure colonic transit time
  - Diagnostic tests for defecatory disorder

- Tests for defecatory disorders

- Give 5 tests to investigate disordered defecation.
  - Defecography
  - Balloon expulsion test
  - Anorectal manometry
  - EMG testing of striated muscle activity
  - Rectal sensitivity and sensation testing
  - Defecography: provides measures of :
    - Rate and completeness of rectal emptying
    - Anorectal angle
    - Amount of perineal descent

- Structural abnormalities
  - Large rectocele
  - Internal mucosal prolapse
  - intussusception
- Limitation:
  - Subjective
  - Patient embarrassment (produces normal inhibition of normal rectal emptying)
  - Differences in texture between barium paste and stool

- Balloon expulsion test
  - Distention of rectum is with a balloon → relaxation of internal anal sphincter
  - Inability to evacuate a 50 to 60 mL inflated ballon in the rectum while sitting on the toilet for two minutes, with the addition of 200 g of weight to the end of the balloon → diagnosis of a defecatory disorder

- Anorectal manometry
  - Resting and maximum squeeze pressure of the internal and external anal sphincters
  - Relaxation of the anal sphincter during balloon distention of the rectum (rectoanal inhibitory reflex)
  - Rectal sensation
  - Ability of the anal sphincter to relax during straining

- EMG testing of striated muscle activity
  - Rarely indicated
  - Used in suspected spinal cord or cauda equine lesions
  - Bilateral or unilateral dysfunction of the external anal sphincter can be demonstrated

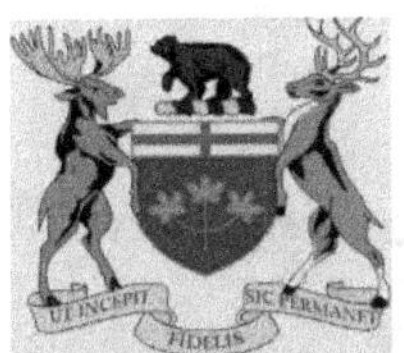

- Rectal sensitivity and sensation testing
  - Introducing successive volumes of air into a rectal balloon allows for the measurement of the
    - Volume at which the stimulus is first perceived
    - Volume that produces an urge to defecate
    - Volume above which further addition of air can no longer be tolerated
  - Absence of the rectoanal inhibitory reflex suggests the possibility of Hirschsprung's disease
  - A high resting anal pressure suggests the presence of an anal fissure or anismus
  - Rectal hyposensitivity suggests a neurologic disorder

Chronic Ideopathic Constipation (CIC)

- Definition
  - Rome III criteria for functional constipation
    - Two or more of the following:
      - Straining during at least 25% of defecations
      - Lumpy or hard stools in at least 25% of defecations
      - Sensation of incomplete evacuation for at least 25% of defecations
      - Sensation of anorectal obstruction/ blockage for at least 25% of defecations
      - Manual maneuvers to facilitate at least 25% of defecations (e.g., digital evacuation, support of the pelvic floor)
      - Fewer than three defecations per week
    - Criteria fulfilled for the previous three months with symptom onset at least six months prior to diagnosis

- Loose stools should rarely be present without the use of laxatives
- Insufficient criteria for irritable bowel syndrome

➢ Rome III diagnostic criteria for functional defecation disorders using criteria fulfilled for the last 3 months with symptom onset at least 6 months before diagnosis.

- The patient must satisfy diagnostic criteria for functional constipation

- During repeated attempts to defecate must have at least two of the following

- Evidence of impaired evacuation, based on balloon expulsion test or imaging

- Inappropriate contraction of the pelvic floor muscles (i.e. anal sphincter or puborectalis) or < 20% relaxation of basal resting sphincter pressure by manometry, imaging, or EMG

- Inadequate propulsive forces assessed by manometry or imaging

Source: Bharucha AE, et al. *Gastroenterology* 2006; 130: 1510-8, Table 2.

- What "constipation" means to the patients:
  - Straining (52%)
  - Hard stools (44%)
  - Inability to have a bowel movement (34%)
  - < 3 bm/ week
  - Bristol stool chart

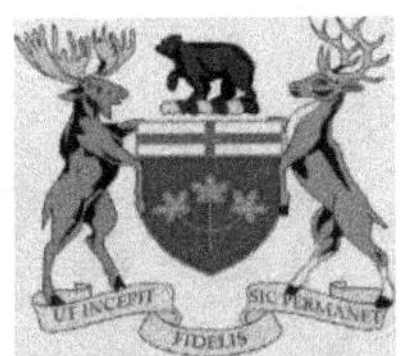

- Stool Gazing: The Bristol Stool Chart

Whole gut transit time	Stool type	Description	Pictorial representation
Long transit (100 hr)	Type 1	Sepatraet hard lump, like nuts, hard to pass	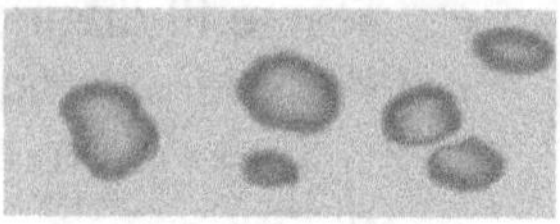
	Type 2	Sausage shaped but lumpy	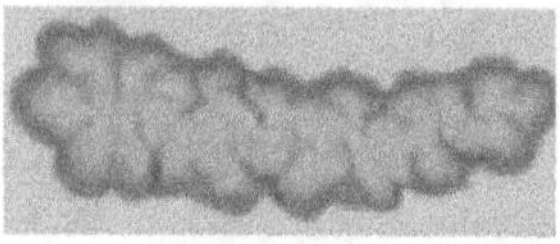
	Type 3	Like sausage but with cracks on its surface	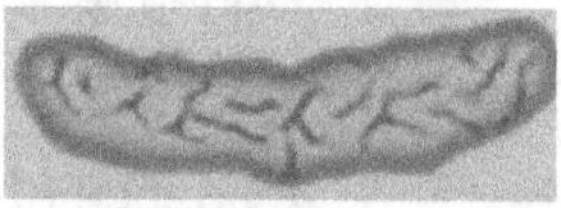
	Type 4	Like sausage or snake, smooth and soft	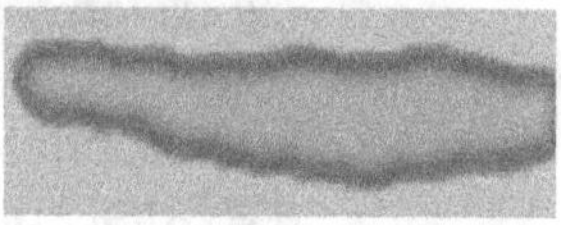
	Type 5	Soft bolbs with clear-cut edges (passed easily)	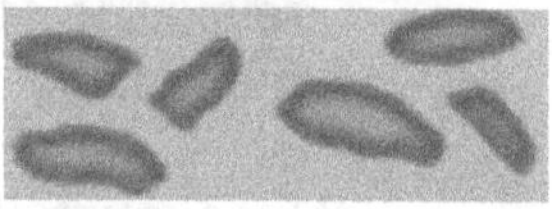
	Type 6	Fluffy pieces with ragged edges, a mushy stool	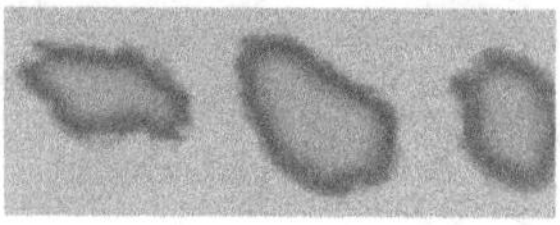
Short transit (10 hours)	Type 7	Watery, no solid pieces	Entirely liquid

- Demographics
  - Prevalence
    - Constipation affects between 2% and 28% If the population

- Risk factors
  - Advanced age
  - Female gender
  - Low level of education
  - Low level of physical activity
  - Low socioeconomic status
  - Non-white ethnicity
  - Use of certain medications

➢ Normal Colonic Function

- Motor
  - Colonic propulsion
    - Low-amplitude propagated contractions (LAPCs)
    - High-amplitude propagated contractions (HAPCs)
  - Colonic muscle function
    - Mixes the contents → enhances contact with the mucosa
    - Slows passage of luminal contents → time for absorption of water
    - Propels the contents toward the anus
    - Stores feces between defecations
  - Mean colonic transit time
    - Normal mean 35 hours

- Absorption
  - Luminal content
    - Food residue
    - Water and electrolytes
    - Bacteria
    - Gas

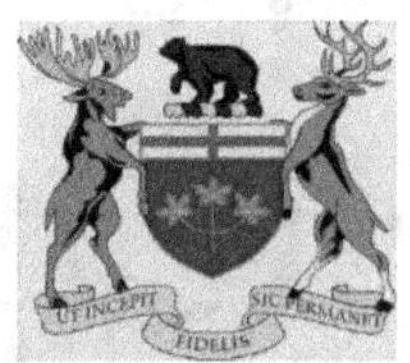

- Most of the colonic water is absorbed, leaving only 100- 200 mL of fecal water from an input of about 1500 mL (90% absorptive efficiency)
- Mechanism: Na^+/Cl^- exchange short-chain fatty acid transport

- Pathophysiology of Constipation
  - Slow proximal colonic transit put normal distal transit suggests slow transit constipation. Normal proximal colonic transit but slow distal transit suggests pelvic dyssynergy or anorectal dysfunction
  - Only slow transit constipation will respond to subtotal colectomy with ileorectal anastomosis
  - With dilation of both the colon and rectum, as well as normal anal sphincter function proctocolorectomy and an ileoanal anastamosis may be suitable; if anal sphincter function is abnormal, an ileostomy needs to be performed
  - Normal-transit constipation
    - Patient may have misperceptions about their bowel frequencies
    - Often exhibit psychosocial distress
    - Abnormalities of anorectal sensory and motor function are similar to those in patients with slow-transit constipation
    - Normal physiologic test results
      - Incomplete evacuation
      - Abdominal pain may be present, but is not a predominant feature
  - Slow-transit constipation
    - Disordered colonic motor function
    - Delayed emptying of the proximal colon and fewer HAPCs after meals
    - Infrequent stools (e.g., ≤ 1/wk)

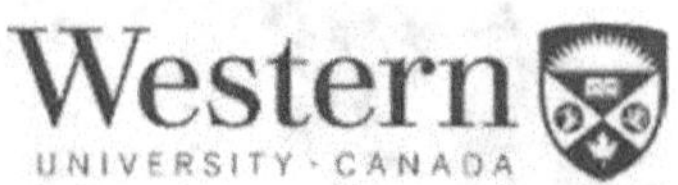

- Lack of urge to defecate
- Poor response to fiber and laxatives
- Generalized symptoms, including malaise and fatigue
- More prevalent in young women
- Relation in colon of > 20% of radiopaque markers five days after ingestion

- Give the manometric changes in the colon which occur with severe slow-transit constipation.

    - ↓ high-amplitude of propagating pressure waves
    - ↑ frequency of low-amplitude antegrade and retrograde propagating sequences
    - ↓ nighttime suppression of propagating sequences
    - ↓ colonic response to a high-calorie meal

- Colonic inertia
    - Severe symptoms of slow transit constipation
    - Colonic motor activity fails to increase after
        - A meal
        - Ingestion of bisacodyl
        - Administration of a cholinesterase inhibitor (such as neostigmine)
- Defecatory disorders (pelvic floor dysfunction, anismus, descending perineum syndrome, rectal prolapse)
    - Frequent straining
    - Sense of incomplete evacuation
    - Need for manual maneuvers to facilitate defecation

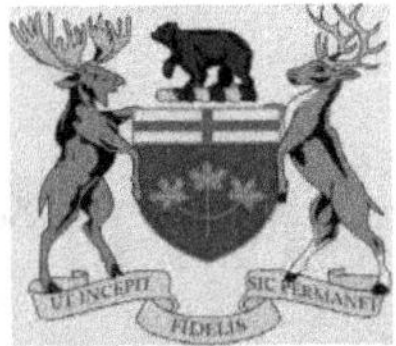

- Abnormal balloon expulsion test and / or rectal manometry

➢ Classification of Functional (non-obstructive) Constipation

Category	Features	Characteristic Findings
○ Normal-transit constipation	– Incomplete evacuation; – Abdominal pain may be present, but is not a predominant feature	▪ Normal physiologic test results
○ Slow-transit constipation	– Infrequent stools (e.g., ≤1/wk) – Lack of urge to defecate – Poor response to fiber and laxatives – Generalized symptoms, ▪ Malaise and fatigue ▪ More prevalent in young women	▪ Retention in colon of >20% of radiopaque markers five days after ingestion
○ Defecatory disorders (pelvic floor dysfunction, anismus, descending perineum syndrome, rectal prolapse)	– Frequent straining – Incomplete evacuation; – Need for manual maneuvers to facilitate defecation	▪ Abnormal balloon expulsion test and/or rectal manometry

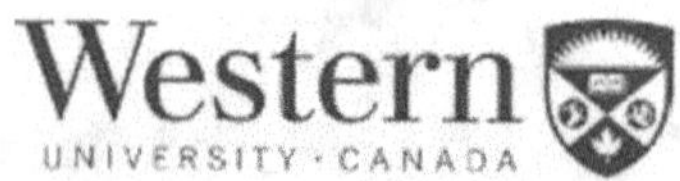

- Causes and associations (4 M's)
  - Mechanical obstruction
    - Anal atresia in infancy
    - Anal stenosis
    - Anal stenosis (atresia in infant)
    - Colorectal cancer
    - Extrinsic compression
    - Rectocele or sigmoidocele
    - Small or large bowel obstruction
    - Stricture
  - Medications
    - 5-hydroxytryptamine3 antagonists (e.g., alosetron)
    - Antacids
    - Anticholinergic agents (e.g., antiparkinsonian drugs, antipsychotics, antispasmodics, tricyclic anti-depressnats)
    - Anticonvulsants (e.g., carbamazepine, Phenobarbital, phenytoin)
    - Antineoplastic agents (e.g., vinca derivatives)
    - Calcium channel blockers (e.g., verapamil)
    - Diuretics (e.g., furosemide)
    - Iron supplements
    - Mu-opioid agonists (e.g., fentanyl, loperamide, morphine)
    - Non-steroidal anti-inflammatory drugs (e.g., ibuprofen)
  - Metabolic and endocrinologic disorders
    - Diabetes mellitus
    - Heavy metal poisoning (e.g., arsenic, lead, mercury)
    - Hyper- hypothyroidism
    - Hypercalcemia

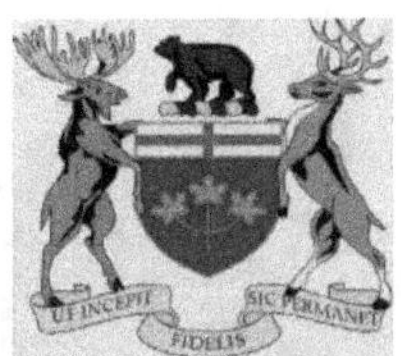

- Hypokalemia
- Panhypopituitarism
- Pheochromocytoma
- Porphyria
- Pregnancy

- Myopathic and neurologic disorders
  - Amyloidosis
  - Autonomic neuropathy
  - Chagas' disease
  - Dermatomyositis
  - Intestinal pseudo-obstruction
  - Multiple sclerosis
  - Parkinsonism
  - Progressive systemic sclerosis
  - Shy-Drager syndrome
  - Spinal cord injury
  - Stroke
  - Congenital or acquired myopathy of the colon
  - Hereditary internal anal sphincter myopathy
  - Muscular dystrophies

- Examples of specific causes of constipation
  - Diabetes mellitus
    - Autonomic neuropathy
    - ↑ colonic transit time
    - ↓ colonic myoelectrical and motor responses after meals

  - Hypothyroidism
    - Infiltration of the intestine by myxedematous tissue
    - ↓ intestinal motor function
    - Myxedema megacolon

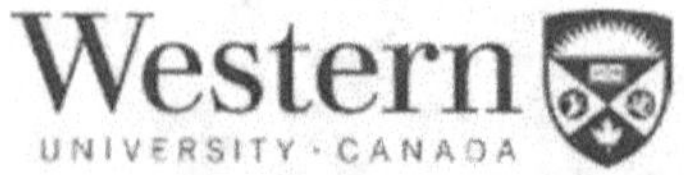

- Multiple sclerosis (MS)
  - Present in 43% of patients with MS
  - ↓ physical activity
  - Medications with constipating side effects
  - Disease in the lumbosacral spinal cord
  - Visceral neuropathy
  - ↓ colonic motor activity after meals
  - Pelvic floor muscular and anal sphincter dysfunction
- Parkinson disease
  - ↓ dopaminergic neurons in the enteric nervous system
  - ↓ colonic transit
  - ↓ phasic rectal contractions
  - Weak abdominal wall muscle contraction
  - Paradoxical anal sphincter contraction
  - ↓ relaxation of the striated muscles of the pelvic floor (as part of extrapyramidal motor disorder)

➢ Spinal cord lesions

- Lesions above the sacral segments (UMNL)
  - ↓ colonic transit
  - ↓ rectal sensation
  - ↑ anal relaxation on rectal distention
  - ↓ rectal pressue on straining
  - Loss of conscious external anal sphincter control

- Lesions of the sacral cord, conus medullaris, cauda equine, and nervi erigentes (S2 to S4; LMNL)
  - ↓ progression of contractions in the left colon
  - Distal colon and rectum dilate,
  - Feces accumulates in the distal colon
  - Rectal sensation may be diminished
  - Spasticity of the anal canal

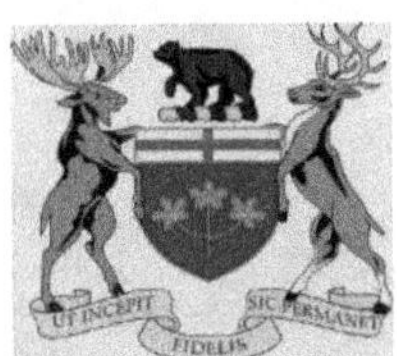

Abbreviation: LMNL, lower motor neuron lesion; UMNL, upper motor neuron lesion

➢ Another approach to the causes of constipation

The causes of constipation may be classified as neurogenic, drug associated, and metabolic.

- Give 8 causes of constipation in each category.

- Psychological
  - Depression
  - Eating disorders
    - Prolonged whole-gut transit time (reversible)
    - Pelvic floor dysfunction (irreversible)
  - Denied bowel movement

- Neurogenic
  - Central
    - Cerebral infarction (CVA)
    - Medullary trauma
    - Multiple sclerosis
    - Parkinson's disease
  - Spinal
    - Cauda equina lesions
    - Cognitive challenge
    - Dementia
    - Meningocele
    - Spinal cord lesions (trauma, tumour)

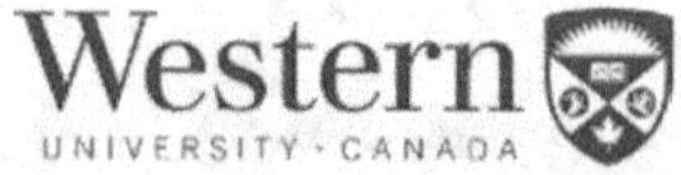

- Gut
  - Aganglionosis: congenital (Hirschsprung's) or acquired
  - Autonomic neuropathy (paraneoplastic, pseudoobstruction, diabetes)
  - Cathartic colon (laxative abuse)
  - Narcotic bowel syndrome

- Enteric nerves
  - Congenital aganglionosis or hypoganglionosis
    - Hirschsprung's disease
      - ↓ ganglion cells in the distal colon
      - Can present later in life (short segment)
      - Colon narrows at the area that lacks ganglion cells, with proximal bowel dilatation
    - Congenital hyperganglionosis (intestinal neuronal dysplasia)
      - Hyperplasia of the submucosal nerve plexus
      - Clinical manifestations similar to Hirschsprung's disease
    - Acquired neuropathics
      - Chagas' disease
      - Paraneoplastic visceral neuropathy
    - Neuropathies of unknown cause

- Drug-associated
  - 5-HT3 antagonists
  - Analgesic: narcotics e.g. opiates ("cathartic colon"), non-narcotics
  - Antacid (aluminum)

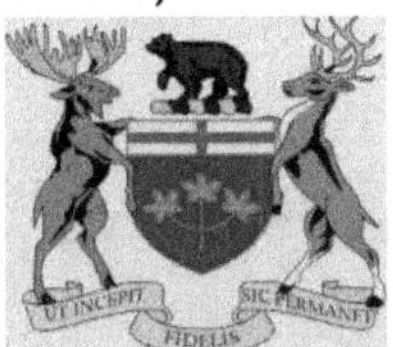

- Anti-Parkinson drugs
- Anticholinergics (dopaminergics)
- Antidepressants (tricyclics, but not SSRIs – serotonin reuptake inhibitors)
- Antidiarrheals
- Antihypertensives (calcium channel blockers, clonidine)
- Antipsychotics
- Antiseizure medications
- Bile acid sequestrants
- Chemotherapeutic agents
- Nutrient supplements: calcium, iron
- Somatostatin analogs

- Metabolic
    - Diabetes mellitus
    - Glucagonoma
    - Heavy metal poisoning
    - Hypocalcemia
    - Hypokalemia
    - Hypomagnesium
    - Hypoparathyroidism
    - Hypopituitarism (panhypopituitarism)
    - Hypothyroidism
    - Low intake of water
    - Porphyria
    - Pregnancy
    - Progesterone level cyclic fluctuation (just before menses)

Printed with permission: Müller-Lissner S. *Best Pract Res Clin Gastroenterol* 2007; 21(3): pg. 475.

- Give the investigations which are appropriate for the investigation of persons with constipation.

    - History and physical– social, laxative and drug use, psychological assessment, stool chart; full examination including digital rectal exam (DRE)
    - Lab tests – Ca^{2+}, glucose, TSH, electrolytes, CBC, Mg^{2+}
    - 3 views of the abdomen
    - Colonoscopy, defecating proctogram (defecogram), colonic transit study, EUS, colonic manometry
    - Diagnostic imaging
    - Manometry, anorectal manometry
    - Functional testing, balloon expulsion

"Mediocrity is metric modulation,
bringing people back (regression) to
the mean."

Grandad

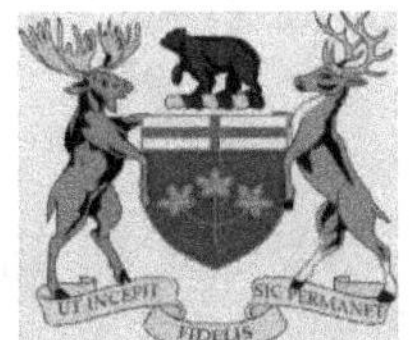

Algorithm for the evaluation and treatment of severe constipation

History and physical examination
Treat secondary causes of constipation
Medicatio n history
Stop/ change medication (s)
Supplement diet with 20 g fiber/d
No
Colonic transit study
Normal transit
Slow transit
Fiber (>20 g/d), osmotic laxative, stimulant laxative
Assess for defecatory disorder (e.g., anorectal manometry, balloon
No
Abnormal
Normal
Assess for defecatory disorder (e.g., anorectal manometry, balloon expulsion test)
Abnormal
Defecograph
Normal
Treat as for irritable bowel syndrome
Evacuation disorder
Rectal anatomic defect
Slow-transit constipation
Biofeedback, physical therapy, consultation with psychologist and/ or dietitian
Repair of prolapsed or rectocele
Osmotic laxative, stimulant laxative, prokinetic agent, rarely colectomy

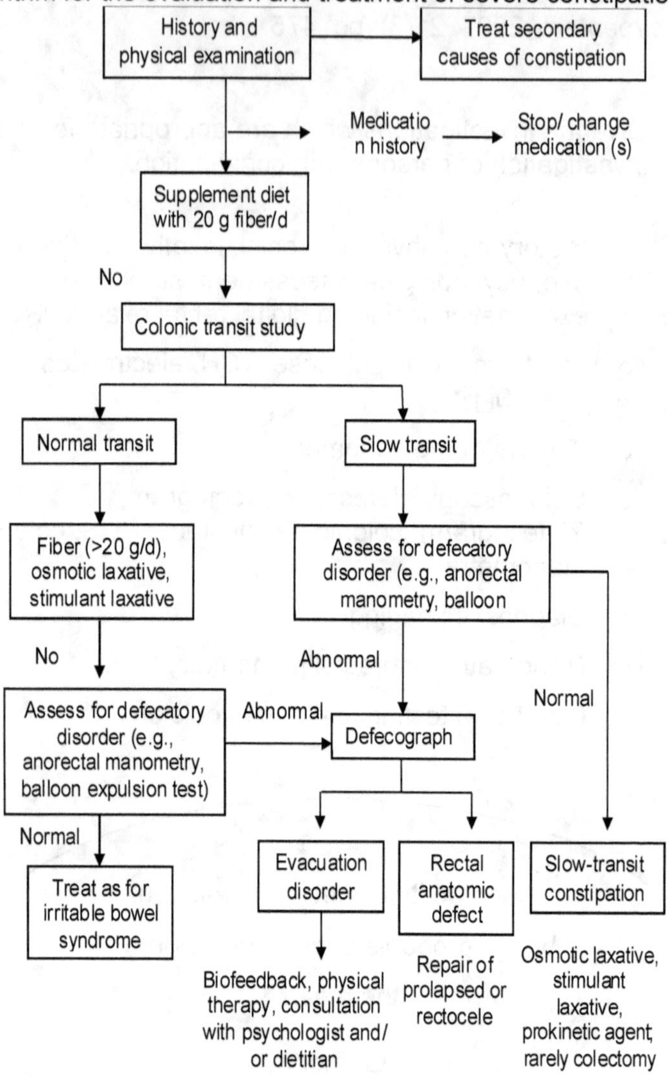

Printed with permission: Algorithm for the evaluation and treatment of severe constipation. Anthony J. Lembo, Sonal P. Ullman. Constipation Sleisenger and Fordtran's Gastrointestinal and Liver Disease. 2010 Elsevier, Philadelphia, page 274, Figure 18-6

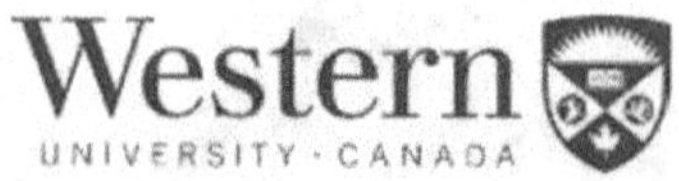

- Measurement of colonic transit time
  - Radiopaque marker test
    - Radiopaque markers in a gelatine capsule are ingested and serial abdominal x-rays are taken
    - Avoid Rx that affect bowel function
    - Normal colonic transit time less than 72 hours
    - Retention of > 20% represents a positive test
    - Slow movement of markers → transit disorder
    - Markers retained in the rectosigmoid → defecatory disorder
    - All the markers move rapidly to the rectum and are retained there → megarectum

  - Wireless motility capsule
    - pH and pressure recording capsule
    - correlates well with the radiopaque marker test
    - allow an assessment of gastric and small bowel transit
    - valuable tool if surgical treatment for severe constipation is being considered
    - abnormal gastric or small bowel motility precludes surgical treatment of constipation

- Treatment

  - Note
    - There is a long menu of choices to treat CIC (Chronic Idiopathic Constipation).
    - Expensive new agents have been developed, but these do not necessarily perform any better than polyethylene glycol, sodium, picosulfate, bisacodyl or lactulose.
    - The NNTs (number needed to treat) to prevent one patient failing to respond to therapy was between 3 and 6.

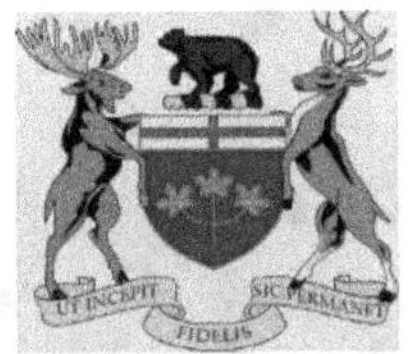

- Dietary fiber
  - Increase dietary fiber in non-constipated persons
    - ↑ stool weight
    - ↑ frequency of defecation
    - ↓ colonic transit time
  - Dietary fiber appears to be effective in relieving mild to moderate but not severe constipation
  - Patients should be encouraged to take about 25 g of NSPs daily
  - Side effects:
    - Abdominal distention
    - Bloating
    - Flatulence
    - Poor taste

- Give 10 non-pharmacological treatments of constipation.
  - Treat underlying conditions
  - Bowel management programs
  - Psychological management
  - Avoid constipating medications
  - Exercise
  - Adequate water intake
  - Dietary measures
  - Biofeedback (pelvic floor retraining)
  - Total colectomy with ileorectal anastamosis

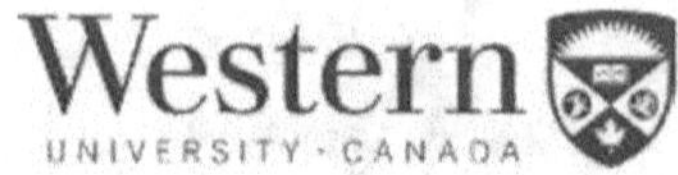

Types of dietary fiber

Agent	Starting daily dose (g)	Comment
○ Methylcellulose	4-6	- Semisynthetic cellulose fiber that is relatively resistant to colonic bacterial degradation - Tends to cause less bloating and flatus than does psyllium
○ Psyllium	4-6	- Made from ground seed husk of the ispaghula plant - Forms a gel when mixed with water, (an ample amount of water should be taken with psyllium to avoid intestinal obstruction) - Undergoes bacterial degradation, which may contribute to side effects of bloating and flatus - Allergic reactions such as anaphylaxis and asthma have been reported but are rare
○ Polycarbophil	4-6	- Synthetic fiber made of polymer of acrylic acid, which is resistant to bacterial degradation
○ Guar gum	3-6	- Soluble fiber extracted from seeds of the leguminous shrub *Cyamopsis tetragonoloba*

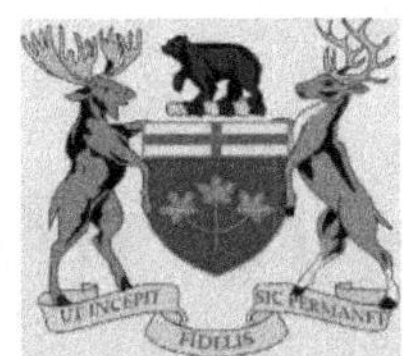

- Note:
  - There is an unproven benefit of fibre to treat constipation, but fiber supplement up to 30 gm per day may be offered on a person-by-person basis.
  - In the absence of dehydration, ↑ water intake does not help constipation

- Give a **classification of laxatives**.

Type of laxatives	Generic name	Dose
➢ Osmotic Laxatives		
o Poorly Absorbed Ions		
– Magnesium	Magnesium hydroxide	15-30 mL once or twice daily
	Magnesium citrate	150-300 mL every day
	Magnesium sulfate	15 g every day
– Sulfate	Sodium sulfate	5-10 g every day
– Phosphate	Sodium phosphate	0.5-10 mL with 12 oz of water
o Poorly Absorbed Sugars		
– Disaccharides	Lactulose	15-30 mL once or twice daily
– Sugar alcohols	Sorbitol Mannitol	15-30 mL once or twice daily15-30 mL once or twice daily
– Polyethylene glycol (PEG)	Polyethylene glycol electrolyte	17-34 g once or twice daily

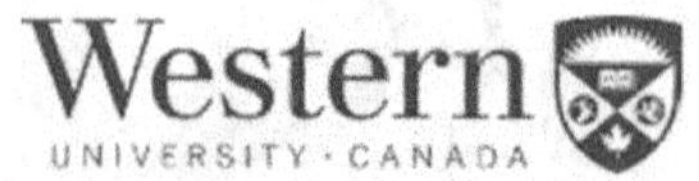

Type of laxatives	Generic name	Dose
➢ Stimulant Laxatives		
○ Anthraquinones	Cascara sagrada	325 mg (or 5 mL) at bedtime
	Senna	1-2 7.5-mg tablets daily
○ Diphenylmethane Derivatives	Bisacodyl	5-10 mg at bedtime
	Phenolphthalein	30-200 mg at bedtime
	Sodium picosulfate	5-15 mg at bedtime
➢ Stool Softeners	Docusate sodium	100 mg twice daily
➢ Emollients	Mineral oil	5-15 mL at bedtime
➢ Enemas, Suppositories	Phosphate enema	120 mL
	Mineral oil retention enema	100 mL
	Tap water enema	500 mL
	Soapsuds enema	1500 mL
	Glycerin suppository	60 g
	Bisacodyl suppository	10 mg
➢ Chloride Channel Activator	Lubiprostone	8-24 µg twice daily
➢ Other agents		
○ Prokinetic agents	Proculpride	2 mg daily
○ Peripheral Mu-opioid antagonists		

Adapted from: Anthony J, et al. Constipation Sleisenger and Fordtran's Gastrointestinal and Liver Disease. 2010 Elsevier, Philadelphia. Table 18-9.

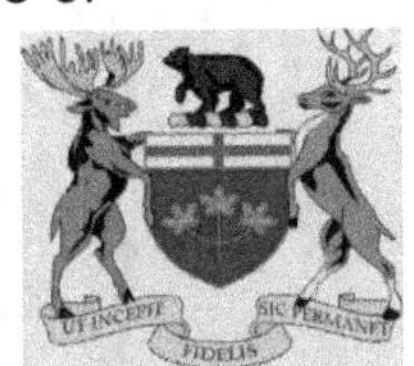

- **Osmotic laxatives** (poorly absorbed ions)
  - Magnesium
    - Osmotic laxative
    - Usually produces a bowel movement within 6 hours
    - Adverse effects
      - Abdominal distension, flatulence, abdominal cramps
      - Renal failure in children
      - Hypermagnesemia-induced
      - Paralytic ileus
      - Coma in kids

  - Sodium Phosphate
    - Adverse effects (AEs)
      - Hyperphosphatemia, especially in patients with renal insufficiency
      - Acute kidney injury (rare)
      - Risk factors for AEs:
        - Hypertension
        - Advanced age
        - Volume depletion
        - ACEI/ NSAID use

  - – Lactulose (poorly absorbed sugars)
    - Undergoes fermentation in the colon to yield short-chain fatty acids (SCFA), hydrogen, and carbon dioxide → lower fecal pH
    - Adverse effect
    - This lowers the pH of stool SCFA stimulate motility
      - Abdominal distention or discomfort
      - Lactulose-induced megacolon

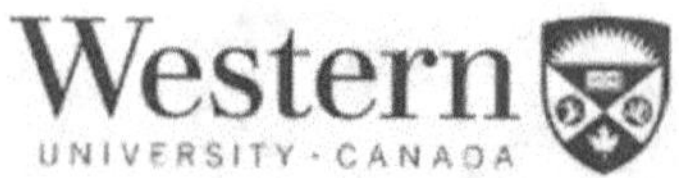

- Polyethylene Glycol (PEG)
  - Osmotic, absorbs water, thereby increasing intraluminal water retention
  - Not metabolized by colonic bacteria
  - Useful for the short-term treatment of fecal impaction
  - Approved for children age 6 months to 15 yrs

- **Stimulant laxatives**
  - ↑ intestinal motility and intestinal secretion
  - Suitable for use in a single dose for temporary constipation
  - Work within hours
  - Adverse effects
    - *Pseudomelanosis coli:*
      - Apoptosis of colonic epithelial cells, which then are phagocytosed by macrophages and appear as a lipofuscin-like pigment
      - Abdominal discomfort
  - Adverse effects
    - Abdominal cramps

  - Anthraquinones
    - Cascara, senna, aloe
    - Pass undigested to the colon
    - Hydrolyzed by colonic bacterial glycosidases to yield active molecules
    - ↑ secretion of electrolytes into the colonic lumen
    - Stimulate myenteric plexuses
    - Start working within 6 hrs

  - Diphenylmethane derivatives
    - Sodium picosulfate is hydrolyzed by colonic bacteria, and thus the action is confined to the colon

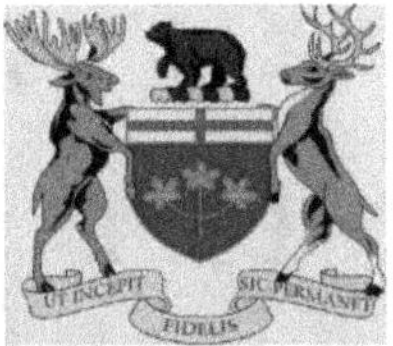

    - Bisacodyl is hydrolyzed by intestinal enzymes and thus can act in both the small and large intestines
    - Bisacodyl induces an almost immediate, powerful, propulsive motor activity
    - Bisacodyl can be used for long term management of severe chronic constipation

- **Stool softeners**
  - Docusate sodium
    - ↑ fluid secretion by the small and large intestines, but no increase in stool weight
    - Docusate sodium is less effective than psyllium for the treatment of chronic idiopathic constipation
  - Mineral oil
    - Emulsification into the stool mass, providing lubrication for the passage of stool
    - Adverse effects – long-term use can cause:
      - Intestinal malabsorption of fat-soluble vitamins
      - Anal seepage
      - Lipoid pneumonia

McRorie JW Daggy BP, Morel JG, et al. Psyllium is superior to docusate sodium for treatment of chronic constipation. Aliment Pharmacol Ther. 1998;12(5):491-7.

- **Enemas and suppositories**

  - Phosphate enemas
    - Cause distention and stimulation of the rectum
    - Superficial damaged to the mucosa appears to heal rapidly
    - Widely used but no conclusive evidence of efficacy

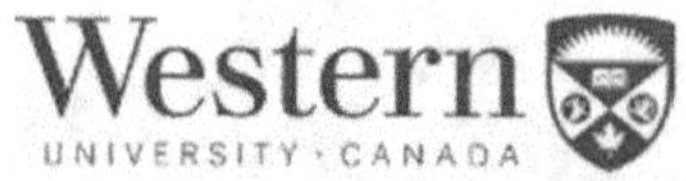

    - If patient can't evacuate phosphate enema, then hyperphosphatemia and hypocalcemic tetany may develop

- Saline, tap water, and soapsuds enemas
    - Water intoxication and electrolyte disturbances if the enema is retained.
    - Soapsuds enemas can cause rectal mucosal damage

- Stimulant suppositories and enemas
    - Glycerine, bisacodyl
    - Bisacodyl suppositories (but not enema) can cause surface epithelial damage

- **Chloride channel activator** (lubiprostone)
  - ↑ intestinal fluid secretion and ↑ transit without altering serum electrolyte levels
  - Used for
    - Chronic constipation
    - Women who have IBS with constipation
  - Adverse effects
    - Nausea
    - Headache
    - Diarrhea

- **Prokinetic agents**
  - Stimulation of 5-HT_4 receptor on afferent nerves in the wall of the gastrointestinal tract induces peristaltic contraction of the intestine
  - Tegaserod and cisapride
    - Withdrawn from the market because of cardiovascular safety concerns
  - Proculpride: recently approved 5-HT4 agonist

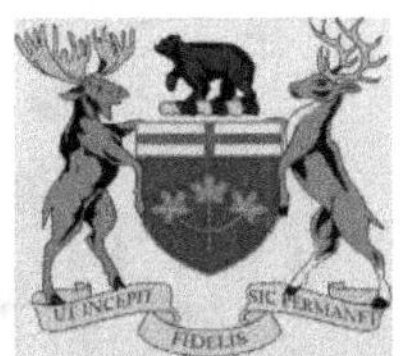

- **Peripheral Mu-opioid antagonists** (methylnaltrexone, alvimopan)
    - Reverses opioid-induced bowel dysfunction without reversing analgesia or precipitating central nervous system withdrawal signs
    - Alvimopan also used to accelerate bowel recovery following surgery

5-HT4 agonists may be used to treat constipation.

- Give the mechanism of the action of 5-HT4 agonists.

    - 5-HT4 agonists "…act on presynaptic receptors and facilitate release of acetylcholine and CGRP (calcitonin gene-related peptide" (Feldman M., et al. Sleisenger and Fordtran's Gastrointestinal and Liver Disease. 9th Edition. Saunders/Elsevier, Philadelphia, 2010, page 1672).

- Other agents
    - Colchicine
    - Misoprostol
    - Cholinergic agents
        - Bethanechol: constipation
        - Neostigmine: used for acute colonic pseudo-obstruction (Ogilvie syndrome)
    - Botulinum toxin
        - Defecatory disorders in which spastic pelvic floor dysfunction causes outlet delay

- Neurotrophins
  - Nerve growth factor (NGF), brain-derived neurotrophic factor (BDNF), and neurotrophin-3 (NT-3)
  - Promote growth of subpopulations of sensory neurons, and modulate synaptic transmission at developing neuromuscular junctions
- Linaclotide
  - minimally absorbed guanylate cyclase C agonist

Efficacy of laxatives

- Give the Grade of Evidence for the Use of Laxatives According to the American College of Gastroenterology Task Force on Chronic Constipation

Laxative	Grade of evidence*
➢ Bulking agents	
Psyllium	B
Calcium polycarbophil	B
Bran	†
➢ Osmotic laxatives	
Milk of magnesia	†
Lactulose	A
PEG	A
➢ Stimulants laxatives	B
➢ Stool softeners	B
➢ Lubricants	C
➢ Chloride channel activator	
Lubiprostone	§
➢ Prokinetics agent	

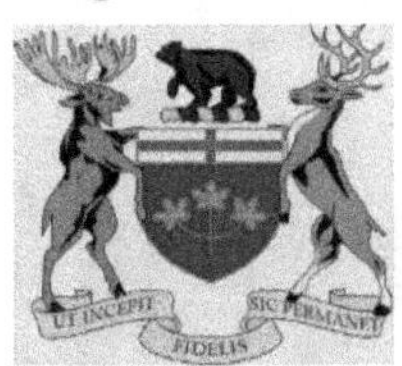

Laxative	Grade of evidence*
Tegaserod[‡]	A

Data from Brandt LJ, Prather CM, Quigley EM, et al. Systematic review on the management of chronic constipation in North America. Am J Gastroenterol 2005; 100(Suppl 1):S5-21.

† Insufficient data.

‡ Removed from the U.S. market.

§ Not yet graded.

	RR	95% CI
○ Older osmotic and stimulant laxatives	0.52	0.46-0.60
○ Newer pharmaceuticals with a big price tag		
- prucalopride	0.82	0.76-0.88
- lubiprostone	0.67	0.56-0.80
- linaclotide	0.84	0.80-0.87

- Note that none of these newer agents were studied against the older laxatives.
- Because of the possible heterogeneity of the studies and the variable placebo response rates, the values of the RR or the NNTs (if they had been reported) cannot be directly compared. However, the osmotic and stimulant laxatives were certainly not "poor second cousins"

- **Surgery for slow transit constipation**
  - Total or subtotal colectomy with ileorectal anastomosis

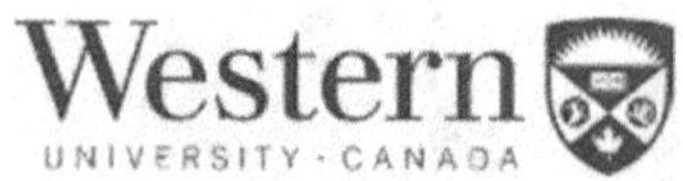

- Chronic, severe, and disabling symptoms from constipation (inertia pattern) that are unresponsive to medical therapy
- Intestinal pseudoobstruction
- Pelvic floor dysfunction
- Abdominal pain as a prominent symptom
- Post – op complications
    - Small bowel obstruction
    - Prolonged ileus
    - Diarrhea
    - Incontinence

- Construction of a stoma, with / without colonic resection
- Operations for defecatory disorders
    - Contrast is retained during defecography
    - Surgical repair may not alleviate symptoms of rectocele or rectal intussusceptions
    - Improved rectal evacuation when pressure is placed on the posterior wall of the vagina during defecation should be demonstrated before considering a rectocele repair

- Give the approximate frequency of 5 undesirable outcomes after colectomy for chronic constipation.

Undesirable outcomes	Approximate frequency (%)
Abdominal pain	40
Small bowel obstruction	15
Reoperation	10
Fecal incontinence	10
Diarrhea	10
Recurrent constipation	10
Stoma dysfunction	5

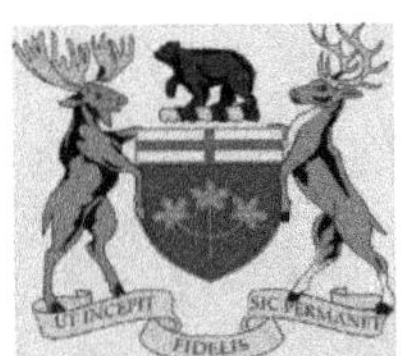

Printed with permission: Müller-Lissner S. *Best Pract Res Clin Gastroenterol* 2007; 21(3):476.
Clinical Challenge

A middle age woman has a normal colonoscopy in association with their constipation. A colonic transit study. Emperic therapy for the constipation has been unsuccessful.

- Give the likely diagnosis and the characteristic findings on anorectal monometry.
    - She likely has pelvic dyssynergy (aka functional anorectal outlet obstruction).
    - Normally, when straining down, as if to have a bowel movement (Valsalva Maneuver), the pressure measured from the rectal lead on manometry increases, and the pressure from the lead in the anus relaxes.
    - With pelvic dyssynergy, with straining, there is a paradoxical increase in the pressure in the anus (failure of relaxation).
- Pelvic dyssynergy and constipation in a middle-aged women is often from obstetrical trauma. When the anal pressure fails to relax with straining (Valsalva) maneuver in a young person, give the more likely diagnosis.
    - She likely has pelvic dyssynergy (aka functional anorectal outlet obstruction).
    - When rectal manometry shows
        - ↑ rectal pressure, plus
        - ↑ anal pressure (failure of relaxation)

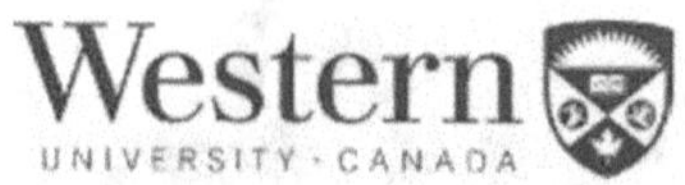

Please see: Chaun H. Chapter 56. In: Therapeutic Choices. Grey J, Ed. 6th Edition, Canadian Pharmacists Association: Ottawa, ON, 2011, Table 3: Constipation, page 741-745.

Clinical Tip

- In a young person, suspect consider the rare possibility of Hirschprung disease (abnormal embryological migration of neural crest cells)

Cathartic Colon

- It has been suggested that long-term use of the anthraquinone (e.g. cascara, senna) and bisacodyl laxatives may cause changes in the colon on diagnostic imaging (barium studies), and on histopathology.
- "there is no evidence that currently used laxatives can produce "carthartic colon" (Feldman M., et al. Sleisenger and Fordtran's Gastrointestinal and Liver Disease. 9th Edition. Saunders/Elsevier, Philadelphia, 2010, page 2246).
- Brown discoloration of the mucosa may occur in ~70% of chronic users of cascara or senna laxatives (melanosis coli).

Malakoplakia

- Malakoplakia may be suspected on colonoscopy by the presence of yellowish, friable mucosal lesions.
- The pigment is lipofuscin within macrophages.

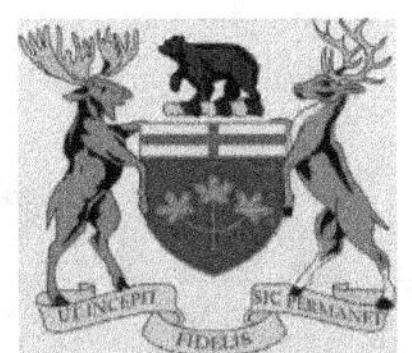

- More common in persons exposed to chemotherapy, immunosuppression for organ transplantation, or with AIDs.

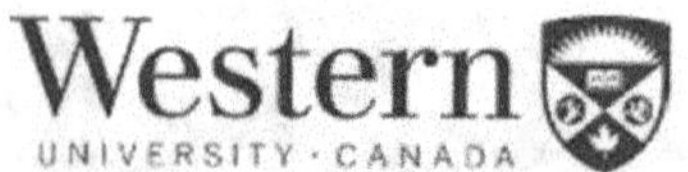

- Give histological features associated with colonic malakoplakia, and indicate (*) which feature is considered to be diagnostic.

  - Macrophages
    - Sheets of large, pale macrophages
    - Cytoplasm may contain coliform bacteria
  - Inclusion bodies*
    - In cytoplasm
    - Laminated
  - For the two standard deviation outlier GI trainee

- In the context of malakoplakia, give the meaning of von Hansemann cells, and Michaelis-Gutmann bodies.

  - Von Hansemann cells
    - Coliform bacteria in the cytoplasm of macrophages in the colonic mucosal biopsies
  - Michaelis-Gutmann bodies
    - Laminated intracytoplasmic inclusion bodies
  - The focal (as compared to the diffuse or isolated [to the rectosigmoid area] form of malakoplakia) may be associated with adenomatous polyps or CRC.

➢ Treatment

  - Dealing with associated risk factors
  - Antibiotics (ciprofloxacin, or trimethoprim-sulfamethoxazole),
  - Surgery for complications (such as bleeding or obstructing strictures)

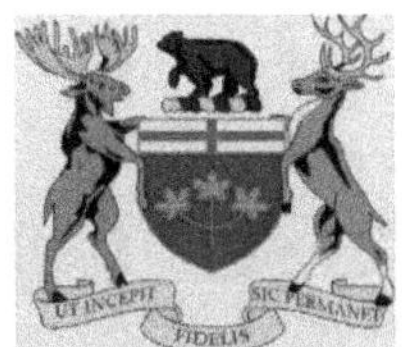

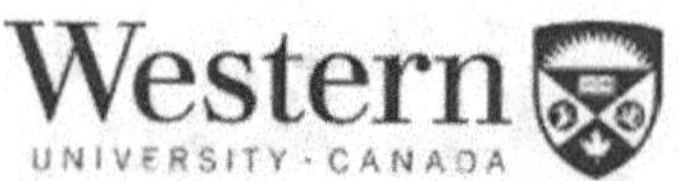
Western
UNIVERSITY · CANADA

Pregnancy

- Give 5 causes of constipation in pregnancy.
    - Reduced exercise
    - Hormonal – slow transit
    - Mechanical
    - Medications
    - Lifestyle
        - Reduced exercise
        - Dietary changes
    - Pre-existing disease:
        - Chronic slow-transit constipation
        - Irritable bowel syndrome
        - Congenital or acquired megacolon
        - Chronic idiopathic intestinal pseudo-obstruction

Adapted from: Quigley EMM. *Best Pract Res Clin Gastroenterol* 2007;21(5): pg. 882.; and Cullen G, and O'Donoghue D. *Best Pract Res Clin Gastroenterol* 2007; 21(5): pg. 810.

- Give the FDA category of laxatives in pregnancy.

Safe (B)	Caution (C)	Unsafe (D)
Lactulose	– Saline osmotic laxatives	-Anthraquinones
Glycerine	– Castor oil	-5HT4 agonists
Polyethylene glycol (PEG)	– Senna	-Prostaglandins (misoprostol)
Bulking agents	– Docusate sodium	
Bisacodyl		

Adapted from: Cullen G, and O'Donoghue D. *Best Pract Res Clin Gastroenterol* 2007; 21(5): pg. 815.; and Thukral C, and Wolf JL. *Nat Clin Pract Gastroenterol Hepatol* 2006; 3(5): pg. 260.

- Give a summary of drugs commonly used for irritable bowel syndrome (IBS) and diarrhea during pregnancy.

Drug	Pregnancy use category	Usual dosage	Additional comments
○ Tegaserod	B	6 mg twice daily	Limited data; should be considered only when other measures fail to control constipation – predominant irritable bowel syndrome
○ Loperamide	B	2-4 mg daily or after each unformed stool	Antidiarrheal agent of choice during pregnancy
○ Diphenoxylate with atropine sulphate	C	1-2 tablets four times daily	Should be avoided during pregnancy. Contains 2.5 mg diphenoxylate plus 0.025 mg atropine per tablet
○ Dicycloverine (dicyclomine)	B	10-20 mg four times daily	Should be reserved for women with refractory symptoms
○ Hyoscyamine	C	0.125-0.250 mg every 6 h as needed	Should be reserved for women with refractory symptoms
○ Tricyclic antidepressants	C/D	Dose differs according to retail brand	Questionable safety in pregnancy; use should be limited to the severely symptomatic

Printed with permission: Thukral, Chandrashekhar., and Wolf, Jacqueline L. *Nat Clin Pract Gastroenterol Hepatol* 2006; 3(5): pg. 261.

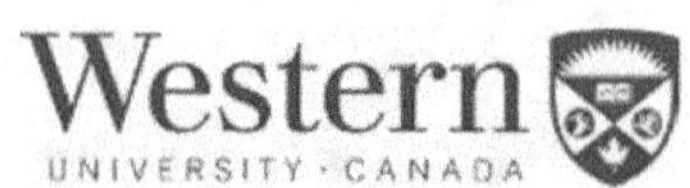

Fecal Continence and Incontinence

- Definition: The recurrent uncontrolled passage of fecal material for at least one month duration

- Subtypes
    - Passive – involuntary release of stool or flatus
    - Urge – release of fecal contents despite voluntary attempts to retain contents
    - Seepage – leakage of small amounts of stool following an evacuation

- Causes

- Give 10 causes of fecal incontinence.

- Rectum
    - Congenital abnormalities of the anorectum
    - Fistula
    - Rectal prolapse
    - Anorectal trauma
    - Fissure – treatment (Botoxin)
    - Childbirth injury
    - Surgery (including hemorrhoidectomy)
    - Sequelae of anorectal infections
    - Crohn disease

- Diarrhea/overflow from constipation

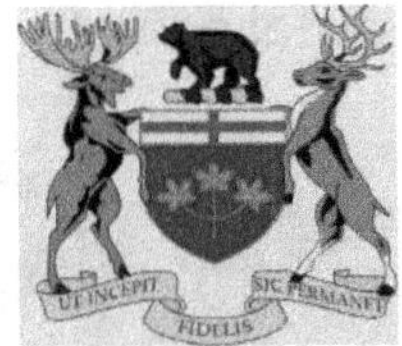

- Central nervous system processes
  - Dementia
  - Encopresis (childhood)
  - Mental retardation
  - Stroke
  - Brain tumour

- Spinal cord injury
  - Multiple sclerosis
  - Tabes dorsalis
  - Cauda equina lesions

- Pudendal nerve damage
  - Polyneuropathies
  - Diabetes mellitus
  - Shy-Drager syndrome
  - Toxic neuropathy
  - Traumatic neuropathy
  - Perineal descent

Printed with permission: Schiller, L. *Sleisenger & Fordtran's gastrointestinal and liver disease: Pathophysiology/Diagnosis/Management* 2006: pg. 202.

- Give 3 **anatomical structures** and the mechanisms by which they contribute to normal fecal continence.
  - Nerves – pudenal nerve/sacral segments S2 – S4/brain: The pudenal nerve has both afferent and efferent limbs, sensing stool entry into the rectum and delivering the impulse through the sacral nerves, spinal cord, to the brain. The

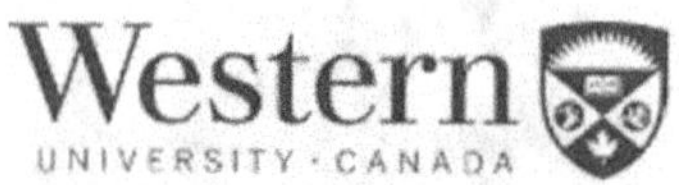

efferent limb carries the sensation of distension, which causes central pathways to send signals via the afferent limb to allow for conscious contraction of external sphincter to maintain continence.

- Muscles
  - Internal anal sphincter (IAS)
  - External anal sphincter (EAS)
  - Levator ani complex:
    - The internal anal sphincter is tonically contracted providing continence at rest.
    - When stool enters the rectum the IAS relaxes, however, continence is maintained if consciously desired by contraction of the EAS.
    - The IAS returns to resting tone, the rectum demonstrates compliance allowing intrarectal pressure to decrease and the urge to defecate to pass.
    - The levator ani muscles provide additional support to the EAS. As well, they form a sling around the anal canal, forming an acute angle during rest, creating a mechanical barrier for continence. Inability to distend without substantial rise in pressure, thus not overwhelming resting anal tone.
    - Rectum - reservoir

Abbreviations: EAS, external anal sphincter; IAS, internal anal sphincter

Adapted from: Schiller LR. *Sleisenger & Fordtran's Gastrointestinal and Liver Disease: Pathophysiology/Diagnosis/Management* 2006: pg. 200-201.

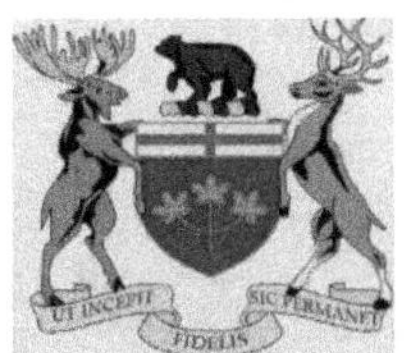

- Give 5 tests/procedures which are useful to investigate the patient with fecal incontinence.

➢ Clinical

- History, physical examination
- Sensory and motor (DRE) testing
- Perianal descent (normally 1.5-3.0 cm)
- Rectal examination
  - Value of rectal examination in the person with fecal incontinence
    - Perianal sensation
    - Sphincter tone at rest or voluntary contraction, and election of perineum
    - Sphincter tone
    - Length of anal canal
    - Anorectal angle

➢ Mucosa

- Endoscopy

➢ Muscle

- Structure
  - EUS
  - MRI/ CT
- Function
  - Colon transit study
  - Contraction pressure: pellet retention test
  - Expulsion pressure: balloon expulsion test
  - Co-ordination: anorectal manometry "defecography"

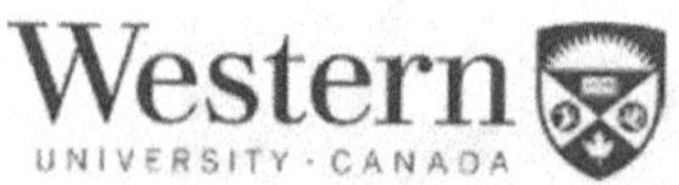

- Nerve
    - Pundendal nerve terminal latency

Abbreviations: DRE, digital rectal examination; EUS, endoscopic ultrasound

- Diagnostic imaging
    - US, CT, MRI, EUA, DRE, EUS (transrectal)

- Treatment

- Give 15 medical and surgical treatments of fecal incontinence.

- Treat underlying cause (s)

- Supportive therapy (the patient)
    - Education/counseling/habit training
    - Trained defecation
    - Diet (fiber; lactose, fructose, reduce caffeine intake
    - Incontinence pad
    - Perianal hygiene/skin care
    - Kegel exercises

- Pharmacological (the stool)
    - Fiber
        - Psyllium has been shown in a RCT to reduce the number of episodes of fecal incontinence by 50%; uncontrolled studies suggest a benefit for cholestyramine or amitriptyline.

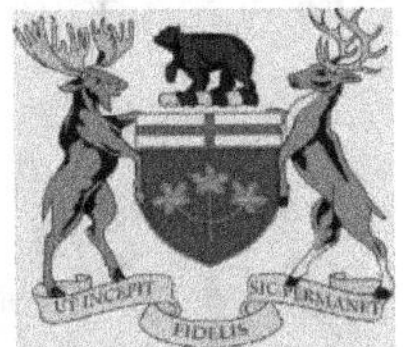

- Loperamide
- Lomotil
- Codeine
- Cholestyramine/colestipol
- Estrogen
- Phenylephrine
- Sodium valproate

- Biofeedback therapy
  - Anal sphincter muscle strengthening
  - Rectal sensory conditioning
  - Recto-anal coordination training
    - The operant conditioning techniques of biofeedback training using visual, auditory or verbal feedback, are meant to improve the strength of the anal sphincter muscles, anorectal sensory perception, and coordination of anal sphincter, gluteal and abdominal muscles following rectal balloon dilation or voluntary squeeze
    - Both biofeedback training and Kegal exercises each produce a 50% reduction in fecal incontinence.
      - One study has shown superior improvement with biofeedback as compared to exercises, on a per protocol but not an intention-to-treat basis.
      - Another study showed 77% of persons with fecal incontinence showing improvement versus 40% treated with Kegal exercises with 66% versus 48%, respectively, being totally content.

- Biofeedback defecation is also of benefit for dyssynergic defecation, providing sustained 12 month improvement in 80% as compared with 22% in the standard care (laxative [PEG] and counseling group), with improved ability to expel a test balloon, and standard care correction of dyssynergy in 79% of the active biofeedback group versus 4% in the sham group
- In a second study, there was 70% improvement at 3 months, with biofeedback vs 23% with diazepam and 28% with placebo
- Biofeedback is also of benefit in persons with solitary rectal ulcer syndrome (Rao SSC, et al. *Clin Gastroenterol Hepatol* 2007:331-8.)

➢ Perianal
  - Anal plugs
  - Pessary
  - Kegal exercises
  - Sphincter bulking (collagen, silicone)
  - Anal electrical stimulation
  - Injection sclerotherapy
  - Sacral nerve stimulation
    - RCTs have shown a benefit for sacral nerve stimulation for fecal incontinence when the anal sphincter is intact
    - The Malone procedure (antegrade continent enema procedure – cecostomy or appendicostomy for antegrade washing of the colon) gives a 61% success rate for fecal incontinence over 39 months

- Surgery
  - Artificial anal sphincter
  - Sphincteroplasty
  - Anterior repair (rectocele)
  - Gracilis/gluteus muscle transposition +/- stimulation
  - Colostomy
  - Pelvic reconstruction
  - Options: rubber band ligation
  - Surgical excision
  - PPH-Stapled Hemorrhoidopexy

Adapted from: Schiller L. *Sleisenger & Fordtran's gastrointestinal and liver disease: Pathophysiology/Diagnosis/Management* 2006: pg. 207.

- Give 3 risk factors for the development of incontinence post-partum.
  - Vaginal delivery
  - Instrumental delivery
  - Emergency cesarean section
  - Epidural anesthesia
  - Perineal laceration

Printed with permission: Quigley EMM. *Best Pract Res Clin Gastroenterol* 2007;21(5): pg. 885.

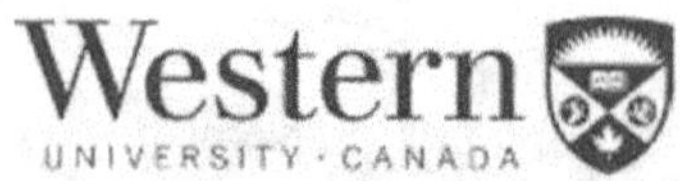

Anorectal and Perianal disease

➢ The Anatomy of the Anal Region

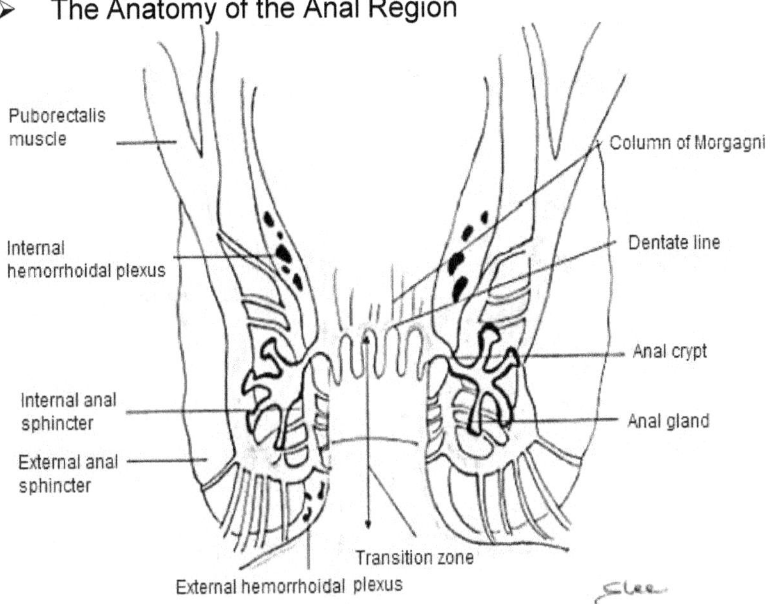

Adapted from: Feldman M., et al. Sleisenger and Fordtran's Gastrointestinal and Liver Disease. 8th Edition. Saunders/Elsevier, Philadelphia, 2006, Figure 122-1, page 2834.

Anorectal ring / sling of puborectalis

Sympathetic and Parasympathetic

Columns of Morgagni

Dentate line

Columnar transitional zone

Squamous mucosa (no hair!)

Somatic innervation

Anal verge / orifice

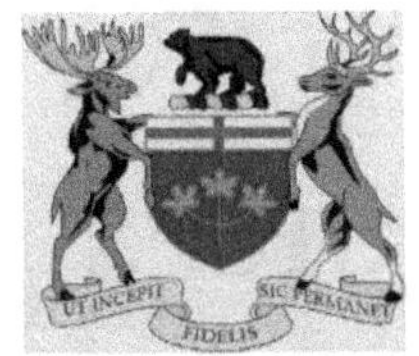

Normal diameters of large bowel

Site	Diameter (cm)
Rectosigmoid, descending	< 6.5
Ascending	8
Cecum	12

supralevator ②
ischial ③
intersphincter ①
levator ani muscle
int ani sphincter
ext ani sphincter
ANUS

- Infection in anal crypts at dentate line → rectal abscess → fistulas
- May be gross / microscopic CD in anal canal → perianal disease
- Why do CD fistula usually not become red – E. Coli bacteroids (anaerobic) don't cause skin damage, as with Staphylococcus or Streptococcus
- When you bear down, the anal sphincter relaxes
- Bowel rest and diversion colostomy for watering can CD perineum
- No effect on inflammation but ↑ throughout – so easier for patient (patient comfort) and ↓ protein loss

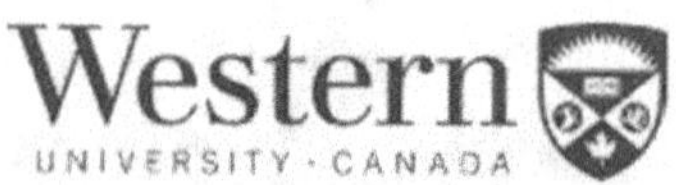

- Recurrence of CD after or – 10% per year → ~100% in 10 yrs!

Proctalgia (rectal pain)

- Solitary rectal ulcer syndrome colitis (SRUS) cystica profunda
- Proctalgia fugax (spasm in levator ani?)
- Intermittent severe rectal pain at night, no Δ BM
- Itch
  - Perianal redness
    - Pinworms (tap test)
    - Yeast infection – cream
    - Cancer
    - Soaps, detergents, dyes underclothes

Anal fissure

- Definition
  - A longitudinal cut in the anoderm
- Position
  - Mid posterior, 90%
  - Anterior, 10%
- Constipation → stretch strains spasm – fissure?
- Anal area "Animus"
- Sharp pain in anus

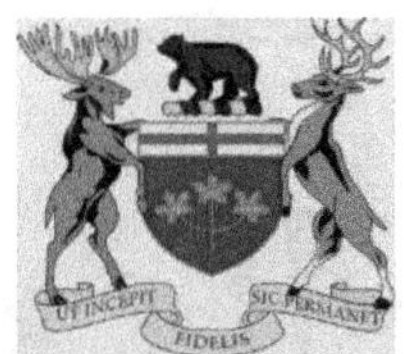

Classification of abscess of Anal region based of their location

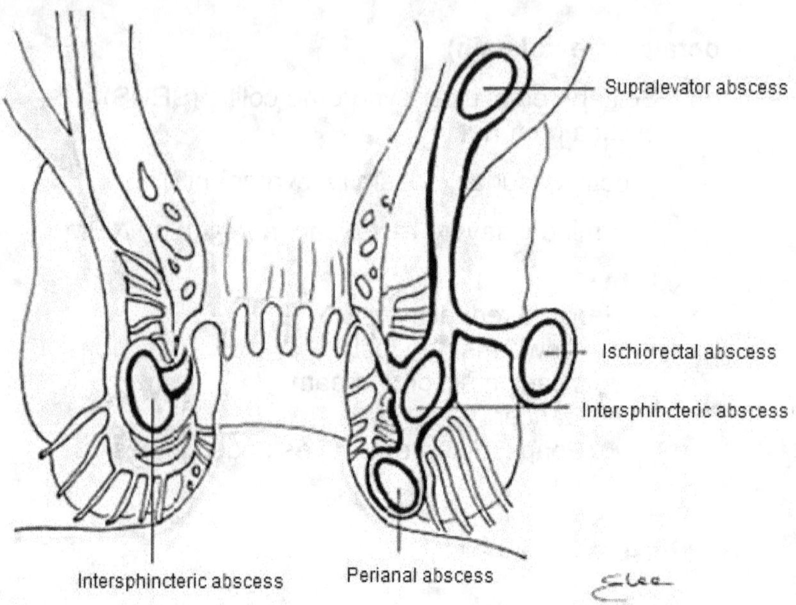

Adapted from: Feldman M., et al. Sleisenger and Fordtran's Gastrointestinal and Liver Disease. 8th Edition. Saunders/Elsevier, Philadelphia, 2006, Figure 122-3, page 2843.

- Give 15 causes of anorectal disease in patients with AIDS, not including non AIDS specific conditions.

➢ Infections

- o Bacteria
  - Chlamydia trachomatis*
  - Lymphogranuloma venereum
  - Neisseria gonorrhoeae*
  - Shigella flexneri
  - Mycobacterium tuberculosis

- Viruses
  - Herpes simplex*
  - Cytomegalovirus*
- Protozoa
  - Entamoeba histolytica
  - Leishmania donovani
- Fungi
  - Candida albicans
  - Histoplasma capsulatum

➢ Neoplasms

- Lymphoma*
- Kaposi's sarcoma
- Condyloma acuminatum
- Squamous cell carcinoma (HPV)
- Cloacogenic carcinoma

➢ Other

- Idiopathic ulcers*
- Perirectal abscess
- Fistula*

* More frequent diagnosis

Abbreviations: AIDS, acquired immunodeficiency syndrome. HPV, human papillomia virus.

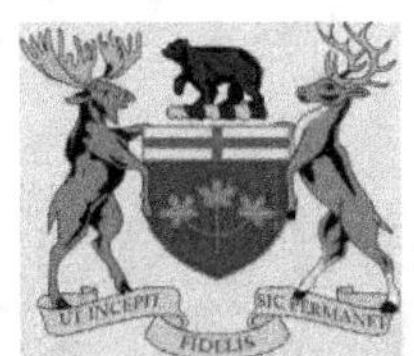

- Give symptoms, investigations and treatment of 4 sexually transmitted infections (STI) of the **anorectal region.**

STI	Symptoms	Investigations	Treatment
Gonorrhea	○ Pruritus ani ○ Mucopurulent anal discharge ○ Rectal pain ○ Tenesmus ○ Bleeding	- Culture and/or NAAT - Anoscopy; rectal friability, erythema, ulceration and mucus	▪ Ceftriaxone (250 mg intramuscularly) ▪ Doxycycline (100 mg orally twice daily) for 1 week
HSV	○ Vesicular lesions ○ Anal pain ○ Tenesmus ○ Discharge ○ Viremic symptoms ○ Lymphadenopathy ○ Pruritus ani ○ Mucoid and/or bloody diarrhea ○ Psychogenic constipation ○ Sacral paraesthesia ○ Impotence	- Viral culture and/or NAAT - Anoscopy; perianal vesicles, rectal ulcers, rectal inflammation	▪ Acyclovir (200 mg orally five times daily) for 5 days
Amebiasis	○ Bloody diarrhea	- Microscopy of stool - Anoscopy; friable rectal mucosa, shallow ulcers with exudates and ring of erythema	▪ Metroidazole (500-750 mg orally three times daily) for 5-10 days

STI	Symptoms	Investigations	Treatment
Shigellosis	○ Abdominal cramps ○ Fever ○ Bloody diarrhea	- Stool culture	▪ Trimethoprim sulfamethox-azole (double strength) orally twice daily for 7 days ▪ Tetracycline 1.5g once and ampicillin 500 mg orally four times daily for 7 days
Non LGV chlamydia	○ Commonly asymptomatic ○ Can cause pruritus ani, mucoid discharge, perianal pain	- NAAT	▪ Doxycycline (100 mg orally twice daily) for 1 week
LGV chlamydia	○ Purulent anal discharge ○ Pain ○ Tenesmus ○ Fever ○ Malaise ○ Genital ulcers /papules ○ Lymph-adenopathy (buboes)	- NAAT - Anoscopy; friable, ulcerated rectal mucosa with or without rectal mass	▪ Doxycycline (100 mg orally twice daily) for 3 week

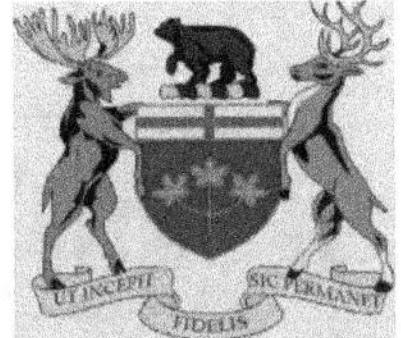

STI	Symptoms	Investigations	Treatment
Primary syphilis	o Anorectal chancres o Anal pain o Discharge o Tenesmus o Itching o Bleeding o Mucus membrane lesions o Maculopapular rash	- Dark field microscopy - Serology tests (eg RPR, TPPA, TPHA)	▪ Procaine penicillin (750 mg intramuscularly once daily) for 10 days or benzothine penicillin (2.4g intramuscularly once) or ▪ Doxycycline (100 mg orally twice daily) for 14 days
Secondary syphilis	o "Snail track" ulcers o Perianal condylomata lata	- Dark field microscopy - Serology tests (eg RPR, TPPA, TPHA) - Anoscopy; painful anal ulcer	▪ Procaine penicillin (750 mg intramuscularly once daily) for 10 days or benzothine penicillin (2.4 g intramuscularly once) or ▪ Doxycycline (100 mg orally twice daily) for 14 days

Abbreviations: HSV, Herpes simplex virus; LGV, lymphogranuloma venereum; NAAT, nucleic acid amplification testing; RPR, rapid plasma regain test; STI, sexually transmitted infection; TPHA, treponema pallidum hemagglutination assay; TPPA, treponema pallidum particle agglutination

Printed with permission: Siew C. Ng & Brian Gazzard. *Nat Rev Gastroenterol. Hepato* 2009;6:592-607, Table 1, page 594.

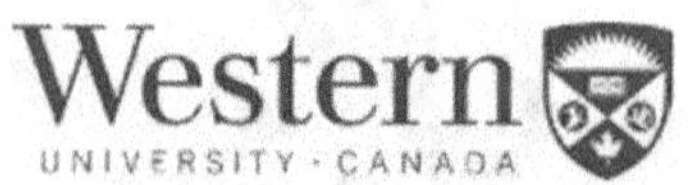

Clinical Challenge

A 78 year old female with severe, poorly controlled Parkinson disease is admitted to a geriatric unit. She has decompensated over the holidays with dysphagia. A gastroscopy was unremarkable. Plans are underway regarding a percutaneous gastrostomy for feeding. In the interim, you are called due sudden onset rectal pain and bleeding. On examination you diagnose an acute anal fissure, in the posterior midline (6 o'clock position).

- Give 3 other causes of bright red rectal bleeding that this patient is specifically at risk for in relation to her underlying disease process (Parkinson's disease).
    - Hemorrhoid
    - Stercoral (ischemic) ulcer
    - Solitary rectal ulcer syndrome

- Give 4 risk factors that this patient has for developing an anal fissure.
    - Age
    - Immobility
    - Constipation
    - Parkinson's Disease related decreased colonic activity
    - Antiparkinsonian drugs L-DOPA, anticholinergics (cogentin)
    - Dehydration/electrolyte imbalance
    - Fecal incontinence (overflow diarrhea)
    - Manual stool extraction
    - Enemas

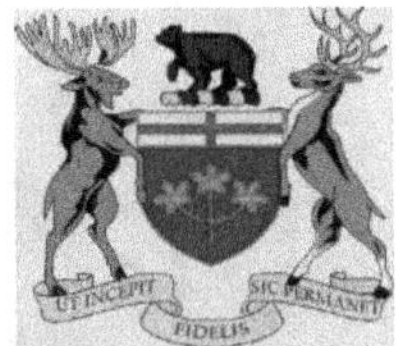

Fistula-in-ano

- Definition: "…… a tunnel that connects an internal opening, usually at an anal crypt at the base of the columns of Morgagni, with an external opening, usually on the anal skin" (Feldman M., et al. Sleisenger and Fordtran's Gastrointestinal and Liver Disease. 9th Edition. Saunders/Elsevier, Philadelphia, 2010, page 2267).

Hemorrhoids

- Definition
  - Dilated vascular channels
- Position
  - 3, 7, 11 o'clock positions
- Surface
  - Internal
    - Above dentate line
    - Covered by columnar or transitional mucosa
  - External
    - Below dentate line
    - Covered by squamous mucosa

- Give the medical and surgical treatment of chronic internal hemorrhoids.
  - Treat underlying associated causes
    - Diarrhea/constipation, prolapse, bleeding, deficient intake of fibre and fluids
  - Supportive therapy
    - Avoid straining and limit time on commode

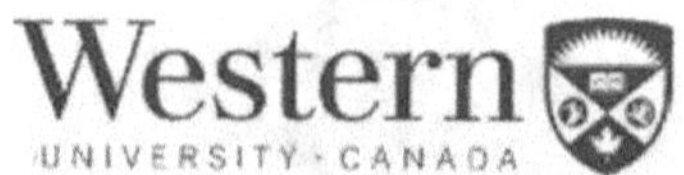

- Pharmacological
  - Barrier creams: zinc oxide, lanolin (limit contact of stool and mucus with sensitive anoderm)
  - Stool softeners, bulk, sitz bath, diet, fluids
  - Topical nitroglycerin(0.2% t.i.d)
    - Hypotension, headache, flushing
  - Diltiazem (calcium channel blocker [CCB]) cream (2%, t.i.d)
    - Flushing, headache, hypotension, bradycardia
  - Botulin toxin injection into the sphincter
    - Fecal incontinence, flatus incontinence (7%); effect wears off
- Surgical
  - Repair fissures to limit further trauma
  - Lateral sphincterotomy
    - Fecal incontinence
    - Recurrence (10%)
- Surgery – rubber band ligation, injection sclerotherapy, surgical excision, PPH-stapled hemorrhoidopexy
- Diverting colostomy

Adapted from: Hull S. *Sleisenger & Fordtran's gastrointestinal and liver disease: Pathophysiology/ Diagnosis/Management* 2006: pg. 2836-9; and 2010, pg. 2263 and 2265.

Solitary Ulcer Syndrome (SRUS)

- Pathology
  - Single or multiple ulcers, polypoid lesion
  - Lamina propria replaced by fibromuscular tissue

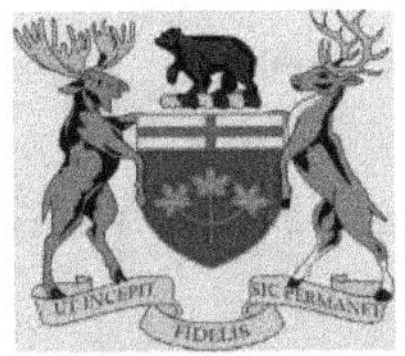

- Usual site of prolapse of rectal mucosa is anterior wall of the rectum, 7 cm to 10 cm above the verge the anus.
- Muscularis mucosa hypertrophied, with muscle fibres extending towards the lumen

➢ Pathogenesis:

- "occult or overt rectal prolapse with paradoxical contraction of the pelvic floor during defecation…." (Feldman M., et al. Sleisenger and Fordtran's Gastrointestinal and Liver Disease. 9th Edition. Saunders/Elsevier, Philadelphia, 2010, page 2080).

➢ Treatment of perianal disease

- Habits
- Obsession with cleaning
- Cleaning
- Sitz bath
- Steroid cream
- Anusol with lidocaine or HC
- Paper
  - Perfume
  - Colouring
- No soap near perineum
- Hot water may make itch worse (histamine release)
- Diet
  - Caffeine r/o
  - Spices
  - Beer is bad

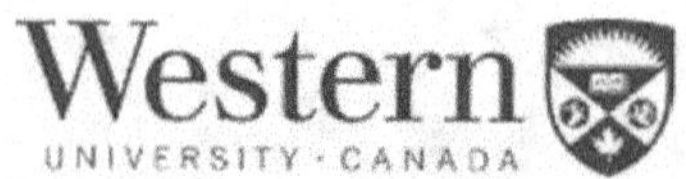

- Gloves, cut nails
- Stretch
  - ↓ spasm
- CCBs (calcium channel blockers), diltiazem 2% qid x 28 days, Anusol HC / Anusol with lidocaine
- GTN 0.2% paste / ointment
- Biofeedback
- Breaks the viscous cycle
  - Botox injection
  - Normal saline dental line, 4 quad using scople or use anoscope
- Surgery
  - Lord's procedure
  - Manual dilation under anesthesia (risk of incontinence)
  - Lateral sphincterotomy (at 3 to 5 o'clock, to relax sphincter)
  - Fissurectomy
  - Tags "extra skin" like a callus on top of your hemorrhoid": hypertrophic squamous epithelium

"A Child's mind is a fire to be kindled,
not a vessel to be filled."

Anonvmous

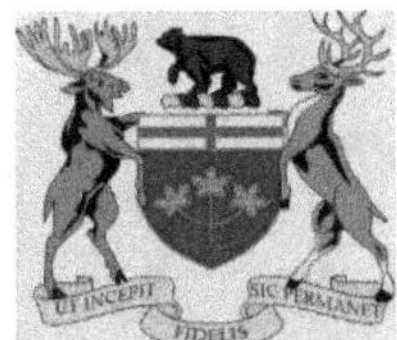

MINI UPDATE

Colorectal Cancer

Mohammed Aljawad

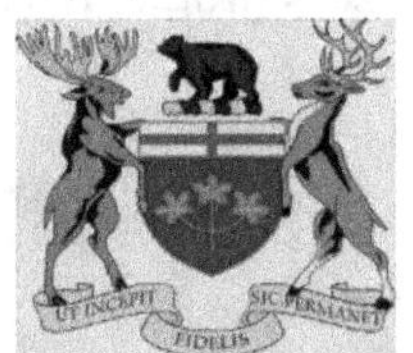

COLORECTAL CANCER

- Demography
  - Constitutes 10% of new cancers in men and women
  - Men = women
  - The age-standardized incidence of CRC (colorectal cancer) in Canada is approximately 25/10^5 persons per year (26.9 for men, 21.3 in women) which means about 6% of the population will develop CRC in their lifetime.
  - Lifetime risk of CRC 6%
  - Lifetime risk of dying form CRC 2.5%
  - Annual CRC mortality ↓ 33% for annual colonoscopy (2.5% → 1.6%, AR 0.8%↓)
  - Conversion rate (CR) to CRC
    - Adenoma, 30%
    - Villous, 17%
    - Dysplasia, 37%
    - Synchronous risk 5%
    - Metachronous risk 5%
  - Miss rate of CRC on colonoscopy, 10%
  - While the lifetime risk of CRC in pancolitis LS ↑ 10x, (pseudopolyps not an ↑ risk of CRC in UC)

Useful background: Approximate incidence of GI cancers (10^5/year)

Years of Age	<49	50-74	>75
Esophagus	<1	12	28
Stomach	<1	22	78
Colon	<1	150	400

Source: Canadian Cancer Surveillance, Health Canada

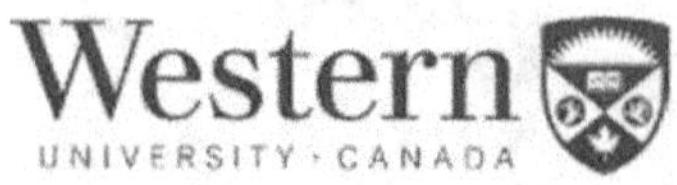

➢ Molecular Genetics

Major Genetics Abnormalities :

- alterations in proto-oncogenes
- loss of tumor suppressor gene activity
- abnormalities in genes involved in DNA mismatch repair (MMR)

Gene	Chromosome	Frequency of Tumors with Gene Alterations (%)	Gene Class
K-ras	12	50	Proto-oncogene
APC	5	70	Tumor suppressor
DCC	18	70	Tumor suppressor
SMAD4 (DPC4, MADH4)	18		Tumor suppressor
TP53	17	75	Tumor suppressor
hMSH2	2		DNA mismatch repair
hMLH1	3		DNA mismatch repair
hMSH6	2		DNA mismatch repair
TGF-β1 RII	3		Tumor suppressor

- There are 3-pathways in the adenoma-CRC pathway: chromosomal instability (CIS) pathway, microsatellite instability pathway (MIS), and the epigenetic pathway.
- With the epigenetic pathway, DNA methylation in the promoter region of genes leads to gene silencing, which is essentially equivalent to inactivating metastasis (Ahnen 09). These epigenetic defects in methylation are replicated through cell division and a defective clone of cells is produced.

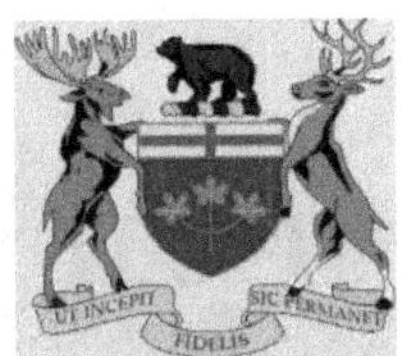

- One of the methylation-induced inactivations is in MLH-1, one of the mismatch repair genes
- Hyperplastic polyps (HP) are the earliest colonic lesion in the epigenetic pathway
- Large hyperplastic polyps (HP) (>10 mm) on the right side of the colon may develop into serrated adenomas, and have a malignant potential
- 15% of all CRCs are thought to develop through this epigenetic pathway of serrated adenomas
- Because both Lynch Syndrome cancers and serrated adenoma cancers make a mismatch repair gene (MLH-1), the tumour morphology may be similar.

- Give 10 examples of **molecular genetic changes** associated with sporatic and familial / hereditary CRC.
    - There are multiple genes, which are altered in at least some patients with CRC, and these gene mutations may become important at different stages in the development of CRC.
    - The gene mutations in CRC occur against a background of CIN
    - CIN occurs in 80% of CRC
    - Candidate genes for CIN include genes responsible for
        - Mitotic spindle checkpoint
        - DNA damage checkpoint
        - Control of number of centrosomes
    - There are three important classes of these sporatic CRC-associated gene
        - Proto-oncogenes
        - Tumor suppressor genes
        - NMR genes

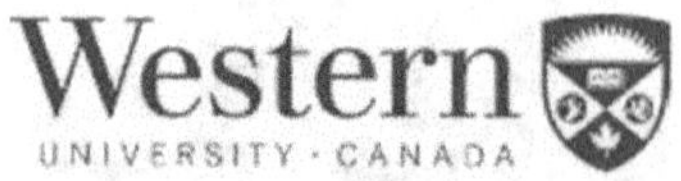

- Other important gene mutations include
  - RAS / RAF / MAPK pathway, with mutation in BRAF gene
  - Expression pattern of micro RNAs

- ↑ proto-oncogenes
  - ↑ activation of proto-oncogenes
    - K-RAS
    - N-RAS
    - H-RAS
  - Role in sporatic CRC
    - Activating point mutations 9especially in K-RAS gene):

Adenomas	< 1 cm	10%
	> 1 cm	58%
Carcinoma		47%

- Loss of tumor suppressive genes
  - APC gene
    - Allelic losses at chromosome locations

      5q

      17p

      18q
  - Truncation of the APC protein
  - Occur in 60% to 80% of sporatic adenomas / carcinomas
  - Loss of DCC (deleted in colon cancer)
  - Low of DPC4 / SAMD4 (loss of activation of TGF-β receptors)

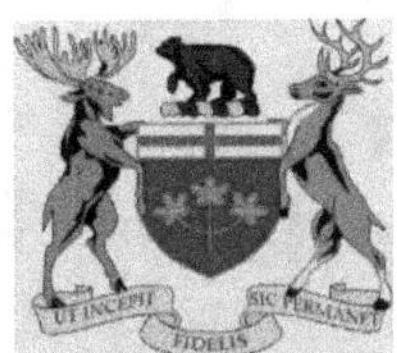

- Loss of p53 tumor suppressor activity from deletion of chromosome 17p leads to loss of cells preventing damaged DNA from going from G1 to S phase of the cell cycle.
- Loss of TP53 gene

- MMR (mismatch repair) genes
  - MSI (microsatellite instability)
  - Alterations in hMLH, hPMS1, hPMS2, hMSH2, hMSH3, hMSH6
  - ↓ repair of mismatches in base pairs → MSI → DNA replication errors → tandem repeat DNA sequences
  - Seen in only 15% of sporatic CRC

- Non-MMR gene changes
  - CIMP (CPG island methylator phenotype)
  - MSI may be caused by mutations in MMR genes, or by epigenetic silencing mechanism
  - Definition: "Epigenetics is the study of clonal changes in gene expression without accompanying changes in DNA coding sequences" (Feldman M., et al. Sleisenger and Fordtran's Gastrointestinal and Liver Disease. 9th Edition. Saunders/Elsevier, Philadelphia, 2010, page 2203).
  - Hypermethylation of the hMLA, promotor, with inactivation of hMLH1.
  - Seen in 70% of sporatic MSI tumors.
  - Common pathway for the development of serrated adenomas.

COLORECTAL CANCER

- Give 5 germline and somatic mutations involved in the initiation and promotion of CRC deleted in colon cancer
    - Familial Adenomatous Polyposis (FAP)
        - FAP – autosomal dominant inheritance of expression of gene changes
        - Only 80% penetrance of ARC gene – large protein, B-catenin pathway is important 2 hit hypothesis for FAP
        - Eye "CHRPE" congenital hypertrophy of the retinol pigment epithelium
    - Attenuated FAP (AFAP)
    - MUTYH-associated polyps (aka MYH-associated polyposis)
        - Suspect if patient has > 10 ad polys
        - Germline mutation in MYH base excision repair gene
        - Occurs in APC region
        - 25% of AFAP with > 15 adenomas have MUTYH mutations
        - May be associated with breast cancer
        - Parents, siblings rarely affected
        - Recessive inheritance
    - HNPCC
        - CRC in 50% - 80%
        - DNA mismatch
        - Younger age when CRC develops
        - Proximal colon
        - Glioblastoma (meduloblastomas in FAP)
        - Clinical criteria to suspect HNPCC
        - In family ⎤ - Amsterdam criteria I, II
        - In individual ⎦ - Bethesda crieria

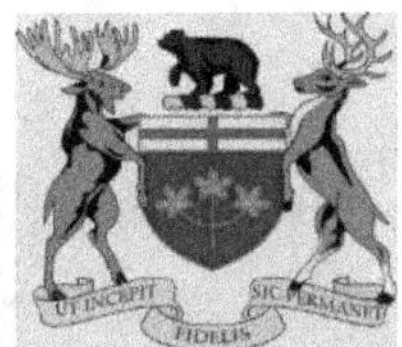

- MSI-histology
  - Lymphocytes infiltrating tumor
  - Crohn-like lymphocytic reaction
  - Mucinous / signet ring appearance
  - Medullary growth pattern
- Genetics
  - Test tumor for MSI
  - MSI (microsatellite instability) analysis, or IHC (immunohistochemistry) 90% of HNPCC tumors are positive
  - Test patient for same gene abnormality as for the index patient (proband)
  - Carrier with mutations need to be screened by colonoscopy

➢ Pathology

- Distribution of CRC within the colon
- 40% of CRCs are distal to the splenic flexus, but the proportion of right-sided tumors may be increasing.

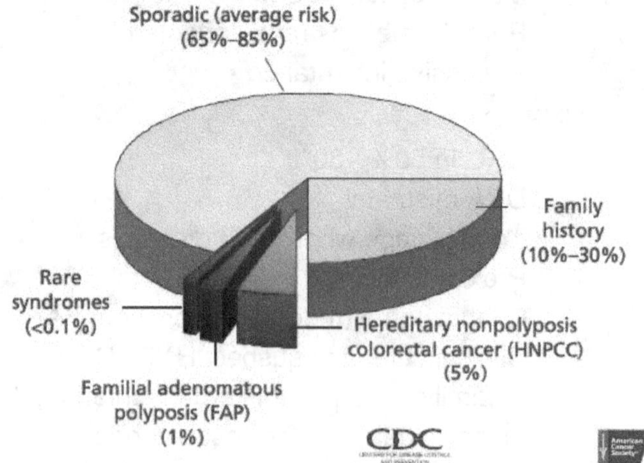

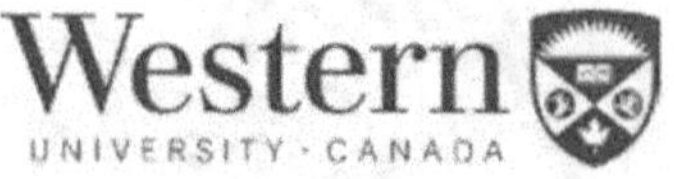

COLORECTAL CANCER

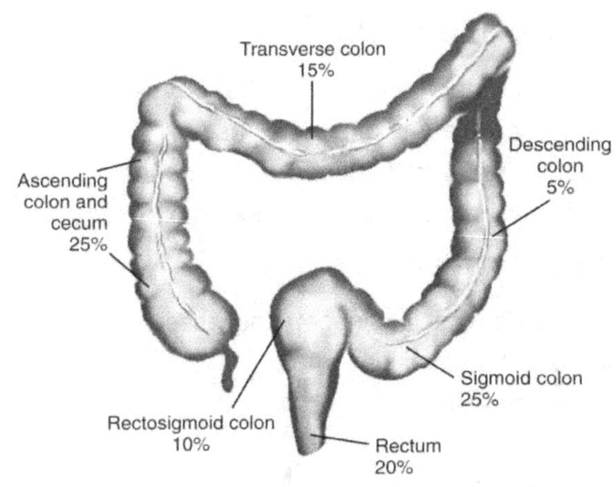

- Site
  - Cecum/Asc. Colon 25
  - Transverse 15
  - Descending 5
  - Sigmoid 25
  - Rectum 20
- About half of CRCs are within reach of flexible sygmoidoscopy

Useful background: The **TNM staging system** for colorectal cancer and published survival rates for different stages

T – Primary tumour (T)

TX	Primary tumour cannot be assessed
T0	No evidence of primary tumour
Tis	Carcinoma in situ: intraepithelial or invasion of lamina propria
T1	Tumour invades submucosa
T2	Tumour invades muscularis propria
T3	Tumour invades through the muscularis propria into subserosa or into non-peritonealised pericolic or perirectal tissues
T4	Tumour directly invades other organs or structures and/or perforates visceral peritoneum

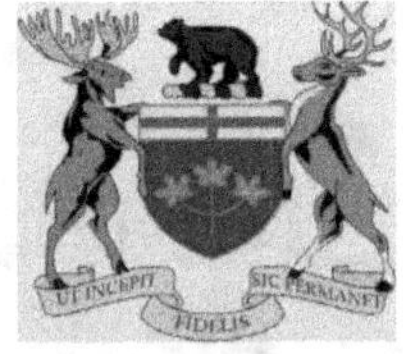

N – regional lymph nodes (N)

NX Regional lymph nodes cannot be assessed
N0 No regional lymph node metastasis
N1 Metastasis in 1 to 3 regional lymph nodes
N2 Metastasis in 4 or more regional lymph nodes

M- Distant metastasis (M)

MX Distant metastasis cannot be assessed
M0 No distant metastasis
M1 Distant metastasis

Stage	T N	M	5-year overall survival
Stage I	T1, T2 N0	M0	80-95%
Stage IIA	T3 N0	M0	72-75%
Stage IIB	T4 N0	M0	65-66%
Stage IIIA	T1, T2 NI	M0	55-60%
Stage IIIB	T3, T4 NI	M0	35-42%
Stage IIIC	Any T N2	M0	25-27%
Stage IV	Any T Any N	MI	0-7%

Printed with permission: Tejpar S. *Best Pract Res Clin Gastroenterol* 2007; 21(6): pg. 1074.

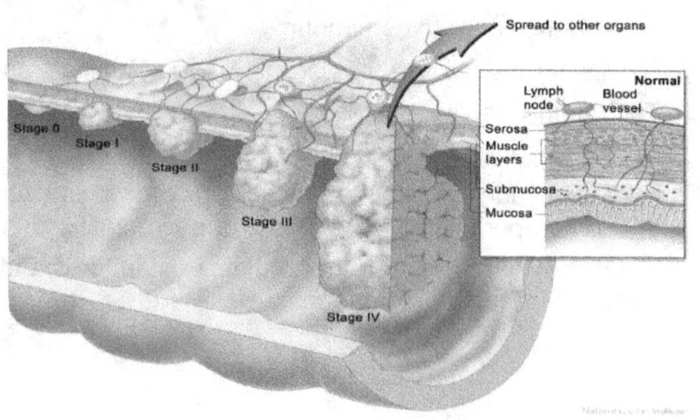

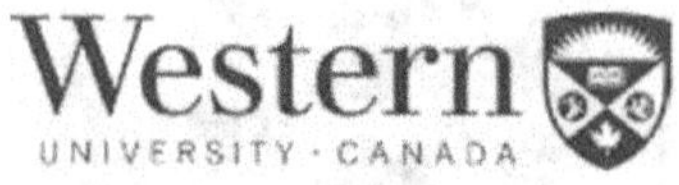

AJCC TNM Staging of Colorectal Cancer

Stage*	Criteria [†]
0	Carcinoma in situ: intraepithelial or invasion of lamina propria[‡] (Tis N0 M0)
I	Tumor invades submucosa (T1 N0 M0) [Dukes A] Tumor invades muscularis propria (T2 N0 M0)
II	Tumor invades through the muscularis propria into subserosa or into nonperitonealized pericolic or perirectal tissues (T3 N0 M0) [Dukes B] Tumor perforates the visceral peritoneum or directly invades other organs or structures and/or perforates visceral peritoneum[?] (T4 N0 M0)
III	Any degree of bowel wall perforation with regional lymph node metastasis N1: metastasis in 1-3 regional lymph nodes N2: metastasis in ≥4 regional lymph nodes Any T N1 M0 [Dukes C] Any T N2 M0
IV	Any invasion of bowel wall with or without lymph node metastasis, but with evidence of distant metastasis Any T Any N M1

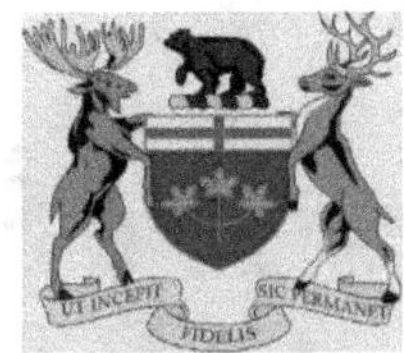

- Poor Prognostic Factors
    - Age < 30 yrs
    - High Preoperative CEA level
    - Depth of colon wall penetration
    - Poorly differentiated
    - Lymphatic or venous invasion
    - More than 4 LN (lymph nodes)
    - Colonic obstruction or perforation
    - Mucinous or signet ring cell histology

Streptococcus Bovis

- Strep. Bovis bacteremia - gram positive cocci, Biotype I
    - Found in blood in 10% - 15% of normal persons
    - Older males
    - When endocarditis occurs with S.bovis, there is usually no typical pre-existing conditions (e.g. artificial valves, IV drug use)
    - S.bovis – in fecal cultures
        - Control 10%
        - CRC 56%
    - Colonic polyps 47%, CRC 16% (no control group)

- Scientific plausibility
    - CRC epithelial cells have receptors for S.bovis
    - S.bovis upregulates COX-2
    - Carcinogenic in rats

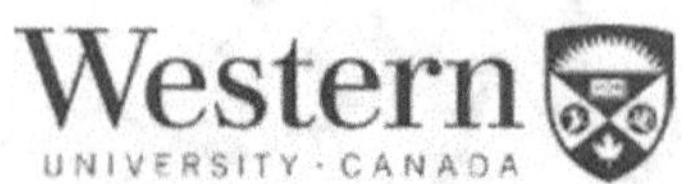

- Recommendation and suggestion
    - Colonoscopy for person with S.bovis in the blood (not if S.bovis is in stool)
    - Think of this issue as finding a source of the S.bovis bacteremia

- Risk factors / causes of CRC
    - Risk factors
        - Age ≥50 years
        - High-fat, low-fiber diet
        - Personal history of
            - Colorectal adenomas (synchronous or metachronous)
            - Colorectal carcinoma (CRC)
        - First-degree relative with CRC
        - Inflammatory bowel disease
        - Family history of a polyposis syndrome or Lynch syndrome
    - Adenomatous / hyperplastic polyps

Adenoma

- Most CRCs arise from pre-existing adenomas
- CRC increases with :
    - number of adenomas
    - size of adenoma (> 1 cm >>> conversion rate 3%)
    - villous histology (CR 17%)
    - nuclear atypia or dysplasia (CR 37 %)
- Risk of synchronous carcinomas 0.7% to 7.6%
- Metachronous carcinomas 1.1% to 4.7%

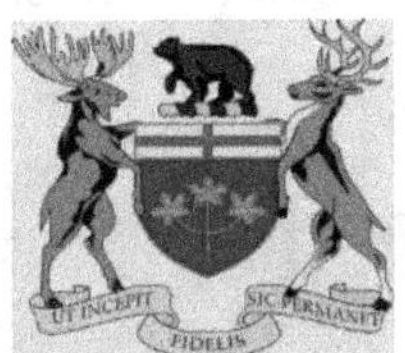

- 50% of metachronous cancers arise within 5-7 years of the index lesion
- Malignant Potential of Colonic Adenomas (%)

		(%)
- Size	< 1 cm	1
	1-2 cm	10
	>2 cm	45
- Histology	Tubular	5
	Tubular Villous	25
	Villous	40
- Dysplasia	Mild	5
	Moderate	20
	Severe	35

Percent of all colorectal cancers: 30, 20, 10

<40 40–49 50–59 60–69 70–79 >80

Age at diagnosis

- From the following table, calculate the absolute risk (AR) of CRC in a 55 year old patient whose father developed proven CRC at age 59, his 50 year old brother had an adenomatous colonic polyp, and a grandmother and an aunt of unknown age had CRC (baseline absolute risk for 50 year old, 6%).

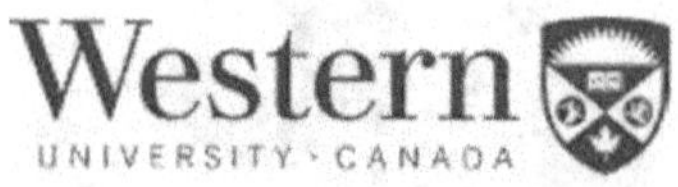

- Family History

Family Hx	RR
One fist degree relative with CRC	2.3
< 45 yrs	3.9
45-59 yrs	2.3
> 59	1.8
Two first degree relatives	3.8
More than two first degree relatives	4.3
One second degree or third degree relative	1.5
Two second degree relatives	2.3
One first degree relative < 60 yrs with an adenoma	2.0

RR=(2.3 x 2.0 x 2.3)= 10.5; Absolute risk for average risk person over age 50, 6%; absolute risk for this person, (10.6 x 6%= RRxAR >60%)

Printed with permission: Winawer SJ. Best Pract Res Clin Gastroenterol. 2007;21(6):1031-48.

- Causative
  - Probable causative
    - High-fat and low-fiber diet
    - Red meat consumption
  - Possible causative
    - Beer and ale consumption (especially for rectal cancer)
    - Cigarette smoking
    - Diabetes mellitus
    - Environmental carcinogens and mutagens
    - Heterocyclic amines (from charbroiled and fried meat and fish)
    - Low dietary selenium

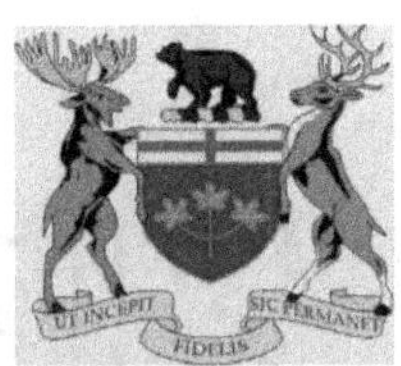

- Protective Factors
  - Probable Protective
    - Aspirin, NSAIDs, and cyclooxygenase-2 inhibitors
    - Calcium
    - Hormone replacement therapy (estrogen)
    - Low body mass
    - Physical activity
  - Possibly Protective
    - Carotene-rich foods
    - High-fiber diet
    - Vitamins C and E
    - Vitamin D
    - Yellow-green cruciferous vegetables

CRC and Inflammatory Bowel Disease (IBD)

- Pancolitis confers a 5- to 15-fold increase in CRC risk
  - Risk begins 8-10 years after diagnosis of IBD
- Limited left sided disease is associated with a 3 fold relative risk (RR)
  - Risk begins 15-20 years after diagnosis of IBD
- Risk not significantly increased with proctitis or proctosigmoiditis alone
- Risk increase with duration
  - Pancolitis: risk up to 30 % after 35 years of disease
- Risk increase with:
  - Primary scleosing cholangitis (PSC)
  - Dysplasia related lesion or mass (DALM)
- Inflammatory pseudopolyps: not dysplastic
  - not risk factor for colon cancer

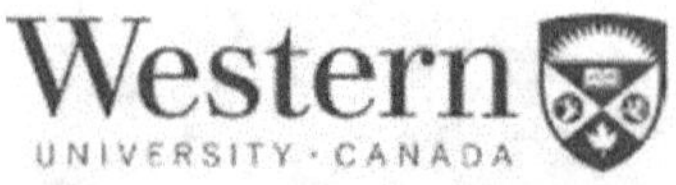

COLORECTAL CANCER

- Clinical presentation
  - Abdominal pain
  - Weight loss
  - Proximal colon tumors grow larger than left colon ones
  - Microcytic anemia: R colon >> Lt
  - Obstruction : L colon >> R
  - Change in bowel habits: L >> R
  - Bleeding per rectum: L >> R

Abbreviation: L, left; R, right
Prevention (screening and surveillance)

- Terms
  - Case finding: the investigation of the patient with symptoms and/or signs suggestive of the diagnosis (such as CRC).
  - Screening: the investigation of an asymptomatic person to find an early pathological lesion or condition.
  - Surveillance: the investigation of a person at regular intervals after and index lesion has been discovered by screening or case finding.
    - Age > 50 years (average risk)
    - Family or personal history history of CRC, adenomatous / hyperplastic polyps, polyposis syndrome
    - Note land marks
      - Cecum
    - Bowel preparation (cleanliness)

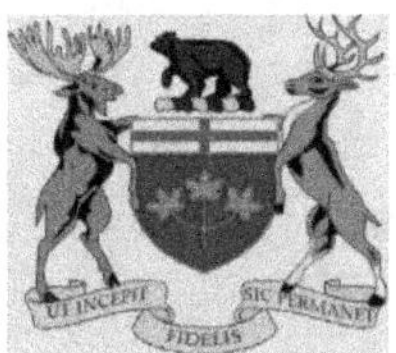

- o Sedation/ patient comfort
- o Withdrawal time (> 6 min)
- o Retroflexion in rectum
- o Miss-rate on consent form
- o Screening polyp detection rate
  - Average risk persons
    - M 25%
    - F 15%
- o Surveillance if screening is positive

Adapted from: *Mayo;*Table 13-2: pg 505.

CRC Screening

- Give new techniques that have been introduced to increase the sensitivity and specificity of endoscopic surveillance.
  - o Chromoendoscopy
    - Dyes to stain the colonic mucosa.
    - Sensitive and so can detect more dysplasia per (targeted) biopsy
    - Effective surveillance method.63-65
  - o Narrow band imaging
    - Interference filters to illuminate the mucosa in narrow red, green and blue
    - Better visualization of the mucosal structure and vascular networks
    - Improve in the detection of dysplasia

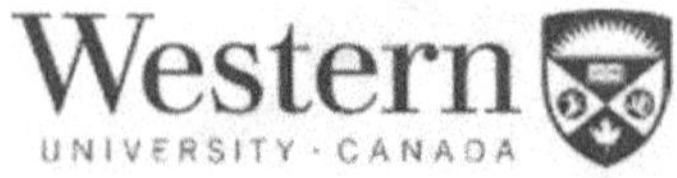

- Autofluorescence imaging
  - Blue light for the excitation of tissue specific autofluorescence.
  - Superior to conventional endoscopy for detecting dysplasia.70
- Endomicroscopy enables
  - Imaging of the microarchitecture of the colonic mucosa and vasculature
  - Using a combination of chromoendoscopy and endomicroscopy, Kiesslich *et al*, reported a 4.75 fold increased detection rate of neoplastic lesions compared with conventional colonscopy alone.72

Source: *Gastroenterology and Hepatology* 2009; 6:672.

- Discuss the ethical issues involved in establishing a colorectal cancer screening program for average risk persons (over age 50 years in Canada).
  - Gain in performance skills of operator.
  - Better bowel cleansing
  - Water instillation
  - Insertion
    - Cap-fit colonoscopy
    - Overtubes
  - Imaging
  - Wide-angle colonoscopy
  - Narrow-band imaging
  - Chromoendoscopy
  - Electronic chromoendoscopy
  - Confocal laser microscopy

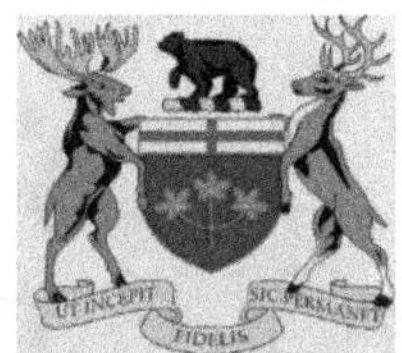

COLORECTAL CANCER

A variety of stool and structure-based tests of the colon are included as options for screening for CRC. In the process of providing your patient with informed consent with regards to their making a choice about these tests, it is necessary for you to know the sensitivity of these investigations.

- Give 5 tests for screening for CRC, and their approximate sensitivities for CRC and AA (advanced adenomas) in average risk persons presenting for colonoscopy.

Test	Sensitivity %	
	CRC	AA
○ Stool-based		
- Guaiac fecal occult		
▪ Standard	33-50	11
▪ "Sensitive"	50-75	20-25
- FIT (fecal immunochemical test), 1-3 stool samples	60-85	20-50
- DNA test, 1 stool sample		
▪ Old	51	18
▪ New	≥ 80	40
○ Structure –based*		
- CT colonography	Probably > 90	90
- Colonoscopy (standard white light)	95	88-98**

* Flexible sigmoidoscopy is not reported here, because it demonstrates less than half of the colon, and its sensitivity will depend upon the distribution of CRC/AA.

** While sensitivities of 88% to 98% are reported, the work of L. Rabeneck as well as others indicates that the miss rate is much higher, especially in the right colon.

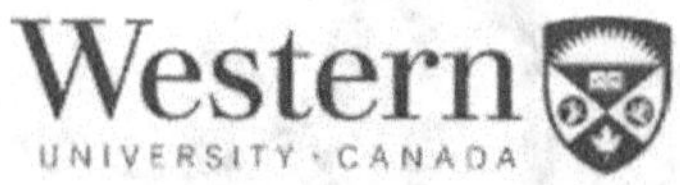

COLORECTAL CANCER

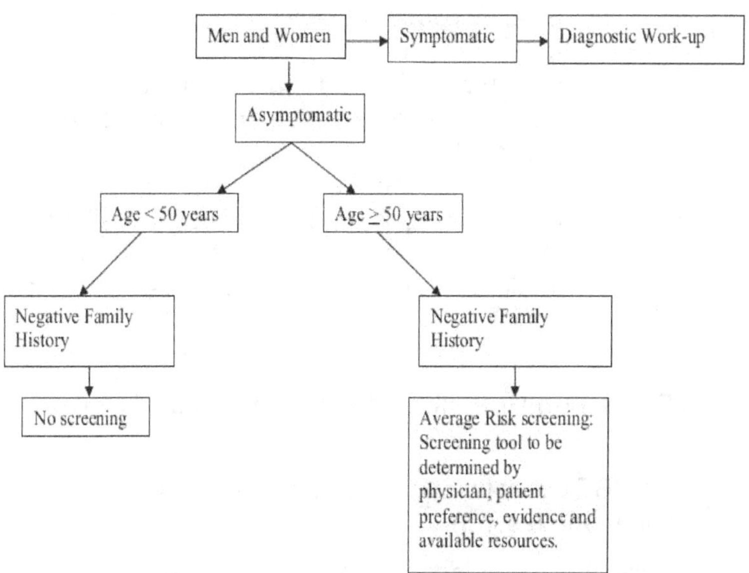

Source: Canadian Association of Gastroenterology (CAG) 2004 Guidelines on CRC screening

- Give 5 factors which must be taken into account when stratifying risk and the need for screening for colorectal cancer (CRC).
  - Age >50 yrs
  - Personal history of colonic polyps or CRC
  - Family history - polyps, CBC, Lynch/FAP-associated tumours
  - High risk groups
    - IBD patients
    - African-Canadians
    - Smokers

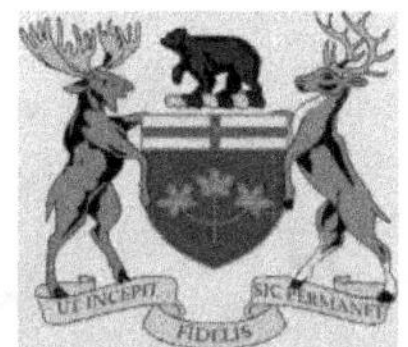

- Obesity (BMI>30, waist circumference>32-34")
- Concurrent PSC (primary sclerosing cholangitis) in conjunction with ulcerative colitis (UC)
- Dietary risk factors – low daily intake of fresh fruit, vegetables and fiber (possible); low intake of calcium and vitamin D; high intake of saturated fatty acids (especially red meat)

CAG Screening Guidelines for Average risk (2004)

- FOBT every two years (needs update on fecal immune testing)
- Flexible sigmoidoscopy every five years
- Flexible sigmoidoscopy combined with FOBT every five years
- Double contrast barium enema every five years (no longer endorsed by most guidelines)
- Colonoscopy every 10 years
- Needs update on CT colonoscopy, role of nurse practitioner colonoscopists)

Surveillance Guidelines in patients with history of CRC, American Society of Clinical Oncology (2005)

- History and physical
  - Every three to six months for the first three years;
  - Every six months during years 4 and 5,
  - Then annually thereafter.

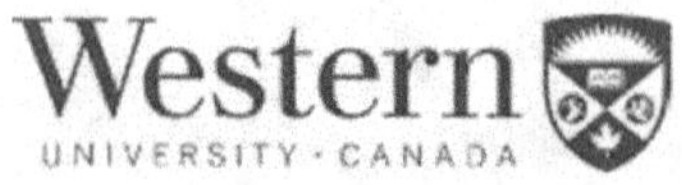

- CEA
  - Serum CEA testing should be performed every three months for at least three years in patients with stage II or III colon or rectal cancer if they would otherwise be candidates for surgery or systemic therapy.
  - Since adjuvant 5-FU-based therapy can falsely elevate the serum CEA, waiting until adjuvant therapy is finished to initiate surveillance is advised.

- CT
  - (stage III or high risk stage II) annual CT of the chest and abdomen for three years
  - Annual pelvic CT for three years should be considered for rectal cancer surveillance

Surveillance Guidelines in patients with history of CRC, ASCO (2005)

- Fecal occult blood test (FOBT)
  - The data are sufficient to recommend against periodic FOBTs in surveillance for colorectal cancer recurrence

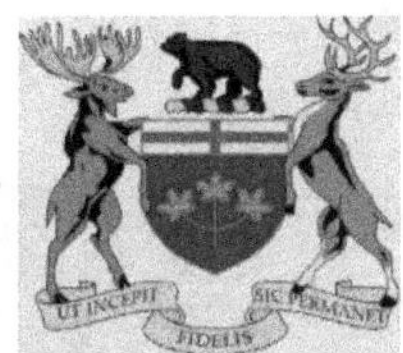

o Colonoscopy	–	Full colonoscopy in the preoperative or perioperative setting to document a cancer-free and polyp-free colon. Patients who present with an obstructing cancer should undergo full colonoscopy within six months of surgery. Repeat colonoscopy is recommended at three years, and if normal, every five years thereafter
o Flexible proctosigmoidoscopy, (rectal cancer)	–	For patients who have not received pelvic radiation therapy, flexible sigmoidoscopy is recommended every six months for five years.

Screening: Average risk

Screening Tool	U.S. Preventive Services Task Force*	American Cancer Society
o High sensitivity FOBT (guaiac-based or immunochemical)	Annually	annually

Screening Tool	U.S. Preventive Services Task Force*	American Cancer Society
○ Flexible sigmoidoscopy	every 5 yr + high-sensitivity FOBT every 3 yr as an option	every 5 yr
○ Colonoscopy	Every 10 yr	Every 10 yr
○ Double-contrast barium enema	Not recommended	Recommended every 5 yr
○ Computed tomographic colonography	Not recommended	Recommended every 5 yr
○ Stool DNA testing	Not recommended	Recommended (interval uncertain)

Screening: Positive Family History

Group	Age	Interval
○ First-degree relative before age 60 yr with CRC or adenomatous polyps or 2 or more first-degree relatives at any age	- At age 40 or 10 yrs before the age of Dx	every 5 years
○ First-degree relative ≥age 60 yr or 2 second-degree relatives with CRC	- At age 40	10 years
○ One second-degree or third-degree relative	- At age 50	10 years

- CRC screening may be stopped at age 70 or 75, or at a time based on serious comorbidities
- Persons of African heritage have a risk of CRC shifted to an earlier age than do Caucasians, and their screening of African Canadians should begin at age 45.
- The performance of screening colonoscopy done by skilled endoscopists or appropriately selected normal risk persons detects adenomas in approximately 15% of women and 25% of men, with 5-10% advanced adenomas (> 10 mm, villous, or with high grade dysplasia), < 1 % cancers, and a complication rate (perforation or bleeding) of about 1 per 1000 colonoscopies

• Give the recommended **follow-up interval** for post-polypectomy colonoscopic surveillance.

Finding on screening	Follow-up interval
< 10 adenomas	
1-2 tubular adenomas < 1 cm	5-10 yrs
3-10 adenomas, or any adenoma with villous elements, high-grade dysplasia or ≥ 1 cm in size	3 yrs
Patients with prior advanced adenomas after normal follow-up examination, or only 1-2 small tubular adenomas	5 yrs
>10 adenomas (possible familial syndrome)	R/ O familial syndromes
Small distal hyperplastic polyps without adenomas	10 yr
Serrated polyps with no dysplasia and < 1 cm	5 years
	3 years

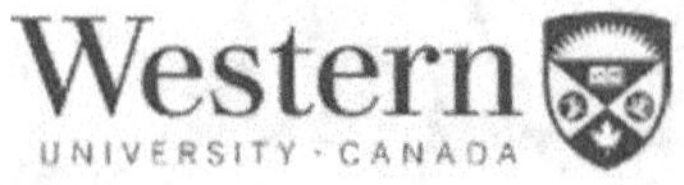

Sessile serrated adenomatous (SSA) polyp with dysplasia or > 1 cm

Adapted from: Liberman DA et al. Gastroenterology 2012; 143(3), 844-857.

- Post polypectomy surveillance recommendations:
  - Patients with small rectal hyperplastic polyps should be considered to have normal colonoscopies, and therefore the interval before the subsequent colonoscopy should be 10 years. An exception is patients with a hyperplastic polyposis syndrome.
  - They are at increased risk for adenomas and colorectal cancer and need to be identified for more intensive follow up on yearly basis.
  - Persons with one or two small tubular adenomas (<1cm) , and with only low grade dysplasia should have their next follow up colonoscopy in 5 to 10 years. The precise timing within this interval should be based on other clinical factors (such as prior colonoscopy findings, family history, and the preferences of the patient and judgment of the physician).

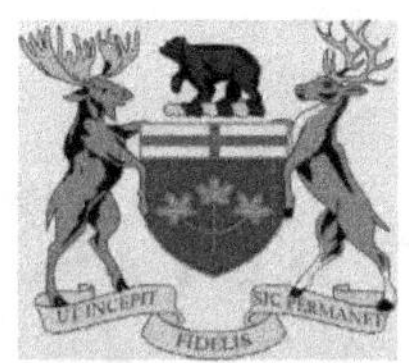

- Patients with 3 to 10 adenomas, or any adenoma 1 cm, or any adenoma with villous features, or high grade dysplasia should have their next follow up colonoscopy in 3 years
- If the follow up colonoscopy is normal or shows only one or two small tubular adenomas with low-grade dysplasia, then the interval for the subsequent examination should be 5 years.
- Persons who have more than 10 adenomas at one examination should be examined at a shorter (<3 years) interval established by clinical judgment, and the clinician should consider the possibility of an underlying familial syndrome.

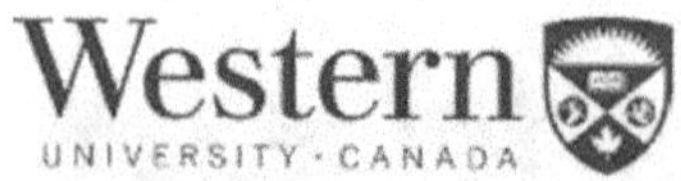

- Patients with Sessile serrated adenoma with size more than 1 cm and/ or with dysplasia should have next follow up in 3 years. In the absence of the mentioned risk factors next follow up should be at 5 year interval.
- Persons with sessile adenomas that are removed piecemeal should be considered for follow up at short intervals (2 to 6 months) to verify complete removal.
- More intensive surveillance is indicated when the family history may indicate hereditary nonpolyposis colorectal cancer.
- Every 5-10 years, except every 3 years for multiple, large, villous and proximal initial lesions.
- Number- for each additional adenoma, OR=1.32
- Size- for each additional 10 mm adenoma size, OR=1.56
- Villous – OR=1.40
- Proximal – OR=1.68

Note: Sessile serrated adenomas and serrated sessile hyperplastic polyps may have malignant potential.

Source: Winawer, Sidney J. Screening and surveillance for colorectal cancer: review and rationale. *2009 ACG Annual Postgraduate Course:*21- 25.

Useful background: From the "Acrin" trial of CT colography (NEJM 2008;359: pp 1207-1219), give the sensitivity (SENS), specificity (SPEC), positive predictive value (PPV) and negative predictive value (NPV) for detecting colonic polyps ranging from 5 to 10 mm

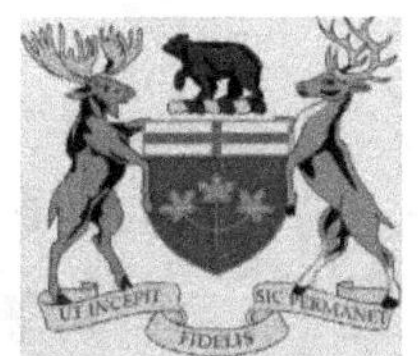

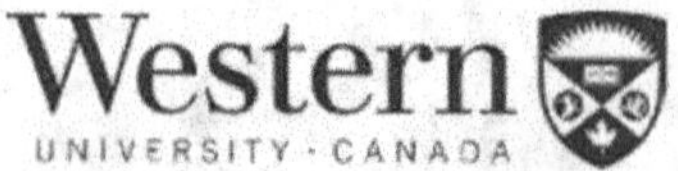

Efficacy and test performance

	>5mm	>6mm	>7mm	>8mm	>9mm	>1cm
SENS	65%	78%	84%	87%	90%	90%
>5mm	>6mm	>7mm	>8mm	>9mm	>1cm	>5mm
SPEC	89%	88%	87%	87%	86%	86%
PPV	45%	40%	35%	31%	25%	23%
NPV	95%	98%	99%	99%	99%	99%

Source: Johnson CD, Chen MH, Toledano AY, et al. Accuracy of CT colonography for detection of large adenomas and cancers. *N Engl J Med.* 2008 Sep 18;359(12):1207-17.

- Give 7 endoscopic techniques or technical improvements which enhance the colonoscopic sensitivity for CRC screening.
  - Improve sedation
  - Improve personal quality assessment
  - Improve performance skills of colonoscopist
    - Documented intubation of cecum (> 90%)
    - Withdrawal time > 7 minutes
    - Personal detection rate of adenomatous polyps on screening colonoscopy of average risk persons > 50 years of age (males, 25%; females, 15%)

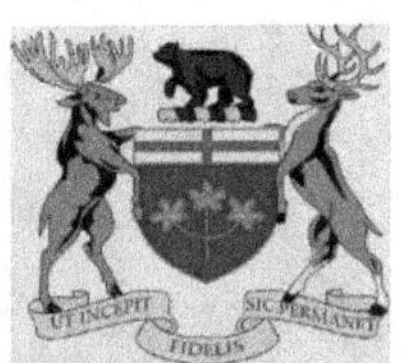

- Improve bowel cleansing

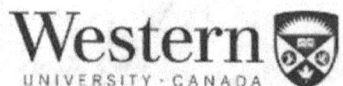

- Improve insertion
  - Cap-fitted colonosocopy
  - Overtubes
- Improve imaging
  - Wide-angle white light colonoscopy
  - Narrow-band imaging
  - Chromoendoscopy
  - Electronic chromoendoscopy
  - Confocal laser microscopy
- Note
  - Narrowing band imaging (NBI) was introduced to overcome the limitations of white light endoscopy (WLE) for adenoma detection.
  - There is difference in detection of polyps or adenomas with NBI and WLE.
  - There is no difference in miss rates of polyps or adenomas with NBI and WLE.

Source: Pasha SF, et al. Am J Gastroenterol 2012; 107: 363-370.

Surveillance: polyps CAG Guidelines (2004)

Risk category	Recommendation
o 1-2 tubular adenoma < 1 cm in size	- Colonoscopy in 5 years
o More than 2 adenomas	- Colonoscopy in 3 years
o Incomplete examination, advanced adenoma, numerous polyps, malignant or large sessile adenoma	- After short interval based on clinical judgment

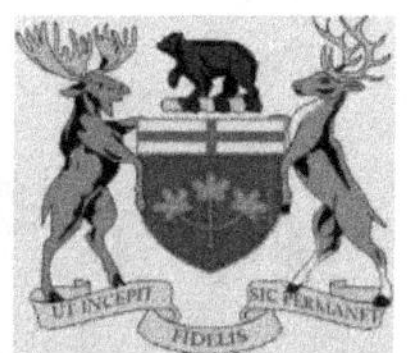

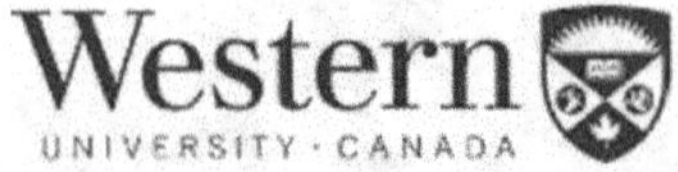

Screening: IBD CAG Guidelines (2004)

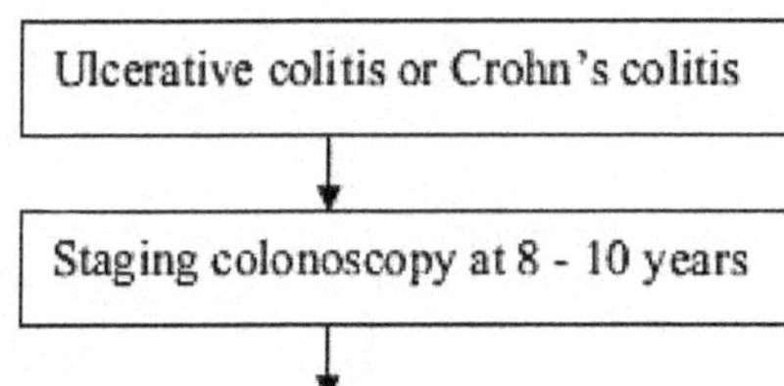

Pancolitis

- First decade: Begin screening at 8 years after onset
- Second decade: Colonoscopy every three years
- Third decade: Colonoscopy every two years
- Fourth decade: Colonoscopy every year

Left sided colitis

- Begin screening at 15 years after onset

- Give the guidelines for surveillance in patients with history of CRC

Risk category	Age to begin	Recommendation	Comment
• **Increased risk – patients with colorectal cancer**			
○ Patients with colon and rectal cancer should undergo high-quality perioperative colonoscopy to ensure there is no synchronous CRC	3 to 6 months after cancer resection, if no unresectable metastases are found during surgery: alternatively, colonoscopy 1 year after the resection, or 1 year following the performance of the colonoscopy that was performed to clear the colon of synchronous disease	Colonoscopy –	In the case of nonobstructing tumours, this can be done by preoperative colonoscopy. In the case of obstructing colon cancers, CTC with intravenous contrast or DCBE can be used to detect synchronous neoplasms in the proximal colon.

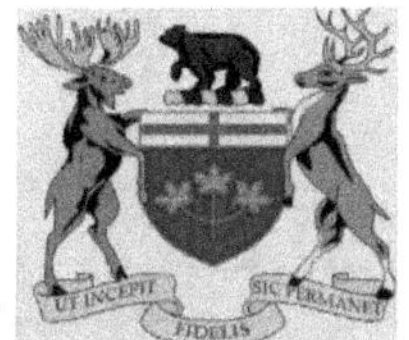

COLORECTAL CANCER

Risk category	Age to begin	Recommendation	Comment
○ Patient undergoing curative resection for colon or rectal cancer		Colonoscopy	– This colonoscopy at 1 year is in addition to the perioperative colonoscopy for synchronous tumours. – If the examination performed at 1 year is normal, then the interval before the next subsequent examination should be 3 years. – If that colonoscopy is normal, then the interval before the next subsequent examination should be 5 years. Following the examination at 1 year, the intervals before subsequent examinations may be shortened if there is evidence of HNPCC or if adenoma findings warrant earlier colonoscopy.
• **Increased risk- patients with a family history**			
○ Either colorectal cancer or adenomatous polyps in a first-degree relative before age 60 years or in 2 or more first-degree relatives at any age	Age 40 years, or 10 years before the youngest case in the immediate family	Colonoscopy	– Every 5 years

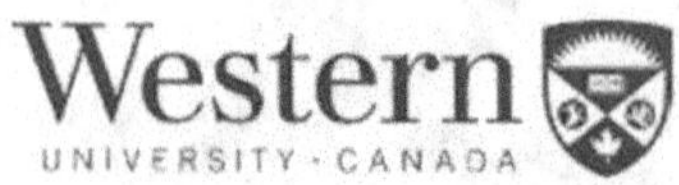

Risk category	Age to begin	Recommendation	Comment
○ Either colorectal cancer or adenomatous polyps in a first – degree relative age 60 or older or in 2 second – degree relatives with colorectal cancer	Age 40 years	Screening options at intervals recommended for average – risk individuals	- Screening should be at an earlier age, but individuals may choose to be screened with any recommended form of testing
High risk			
○ Genetic diagnosis of FAP or suspected FAP without genetic testing evidence	Age 10 to 12 years	Annual FSIG to determine if the individual is expressing the genetic abnormality and counseling to consider genetic testing	- If the genetic test is positive, colectomy should be considered
○ Genetic or clinical diagnosis of HNPCC or individual at increased risk of HNPCC	Age 20 to 25 years, or 10 years before the youngest case in the immediate family	Colonoscopy every 1 to 2 years and counseling to consider genetic testing	- Genetic testing for HNPCC should be offered to first-degree relatives of persons with a known inherited MMR gene mutation. - It should also be offered when the family mutation is not already known, but 1 of the first 3 of the modified Bethesda criteria is present.

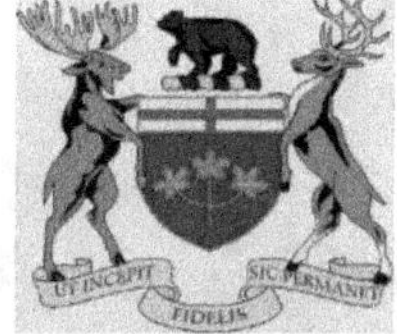

Risk category	Age to begin	Recommendation	Comment
○ Inflammatory bowel disease, chronic ulcerative colitis and Crohn colitis	Cancer risk begins to be significant 8 years after the onset of pancolitis or 12 to 15 years after the onset of left-sided colitis (UC or CC)	Colonoscopy with biopsies for dysplasia	– Every 1 to 2 years – These patients are best referred to a center with experience in the surveillance and management of inflammatory bowel disease

Abbreviations: CC, Crohn colitis; CRC, colorectal cancer; CTC, computed tomographic colography; DCBE, double-contrast barium enema; FAP, familial adenomatous polyposis; FSIG, flexible sigmoidoscopy; HNPCC, hereditary nonpolyposis colon cancer (Lynch syndrome); MMR, mismatch repair; UC, ulcerative colitis.

Printed with permission: Levin B, et al. *Gastroenterology* 2008;134(5): 1570-1595.

Screening modalities

Test	Sensitivity			
	Adenomas ≤5 mm (%)	*Adenomas 6-9 mm (%)*	*Adenomas ≥10 mm (%)*	*Cancer (%)*
○ Hemoccult II	2.0	5.0	12.0	40.0
○ Hemoccult Sensa	7.5	12.4	23.9	70.0
○ Fecal immunochemical test (FIT)	5.0	10.0	22.0	70.0
○ Flexible sigmoidoscopy (within reach)	75.0	85.0	95.0	95.0
○ Colonoscopy	75.0	85.0	95.0	95.0

Source: Zauber AG, et al. *Ann Intern Med 2008;149:659-69.*

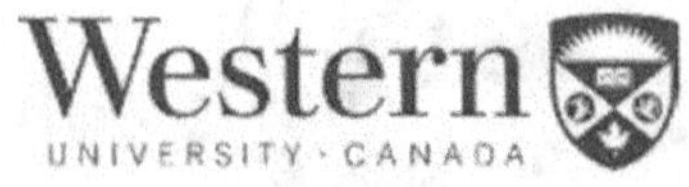

➢ Stool tests

- Guaiac FOBT (gFOBT)

Trial	*Minnesota*	*Nottingham*	*Funen*	*New York*
o Size	46,000	152,850	61,933	22,000
o Compliance	Annual 75% biennial 78%	50%	56%	—
o F/up	18 yrs	7-8 yrs	10 yrs	10 yrs
o Reduction in CRC mortality	33% for the annual group 21% for biennial group	15%	18 %	43 %

False Positive gFOBT

- Red meat
- Uncooked fruits and vegetables
  - Vegetable peroxidase: e.g., broccoli, turnip, cantaloupe, cauliflower, radish
- Any source of GI blood loss
  - Epistaxis, gingival bleeding, upper GI tract pathology, hemorrhoids
- Certain medications (e.g.,
  - Iron supplements, aspirin and other NSAIDs

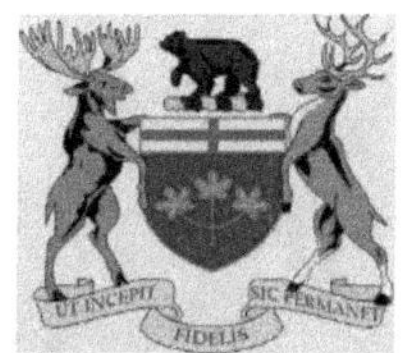

False Negative gFOBT

- Storage of slides for a prolonged period
- Degradation of hemoglobin by colonic bacteria
- Ascorbic acid (vitamin C) ingestion
- Improper sampling
- Non-bleeding lesion at the time of stool collection

- Fecal immunochemical tests(FIT)
    - Specific for human blood and lower GI bleed
    - Not affected by diet or drugs
    - Requiring fewer stool sample
    - More expensive than gFOBT
    - Quantitative Systematic Reviews have shown that guaiac-based fecal occult blood testing (FOBT) reduce CRC mortality by 13-16% on an intention-to-treat basis, and a 25% reduction when adjusted for screening attendance (Source: Hewitson P, Glasziou PP, Irwig L et al. Cochrane systematic review of colorectal cancer screening using the fecal occult blood test (Hemoccult): an update. *Am J Gastroenterol* 2008;103:1541-9.)
    - Three FOBT RCT's performed in 1993 to 1996 demonstrated a 13-21% reduction in CRC mortality (Winawer 09). The performance characteristics (sensitivity and specificity) of FIT (fecal immunochemical test) is comparable to FOBT1, without the need for dietary changes three days before FOBT.

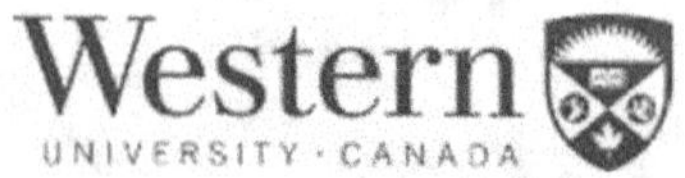

- Diagnostic imaging
  - Double-Contrast Barium Enema

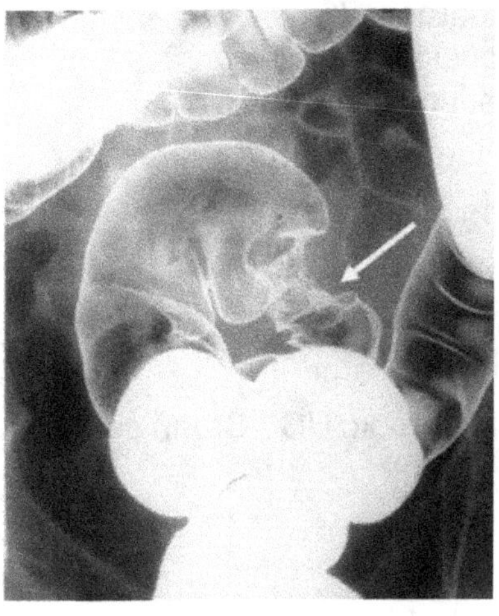

- PROS:
  - Low cost, exam in whole colon, with some blind spots
- CONS:
  - Never studied as a screening test
  - Missed 50% of adenomas < 1 cm in National Polyp Study
  - Sensitivity for cancer in patients with positive FOBT: 50-75%
  - Poor specificity; best interval unknown
- No longer recommended in some practice guideline

Source: Winawer SJ, et al. Gastroenterol 1997;112:594-642;Rex DX. Endoscopy 1995;27:200-2; Lieberman DA, et al. N Engl J Med 2000;343:162-8.

- Endoscopy

- Colonoscopy (standard"white light")
  - PROS:
    - Exams entire colon
    - Therapeutic – polyps removed at time of procedure

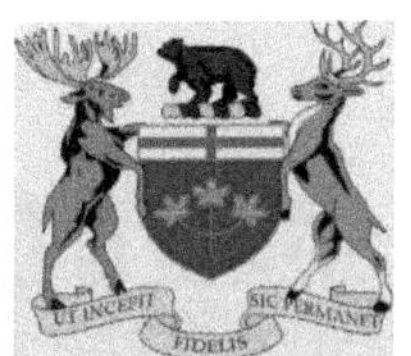

- CONS:
  - Invasive, risk of complications
  - Requires bowel prep, missed work, escort home
  - Incomplete procedures ~5%
  - Miss up to 10 % of significant lesions
  - Randomized trials lacking

- EUS (endoscopic ultrasound) of rectum in CRC
  - Sessile polyp
  - Determine resectability of rectal CRC (surgeon needs 5 mm tumor-free margin)
  - Suspected DALM in chronic UC / Crohn colitis

- Stool DNA Testing
  - Home-based
  - Low sensitivity of current tests for detection of cancers (50-70%) or polyps (27-74%)
  - Cost (? frequency of exam)
  - +ve test and –ve colonoscopy
    - What to do ??

- Flexible Sigmoidoscopy
  - PROS:
    - May be done in the office
    - Inexpensive, cost-effective
    - Mortality from rectal cancer reduced by 60-70% in case-control studies
    - Easier bowel preparation, usually done without sedation

- CONS:
  - Detects only one-half of adenomas
  - 40% of cancers arise proximal to splenic flexure
  - 75% of proximal cancers have no adenomas distal to splenic flexure
  - Often limited by discomfort, poor bowel preparation

Source: Selby JV, et al. N Engl J Med 1992;326:653-7; Stewart BT, et al. Aust NZ J Surg 1999;69:19-21; Rex DK, et al. Gastrointest Endosc 1999;99:727-30; Painter et J, al. Endoscopy 1999;31:227-31; Newcomb PA, et al. J Natl Canc Inst 1992;84:1572-5.

➢ CT colonoscopy (virtual colonoscopy)

Lesion	Sensitivity	Specificity
o Adenoma > 1 cm	90%	86%
o Polyp 6-9 mm	84 %	86-89 %

- PROS
  - No sedation necessary
  - Low risk
  - Fast: 20 min vs. 25 min for colonoscopy (plus 60-min recovery)
  - Detection of extracolonic lesions
  - Option for failed colonoscopy or unsuitable patients
- CONS
  - Preparation still needed: stool and fluid can simulate/obscure polyps
  - Lack of mucosal detail: flat polyps can be missed (same with colonoscopy)
  - Steep learning curve for radiologist
  - Radiation dose

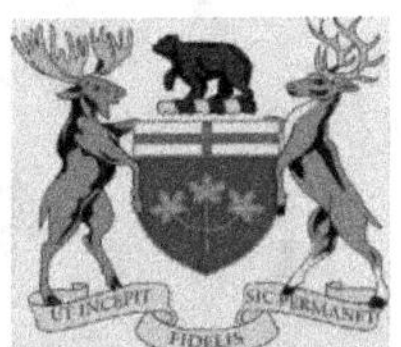

- Prevention
  - Primary prevention "identifying genetic, biological, and environmental factors that are etiologic or pathogenetic and subsequently altering their effects on tumor development" (Feldman M., et al. Sleisenger and Fordtran's Gastrointestinal and Liver Disease. 9th Edition. Saunders/Elsevier, Philadelphia, 2010, page 2219).
  - Secondary prevention "..... identify existing preneoplastic and lesion and to treat them thoroughly and expeditiously" (Feldman M., et al. Sleisenger and Fordtran's Gastrointestinal and Liver Disease. 9th Edition. Saunders/Elsevier, Philadelphia, 2010, page 2219).
  - Numerous environmental factors have been suggested to be associated with the development of adenomas, or their progression of CRC. Despite contrary popular views, dietary fibre supplementation, or the intake of antioxidants have failed to be beneficial when studied in properly designed prospective studies.
  - Initial evaluation before surgery :
    - Pre-operative colonoscopy (if not done already)
    - Staging CT
    - CEA level
  - Rectal Carcinoma
    - EUS or MRI

- Give the pharmacological or nutritional agents, which have been shown to be effective chemoprevention to reduce the risk of development or redevelopment of colorectal adenomas/CRCs.

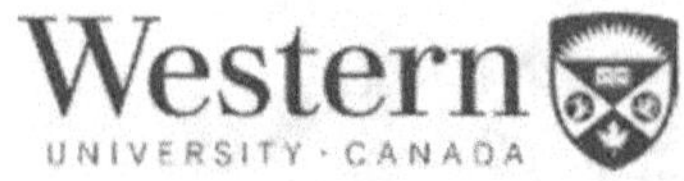

- Drugs
  - ASA
  - Coxibs
  - 5-ASA in IBD
  - Hormone replacement therapy (HRT) in post menopausal women
- Nutrients
  - Selenium
  - Calcium (+ vitamin D)
  - Non-western diet (low intake of saturated fats in red meat)
  - High intake of green leafy vegetables
  - Possibly folate, vitamins C, E, B-carotene
  - Probably not dietary fiber
- Exercise

Adapted from: Arber N, and Levin B. *Gastroenterology* 2008;134(4): 1224-1237; and Meyerhardt JA, et al. *JAMA* 2007;298(7): 754-764.

- Give factors for which there is adequate and appropriate human data to suggest a beneficial effect on reducing adenomas or CRC.

  - Calcium
    - 5% ↓ recurrence of adenomas over 3 y with the small protective effect lasting to 5 years after the calcium was stopp

- Prior to resection for CRC, perform staging diagnostic imaging so that IOUS (intraoperative ultrasonography) does not need to be performed.

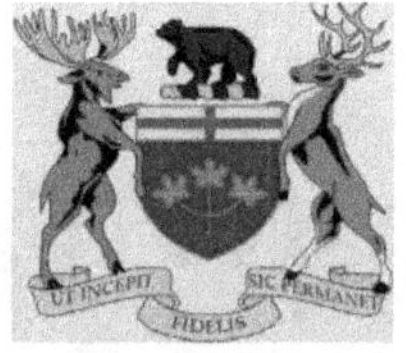

- "in patients whose tumor [CRC] recurs after hepatic resection, the liver is the initial site of recurrence in about 35% (Feldman M., et al. Sleisenger and Fordtran's Gastrointestinal and Liver Disease. 9th Edition. Saunders/Elsevier, Philadelphia, 2010, page 2232).
- Risk of postoperative relapse of CRC
  - Stage II, 20% to 30%
  - Stage III, 50% to 80%

➢ Post-surgical colonoscopic follow-up
- Colonoscopy 0→1→3→5 yr
- CT yearly for 3 yr follow-up 0→1→3→5 yr
- CEA q 3 months for 3 yr
- Adjuvant chemotherapy with 5-FU can ↑ serum CEA (false elevation of CEA)

Post-resection Recurrence of CRC

- Adjuvant therapy within 8 weeks of resection for CRC
  - ↓ recurrence
  - ↑ survival
- 5-FU (5-fluorouracil) plus levamisole (levamisole increases tumor response rates from 12% for 5-FU to 23% for 5-FU + levamisole

Relative	Risk reduction
CRC	Overall
Recurrence	Mortality

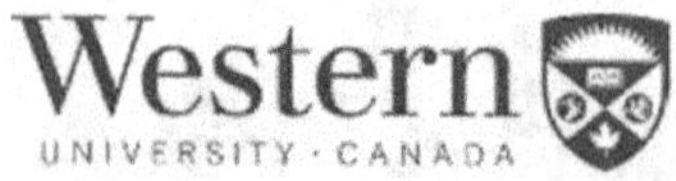

- Dukes C / Stage III 42% 33%
  - 5-FU plus leucovorin > 5-FU plus levamisole in efficacy after curative surgery for CRC
  - 5-FU plus leucovorin plus oxaliplatin in Stage III
    ↑ 3 year disease-free survival
    May also be small benefit in Stage II
  - For rectal CRC Duke B2 / Stage II (transmural extension) or Duke C / Stage III (positive lymph nodes)

5-year rates	Radiation	Radiation plus chemotherapy
No recurrence	35	60
Survival	40	50

- Terminology: **chemotherapy and / or radiotherapy given for CRC**
  - Before curative surgery – Neoadjuvant
  - After curative surgery – Adjuvant
  - There are studies in progress assessing preoperative (neoadjuvant) chemoradiotherapy, curative surgery, followed by 4 months of post-surgery (adjuvant) chemotherapy.
  - The limitation to radiotherapy is its toxicity, but enhances of radiation therapy (e.g. capecitabine) may ↑ benefit without an ↑ toxicity
  - Studies also examining possible benefit of infusion of 5-FU, leucovorin plus oxaliplatin (combination called FOLFOX).

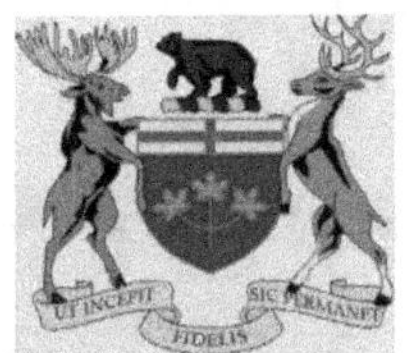

- NSAIDs / ASA / Coxibs
  - ASA
    - Relative risk among users, 0.68
    - ↓ adenoma, 19% to 37%
    - ↓ advanced adenoma, 37% to 41%
  - Sulindac
    - FAP
      - ↓ number 44%
      - ↓ diameter 35%
  - Coxibs
    - FAP
      - ↓ number 28%
      - ↓ number of patients in 3 years with
        - New adenomas ~40%
        - Advanced adenomas ~60%
  - DFMD (ornithrine decarboxylate inhibitor difluomethyornithine) plus sulindac
    - 70% ↓ new adenomas at 3 years
  - Statin use
    - 47% ↓ relative risk for CRC

Adjuvant or neoadjuvant chemotherapy for Stage II or III resected CRC is often given as 5-FU plus leucovorin.

- Give the mechanism of action of these two drugs.

5-FU	Binds to thymidylate synthetase → ↓ methylation of deoxyuridylic acid to

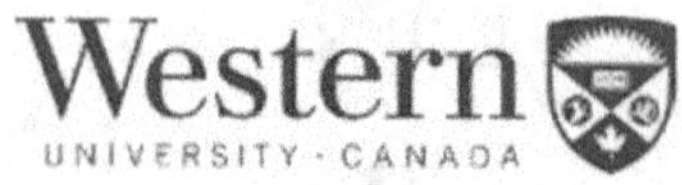

	thymidylic acid → ↓ DNA synthesis
Leucovorin	↑ binding of 5-FU to thymidylate synthetase, thereby ↓ DNA synthesis (please see above)

- Adjuvant chemo-radiotherapy
  - Benefit
    - Stage III MR 33%
    - Colon Ca recurrence 42% ↓
  - Use
    - T3/4 rectal cancer (locally advanced)
    - After resection of liver / lung metastases

- **Surgery**
  - Overview
    - Curative for stage I CRC
    - Wide resection of the involved segment of colon with removal of its lymphatic drainage
    - TME, total mesenteric excision for CRC
    - Resection is performed even in the presence of distant metastases to prevent obstruction or bleeding
    - Rectal cancer
      - Rectosigmoid and upper rectum
        - Transabdominal low anterior resection with primary anastomosis
      - Low rectal lesions
        - Sphincter-saving resection can be performed if a distal margin of at least 2 cm of normal bowel can be resected below the lesion

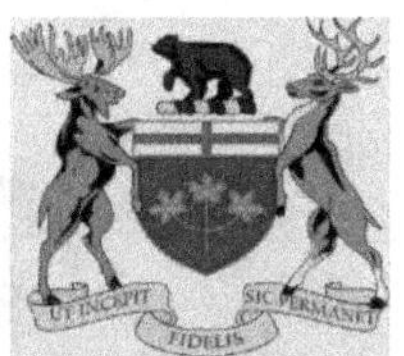

- Abdominoperineal resection (APR) of distal sigmoid, rectum, and anus and a permanent sigmoid colostomy is performed

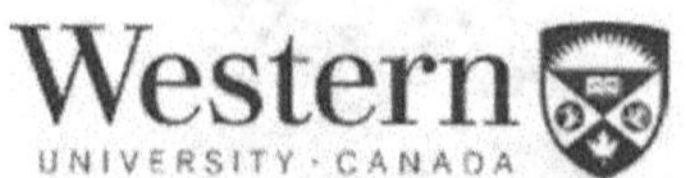

- Patient not fit for surgery
  - Palliative approach: laser photoablation, APC or stent placement

- Surgical resection for liver metastases
  - 10% to 25% at presentation
  - Resection
    - < 5 metastases in liver
    - No extrahepatic metastases
    - No extensive liver involvement (< 70%)
- Non-operable, metastatic CRC
  - Chemotherapy
  - Stent
  - Photoabalation

- **Adjuvant Chemotherapy Colon Cancer**
  - Stage III colon Ca
    - Reduce recurrence by 42%
    - Reduce death rate by 33%
  - High risk stage II (controversial)
    - Not recommended routinely
  - Post complete resection of liver or pulmonary mets
  - Adjuvant Therapy Rectal Cancer
    - Neoaduvant chemo-radiotherapy is recommended in locally advanced (T3/4) rectal cancer
    - Adjuvant chemo-radiotherapy reduce recurrence and mortality
      - Stage II and stage III cancer
  - Metastatic CRC
    - Liver is the most common site of distant metastases from CRC

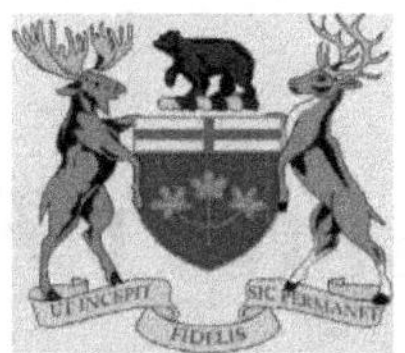

- 10% to 25% of patients have liver mets at initial presentation
- Survival rate after resection is 40 %
- Resection is recommended if :
    - 4-5 mets or less
    - No extrahepatic mets
    - No extensive liver involvement
- Chemotherapy is mainly palliative
    - Prolong overall survival and
        - Median survival is 2 years with chemo
        - 5-6 months with best supportive care
    - Maintain quality of life (QOL)
- Palliative treatment
    - Stent
    - Photoablation or APC

- Prognosis
    - The original Dukes staging system for CRC has been modified at least 6 times over the past 80 years (Feldman M., et al. Sleisenger and Fordtran's Gastrointestinal and Liver Disease. 9th Edition. Saunders/Elsevier, Philadelphia, 2010, Table 123.9, page 2214).
    - This has been largely replaced by the now ten year old AJCC (American Joint Committee on Cancer), TNM (tumor-node-metastasis) classification (Feldman M., et al. Sleisenger and Fordtran's Gastrointestinal and Liver Disease. 9th Edition. Saunders/Elsevier, Philadelphia, 2010, Table 123.10, page 2215).
    - Generally speaking, CRC of the left (distal) colon have a better prognosis than these of the right (proximal) colon, and CRC of the colon has a better prognosis than the rectum.

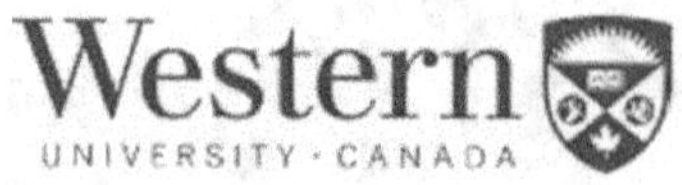

- Give the 5 year **survival rates** for CRC base on the Duke Stage

Dukes stage		Approximate 5 year survival rate
A	Limited to mucosa	
B1	Into muscularis propria (MP)	80
B2	Through MP	60
C	Regional node metastasis	40
C1	B1 plus regional node metastasis	
C2	B2 plus regional node metastasis	
C	1 to 3 nodes (N1)	50
	≥ 4 nodes (N2)	25
D	Distant metastases	0

- Give 4 complications for **colorectal self-expandable metal stents**. The mean % incidence is shown for your interest.

Complication	Mean incidence (%)
o Re-obstruction	10
o Migration	10
o Bleeding	5
o Pain	5
o Perforation	4
o Death	1

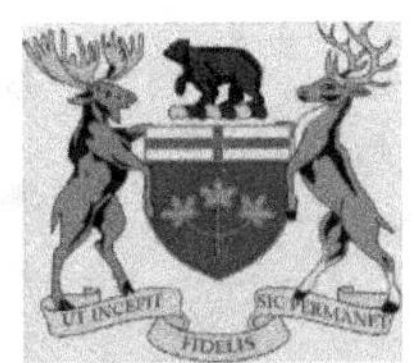

Printed with permission: Baron, Todd H., et al. *Best Pract Res Clin Gastroenterol* 2004: pg. 220.

- Suggest 10 quality assurance measures that you should consider to continuously monitor in your clinical practice.

Clinical Condition	Selected Quality Measures
○ Acute coronary syndrome	– Aspirin at arrival & discharge – B-blocker at arrival & discharge – ACE inhibitor for LVSD – Assessment for hypertension, hyperlipidemia, metabolic syndrome, smoking cessation, exercise program
○ Congestive heart failure	– Left ventricular function assessment – ACE inhibitor for LVSD – Smoking cessation advice & counseling
○ Community-acquired pneumonia	– Oxygenation assessment within 24 h – Pneumococcal screening & vaccination – Antibiotic timing (first dose in < 4 h) – Smoking cessation advice & counseling

Abbreviation: ACE, angiotensin-converting enzyme; LVSD, left ventricular systolic dysfunction

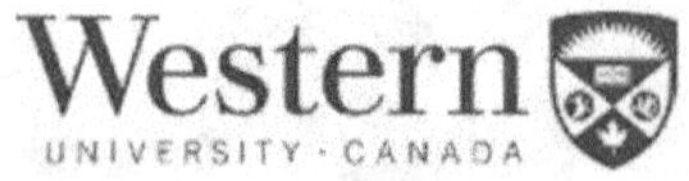

COLORECTAL CANCER

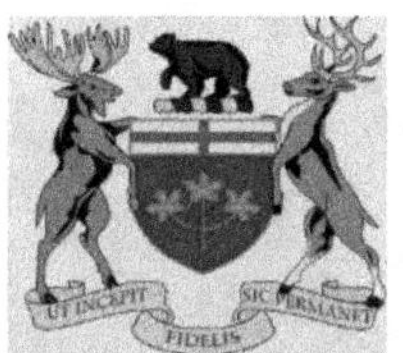

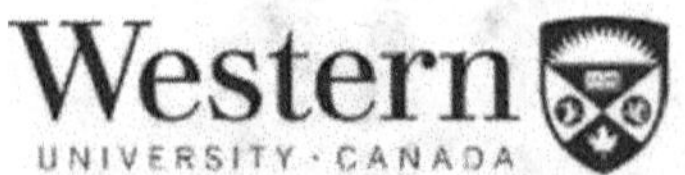

Diminutive Colonic Polyps

Aze Wilson

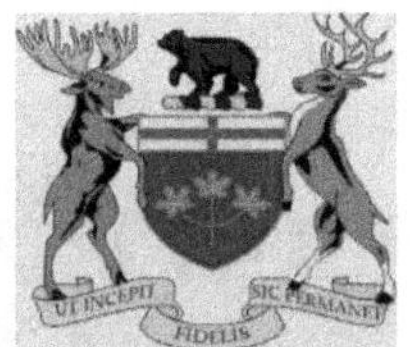

DIMINUTIVE COLONIC POLYPS

- **Definition of Polyps by Size**
  - "Large" > 10 mm (35% of detected polyps)
  - "Small" 6-10 mm
  - "Diminutive" < 5 mm
  - Over/underestimation of polyp size can lead to misappropriation of the correct surveillance interval without pathologic assessment
  - Compare size of polyp with biopsy forceps

- **Polyp progression**
  - Adenoma-carcinoma sequence was first reported in 1976 by Morson (Clin Gastroenterol 1976).
  - The formation of colorectal cancer (CRC) from adenoma increases with adenoma size, number, and histology.
  - The removal of adenomatous polyps prevents CRC (National Polyp Study, Winauer, NEJM 1993).
  - But what about the diminutive polyp?
    - 35% of detected polyps >1cm (reference populations included ONLY patients with polyps >1 cm)
  - Retrospective trial evaluating the risk of CRC progression in small polyps vs diminutive polps (DPs)
  - 1369 polyps <1cm retrieved at colonoscopy

(Unal et al. Dig Dis & Sci 2007;52(10):2796-9)

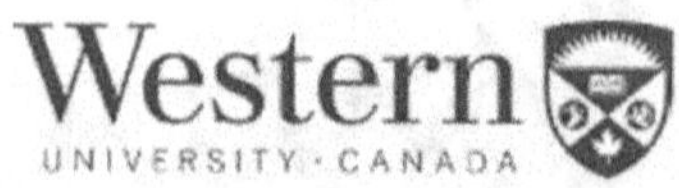

➢ The Value of Polypectomy

SO YOU WANT TO BE A GASTROENTEROLOGIST!

- Give the importance of the **National Polyp Study**, 1993.
  - The National Polyp Study (NPS) was a longitudinal study that provided prospective data on the adenoma-carcinoma sequence and the effect of colonoscopic polypectomy.
  - Its purpose was to evaluate more frequent and less frequent follow-up surveillance intervals in patients in whom newly diagnosed adenomas were removed.
  - The study cohort consisted of 1418 patients who had a complete colonoscopy during which one or more adenomas of the colon or rectum were removed.
  - The polyp-patients subsequently underwent periodic colonoscopy during an average follow-up of 5.9 years, and the incidence of colorectal cancer was ascertained.
  - The incidence rate of colorectal cancer was compared with that in three reference groups, two cohorts in which colonic polyps were not removed, and one general-population registry, with adjustment for sex, age, and polyp size.
  - Removal of these adenomas resulted in a colorectal cancer incidence that was markedly lower than expected without polypectomy.
  - These results support the view that colorectal adenomas progress to adenocarcinomas, as well as the current practice of searching for and removing adenomatous polyps to prevent colorectal cancer.

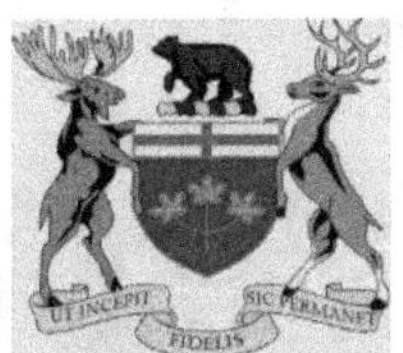

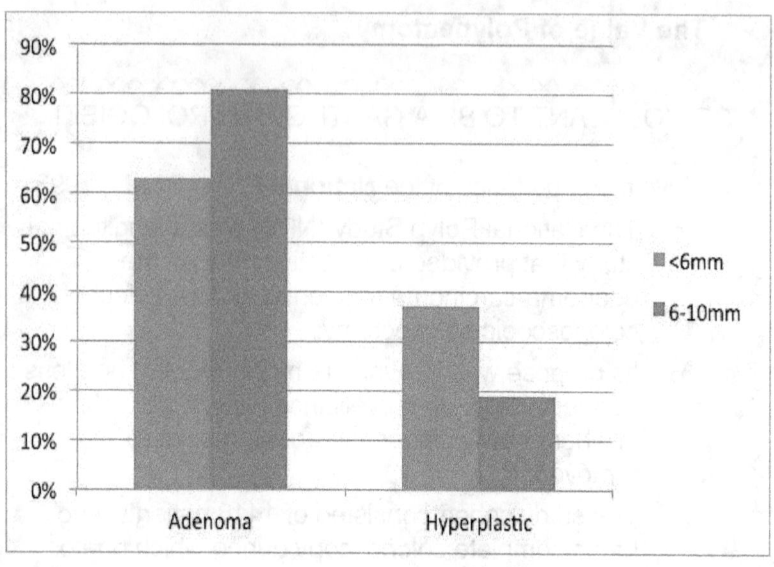

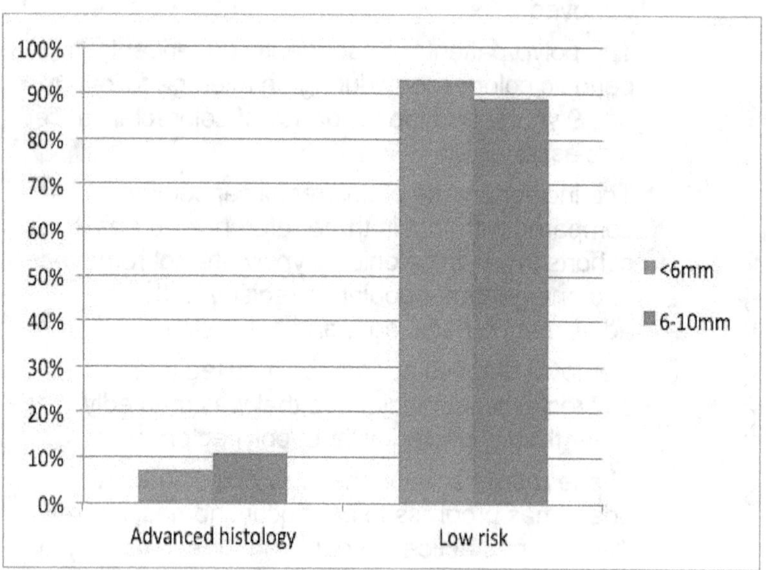

- Above the recto-sigmoidal junction (RSJ), the proportion of diminutive polyps (< 6 mm) which are

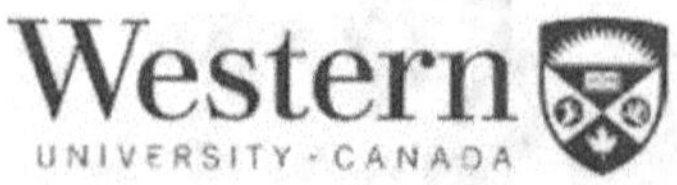

adenomas was found to be about 67%, versus ~ 75% for "small" polyps (SP; 6-10 mm in size)

- Below the RSJ, the proportion of DPs tha are adenomas is small
- The larger the polyp, the higher the risk of advanced histology; polyps 5 mm in size
- Polyps 5 mm in size have an extremely low prevalence of invasive cancer, or of advanced histology
- Infuence of polyp size on presence of advanced histological features:
  - DPs – 0.5%
  - SPs – 1.5%
  - LPs – 15%

Abbreviations: DP, piminutive polyp; LP, large polyp > 10 mm; SP, small polyp, 6 to 10 mm;
Gupta A et al. Gastrointest Endosc. 2012;75(4):705-11.

- Removal
  - 6% of DPs are incompletely removed by biopsy foreceps
  - Use EMR, 1-2 mm margin, and resect until no further polyp tissue

(Efthymiou et al. Endoscopy 2011;43(4):312-6)

- Option-biopsy DP, or use real-time endoscopic assessment of the histology using narrow band imaging (NBI; 90% accurate) (Ad hoc committee of the ASGE Technology and Standards of Practice Committee Chairs)
- Resect and discard strategy is acceptable
- Assessment for distinguishingbetween hyperplastic
  - Only 95% accuracy of pathology imperfect

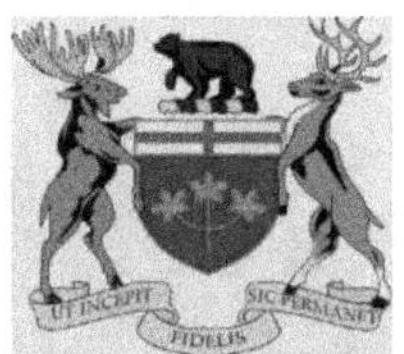

- Cost
    - To detect one advanced adenoma or prevent 1 CRC over 10yrs:
        - DPs – 562
        - SPs – 71
        - LPs – 2.5
    - Estimated 5-yr risk of CRC in unresected polyps: DPs (0.08%); SPs (0.7%); LPs (15%)
    - Cost effectiveness ratio of removing DPs and SPs: $464,407 (USD) and $59,015 per year-of-life-gained
    - Note: Polypectomy for LPs yielded a cost-savings of $151 per person screened

(Pickhardt PJ, et al. Radiology. 2008;249(1):151-9)

- 2010: Hassan et al evaluated the cost-effectiveness of a 'resect/discard' strategy in the setting of DPs

Cost-effectiveness characteristics	No screening	Colonoscopy	Colonoscopy with resect and discard policy
Cost/person	$3,390	$3,222	$3,197
Relative efficacy	—	51 days/person	51 days/person

- A markov model was used to predict cost-effectiveness of the "resect / discard strategy.
- Narrow band imaging (NBI) was used to distinguish hyperplastic and adenomatous polyps assuming a rate of 84% of high confidence classification, and a sensitivity (94%) and specificity (89%) of adenoma detection.

(Hassan C, et al. Clin Gastroenterol Hepatol. 2010;8(10):865-9)

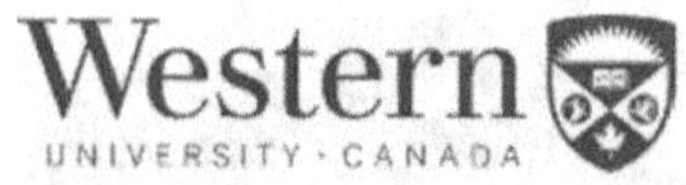

- Recommendation for DPs
  - Rectum — No need to resect
  - Above the rectum — Resect and discard

Preservation and Incorporation of Valuable Endoscopic Innovations (PIVI) 2011

Cancer prevalence by size

Author (year)	≤ 5 mm	6-9 mm	≥ 10 mm
Odom (2005)**	1/2851 (0.03%)	1/152 (0.65%)	9/222 (4.05%)
Church (2004)**	2/4381 (0.05%)	1/666 (0.15%)	21/675 (3.11%)
Aldridge (2001)**	0/182 (0%)	2/132 (1.5%)	23/226 (10.2%)
Butterly (2006)*	1/1305 (0.08%)	2/487 (0.4%)	
Gschwantler (2002)#*	0/3016 (0%)	26/2789 (0.9%)	156/1785 (8.7%)
Lieberman (2008)	1/3744 (0%)	2/1198 (0.17%)	25/949 (2.6%)
Pickhardt (2003)	0/966 (0%)	0/262 (0%)	2/82 (2.4%)
Kim (2007)^	0/2006 (0%)	0 (0%)	18
Graser (2009)	0/418 (0%)	0/56 (0%)	1/37 (2.7%)
Yoo (2007)*	1/3303 (0%)	7/1432 (0.49%)	20/1261 (1.6%)
Kapsoritakis (2002)@	0/293 (0%)		
Rex (2009)	4/8798 (0.05%)	0/1282 (0%)	

Printed with permission: Rex DK, et al. Gastrointestinal Endoscopy 2011;73(3), 419–422

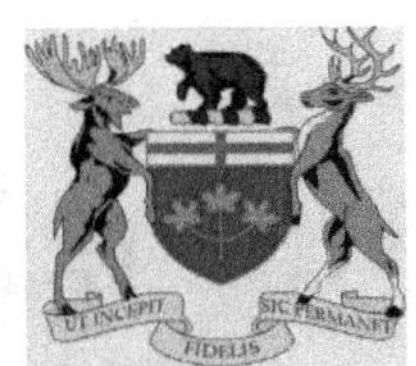

Advanced adenoma prevalence by polyp size (denominator polyps in same size range unless otherwise specified)

Author (year)	Advanced adenoma definition	≤ 5 mm	6-9 mm	≥ 10 mm
Church (2004)**	> 25% villous architecture, severe dysplasia	89/4381 (2.0%)	65/666 (9.8%)	305/675 (45.2%)
Butterly (2006)*	> 25% villous elements, HGD	34/1305 (2.6%)	38/487 (7.8%)	
Aldridge (2001)**	Severe dysplasia	2/182 (1.1%)	9/132 (6.8%)	13/226 (5.8%)
Bretagne (2010)**	TVA, VA, HGD, intramucosa l CA	15/535 (2.8%)	34/219 (15.5%)	248/530 (46.8%)
Gschwantle r (2002)#*	HGD	104/301 6 (3.4%)	350/278 9 (12.5%)	531/178 5 (29.7%)
Lieberman (2008) $	TVA, VA, HGD, Serrated	62/3744 (1.7%)	77/1198 (6.4%)	265/949 (27.9%)

Printed with permission: Rex DK, et al. Gastrointestinal Endoscopy 2011;73(3), 419–422

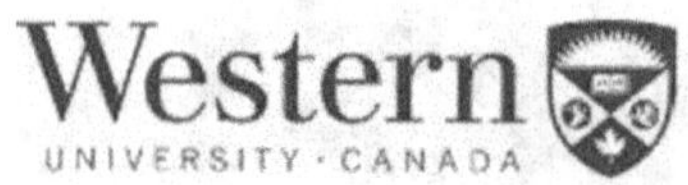

Histology of polyps by colon subsite (% adenomatous)

Aurthor (year)	< 6 mm	6-9 mm	10 mm or more	Any
Pickhardt (2003)**	**Rectum 14%** **Sigmoid 28%** Descending 43% Splenic Flexure 29% Transverse colon 44% Hepatic flexure, 51% Ascending 55% Cecum 53%	Rectum 41% Sigmoid 60% Descending 69% Splenic Flexure 50% Transverse colon 85% Hepatic flexure, 61% Ascending 53% Cecum 72%	Rectum 71% Sigmoid 47% Descending 86% Splenic Flexure 50% Transverse colon 42% **Hepatic flexure, 0%** Ascending 66% Cecum 70%	**Rectum 22%** Sigmoid 36% Descending 51% Splenic Flexure 35% Transverse colon 53% Hepatic flexure, 52% Ascending 53% Cecum 58%
Graser** (2009)	**Rectum 6%** **Sigmoid 30%** Descending 48% **Transverse colon 38%** Ascending 64% Cecum 48%	Rectum 40% Sigmoid 94% Descending 75% Transverse colon 57% Ascending 82% Cecum 67%	Rectum 83% Sigmoid 100% Descending 100% Transverse colon 80% Ascending 67% Cecum 75%	Rectum 13% Sigmoid 44% Descending 55% Transverse colon 43% Ascending 67% Cecum 51%
Church (2004)	Left: 2.3% advanced Right 2.4% advanced	Left: 13.9% advanced Right 14.1% advanced		

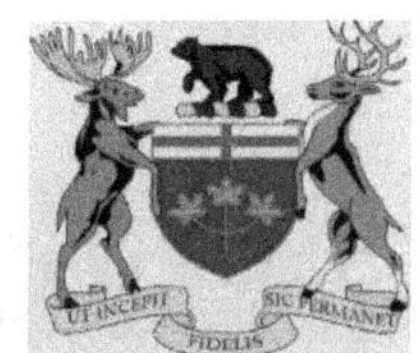

DIMINUTIVE COLONIC POLYPS

Aurthor (year)	< 6 mm	6-9 mm	10 mm or more	Any
Lieberman (200*)	Distal 1.6% advanced Proximal 2.1% advanced Both 0.5% advanced	Distal 8.4% advanced Proximal 5.0% advanced Both 0.5% advanced	Distal 33.9% advanced Proximal 28.2% advanced Both 9.8% advanced	

Low prevalence of adenomas below the recto-sigmoid junction

Printed with permission: Rex DK, et al. Gastrointestinal Endoscopy 2011;73(3), 419–422.

> "Be an advocate, seek something good for everyone: seek justice and love."
>
> Grandad

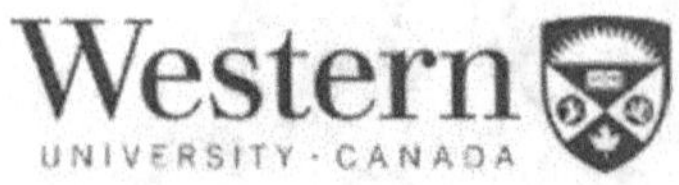

MINI UPDATE

Irritable Bowel Syndrome

Malcolm Wells

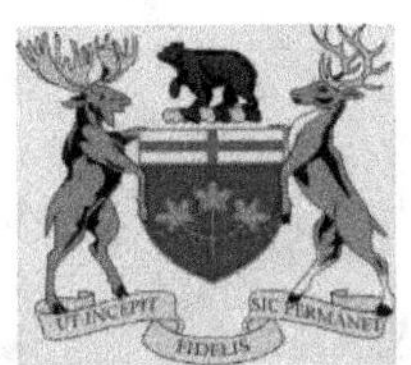

IRRITABLE BOWEL SYNDROME

- Demography
  - 2:1 F:M ratio
  - Prevalence comparable in all countries it's been studied
  - 10-20% of individuals in the general population have symptoms consistent with IBS
  - Most commonly diagnosed gastrointestinal disorder
  - Accounts for 12% of visits to primary care providers
  - Accounts for 30% of GI referrals
  - IBS often overlaps with other functional disorders

- Clinical diagnostic criteria

Rome III Disorders and Criteria

Rome Foundation copyright policy and licensing fee schedules for translations and usage of these items and products are now available. Please contact Michele Pickard at mpickard@theromefoundation.org

The Rome criteria is a system developed to classify the functional gastrointestinal disorders (FGIDs), disorders of the digestive system in which symptoms cannot be explained by the presence of structural or tissue abnormality, based on clinical symptoms. Some examples of FGIDs include irritable bowel syndrome, functional dyspepsia, functional constipation, and functional heartburn. The most recent revision of the criteria, the Rome III criteria, were published in 2006 in book form, and in a shorter Journal supplement in Gastroenterology.

Rome III Diagnostic Criteria for Functional Gastrointestinal Disorders

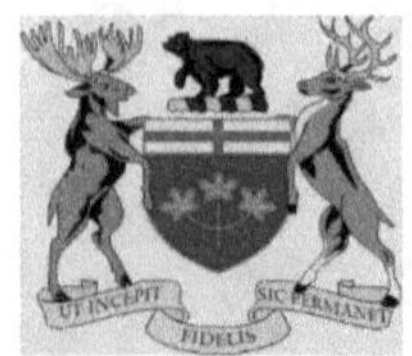

Comparision Table of Rome II & Rome III Adult Diagnostic Criteria

- **Rome III Diagnostic Criteria for Functional Gastrointestinal Disorders**

  *Diagnostic criteria**

- Recurrent abdominal pain and discomfort** at least 3 days/month in the last 3 months associated with two or more of the following:
  1. Improvement with defecation
  2. Onset associated with a change in frequency of stool
  3. Onset associated with a change in form (appearance) of stool

*Criterion fulfilled for the last 3 months with symptom onset at least 6 months prior to diagnosis

**"Discomfort" means an uncomfortable sensation not described as pain.

In pathophysiology research and clinical trials, a pain / discomfort frequency of at least 2 days a week during screening evaluation is recommended for subject eligibility.

- **Additional Features (occur in ~ 1 in 3 patients with IBS)**
  - Bloating
  - Nausea
  - Dyspepsia
  - Associated conditions:
  - Depression
  - Anxiety
  - Fibromyalgia
  - IBD

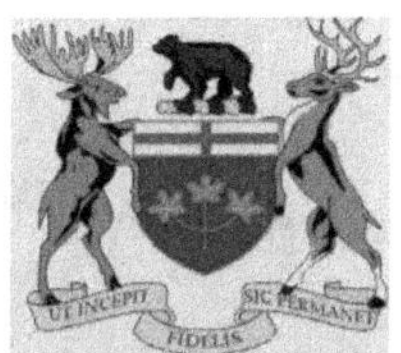

- **Subtypes**
  - IBS with constipation (IBS-C) -- is defined as the presence of hard or lumpy stools with ≥25 percent of bowel movements and loose or watery stools with <25 percent of bowel movements.
  - IBS with diarrhea – IBS with diarrhea (IBS-D) is defined as the presence of loose or watery stools with ≥25 percent of bowel movements and hard or lumpy stools with <25 percent of bowel movements.
  - Mixed IBS – Mixed IBS (IBS-M) is defined as hard or lumpy stools with ≥25 percent of bowel movements and loose or watery stools with ≥25 percent of bowel movements.
  - Unsubtyped IBS – IBS is termed unsubtyped if there is insufficient abnormality in stool consistency to meet the above subtypes.
  - Physical Examination
    - Usually normal
    - Deep tenderness over colon
    - Must exclude abdominal wall pain

- **Proposed pathophysiology**
  - Several pathphysiologic mechanism proposed
  - None confirmed; etiology unknown
  - Brain
    - Altered perception
    - Central dysregulation
    - Stress
    - Upbringing

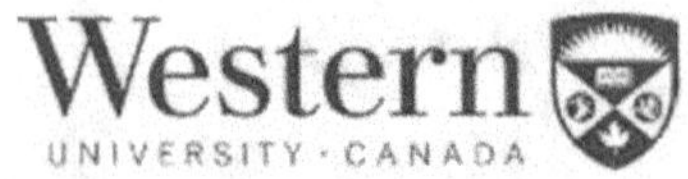

- Gut
  - Altered colonic and SB motility
  - Visceral hypersensitivity
  - Altered gut flora
  - Previous acute enteric infection
  - Mast cell activation and inflammation
  - Increased intestinal permeability
  - Cytokine release
  - Food allergies
  - Genetic factors
- Central Dysregulation
  - Cerebral blood flow changes, functional brain imaging studies (PET) suggest alterations in the brain response to visceral stimuli in IBS
    - Greater activation of mid-cingular cortex (area that processes visceral signals) following delivered or anticipated rectal distention
  - This may explain why anxiety/stress may enhance perception of visceral pain – and why relaxation/distraction decreases pain in IBS
  - Gender differences in brain networks in IBS patients have been observed
- Psychological factors
  - Psychiatric comorbidity is higher in IBS patients
    - History of sexual, physical, emotional abuse (may modulate central brain responses to pain)
    - More likely to report greater lifetime and daily stressful events, may be more susceptible to stress-altering gastrointestinal function

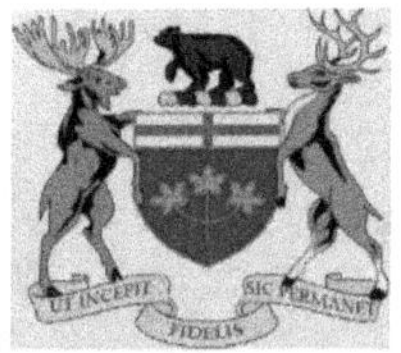

- Genetics
  - Limited but increasing evidence for small hereditary component of IBS
  - Clustering of IBS in families
  - Greater concordance of IBS in monozygotic compared with dizygotic twins
  - Specific genes not yet identified with certainty
- Altered colonic and small bowel motility
  - Extensively studied, but no motility pattern is diagnostic of IBS
  - Diarrhea
    - Increased HAPCs, enhanced gastrocolic response, rectal hypersensitivity
  - Constipation
    - Increased nonpropulsive contractions, decreased HAPCs
  - Colonic and SB transit has correlated with diarrhea and constipation, but not in all studies
  - Colonic motility can be increased by stress/anger, but not a specific finding
  - Pain may be associated with HAPCs
- Visceral Hypersensitivity
  - Recognized in IBS for >30 years
    - Balloon distention in rectum induced pain at lower volumes in IBS patients than controls
  - Visceral hypersensitivity in 60% of IBS patients,
  - Some IBS patients with normal baseline visceral hypersensitivity may have rectal hypersensitivity induced by repeated sigmoid distention

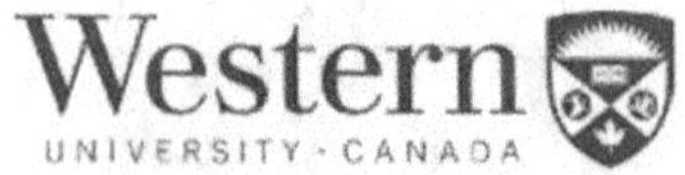

  - This implicates abnormal sensitization within dorsal horn of spinal cord or higher
    - Putative neurotransmitters: serotonin, neurokinins, calcitonin gene-related peptide
    - NMDA receptor may be important (modulates central neuronal excitability) □ NMDA receptor antagonists can reduce visceral sensitivity in the esophagus

- Abnormal gas propulusion/expulsion
  - Abdominal girth normally increases during the day, decreasing with lying down – exaggerated in IBS
  - Retention of gas is greater in IBS patients in studies of gas infusion into SB
  - Gas infusion causes more discomfort in IBS patients than controls
  - IV neostigmine has been demonstrated to clear retained intestinal gas and reduce abdominal symptoms, functional bloating in IBS patients

    Physical activity may also enhance gas transit

- Food intolerance & allergy
  - 10-15% of wheat in diet not digestible by human enzymes; subtle forms of gluten intolerance may exist
    - In absence of diagnosis of celiac disease, gluten-free diet is NOT recommended
  - Differentiate IBS from lactose intolerance, fructose/sorbitol malabsorption

- Abnormal colonic flora & SIBO
  - Abnormal colonic flora could lead to increased colonic fermentation □ excess gas
    - Recent interest in probiotics, FODMAPs approach

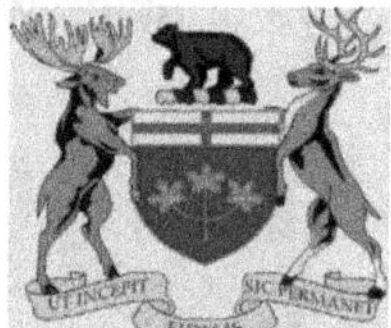

- Some studies report high prevalence of SIBO in IBS with H2 breath testing and clinical response to Abx
    - Caveats – transit abnormalities can give abnormal hydrogen breath tests, studies did not confirm with cultures
- Local Inflammation
    - Inflammatory cells (mast, T cells) are increased more than normal in mucosa in some patients with IBS
        - Infections, abnormal bacterial flora, bile, food antigens implicated
    - 7-30% of patients with bacterial enteritis develop IBS
        - Increased risk in those with psychological distress; illness lasting >3 weeks; organisms that are toxigenic
    - In post-infectious IBS, increases in CD3, CD4, CD8, T cells, macrophages, enteroendocrine cells
    - Colonic inflammation increases production of key mediators □ prostaglandins, 5-HT have central role in IBS manifestations
- Post-infections IBS
    - Prevalence of IBS: 28% at 2 yrs, 15% at 8 years
    - Both significantly higher than unaffected individuals: 5%
    - Well recognized disorder
    - Walkerton study the largest and longest (8 years) prospective study
        - May 2000: E. coli O157:H7 outbreak due to contaminated drinking water

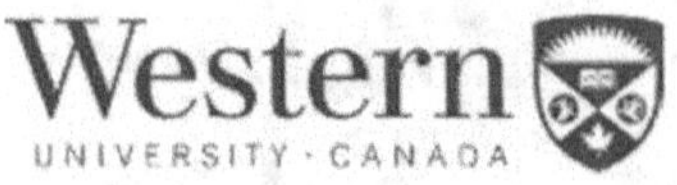

    - 7 died from E-coli sepsis and another 14 people died from E-coli related illnesses
    - 2600 people were ill
  - Several potential mechanisms:
    - Altered gut flora
    - Local inflammation
    - Genes that encode proteins involved in epithelial cell barrier function and the innate immune response to enteric bacteria

- Diagnosis
  - Please see Rome III diagnostic criteria definition of IBS
  - Systematic review
    - In absence of alarm features, patients who meet ROME criteria are unlikely to have another cause for their symptoms
  - Alarm features
    - Bleeding, Anemia
    - Unexplained weight loss, Fever
    - Unexplained vomiting
    - Progressive dysphagia
    - Family History of malignancy
    - New-onset symptoms in elderly
    - Night-time symptoms
  - How much testing is reasonable?
    - CBC, renal and liver function testing, thyroid function, stool for O&P, CRP are likely low yield – but cheap, and may be reassuring to the patient

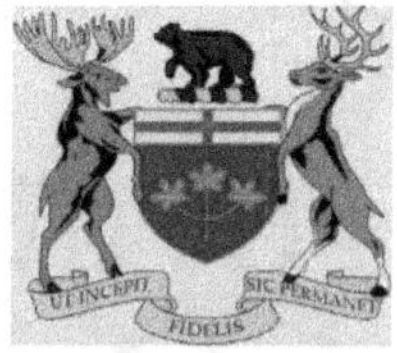

- UK data suggest that celiac testing may be cost-effective – 5% of patients with symptoms c/w IBS had celiac sprue compared with 0.5% of controls (though much lower rates reported in US)
- Tests that may be less cost-effective (no alarm symptoms): capsule endoscopy, colonoscopy with biopsy, H2-breath testing

➢ Management
  - Education and support
  - Diet
  - Medications
    - Bulking agents
    - Antispasmodics
    - Laxatives
    - Antidiarrheals
    - Newer therapies
  - Psychological treatments
  - CAM
    - Probiotics

- Education and support
  - IBS tends to be a life-long disorder
  - A good physician-patient relationship has been associated with reduced use of medical services
  - Listen to the patient – Why now? Are there any particular concerns? What are the expectations of the encounter?
  - Reassure the patient. Validate their concerns

- Diet
  - Fiber (RCT evidence)
    - May benefit constipation and provide some global symptom benefit
    - Not helpful for pain or diarrhea
  - Exclude lactose intolerance
  - Reduce excess fructose, fatty foods, gas-producing foods, caffeine, alcohol
  - Exclusion diets
    - Can measure IgG antibodies to foods
  - Probiotics
    - Variable findings for a wide spectrum tested
  - Low FODMAP diet
    - **F**ermentable **O**ligo- **D**i- and **M**ono-saccharides **a**nd **P**olyols
    - E.g. fructose, corn syrup
    - These short chain carbohydrates are poorly absorbed and are osmotically active in the intestinal lumen where they are rapidly fermented resulting in symptoms of abdominal bloating and pain.
    - A low FODMAP diet involves elimination of a larger number of high FODMAP foods that would not be excluded in a diet that only required avoidance of gas producing foods (e.g., foods that contain fructose including honey, high fructose corn syrup, apples, pears, mangoes, cherries or oligosaccharides including wheat).
    - Studies have demonstrated an improvement in IBS symptoms with FODMAP restriction

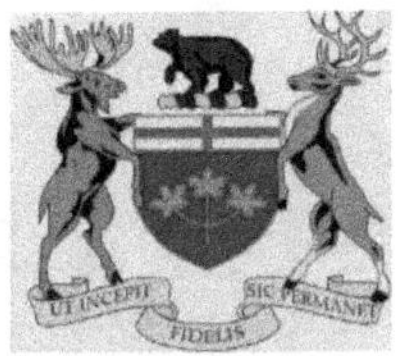

IRRITABLE BOWEL SYNDROME

- Antispasmodics and anticholinergics
  - Anticholinergic vs. non-anticholinergic antispasmodics
  - Meta-analysis of 23 RCTs: antispasmodics superior to placebo, but paper of questionable quality
  - Anticholinergic anti-spasmodics do not have well-established efficacy
    - More useful for postprandial pain if taken 30 mins prior to eating
  - Non-anticholinergic antispasmodics (mebeverine – smooth muscle relaxant, selective CCB [pinaverium], opiate agonists [trimebutine]) unavailable in NA

- Laxatives
  - No RCTs of laxatives in IBS, efficacy uncertain
  - PEG likely better tolerated than osmotic laxatives
  - Similarly, stimulant laxatives can also induce abdominal cramping and pain; generally unsatisfactory for pts with IBS.

- Antidiarrheals
  - Loperamide efficacious in RCTs for IBS with diarrhea
    - Does not improve abdo pain or bloating
    - Best if taken regularly/prophylactically
    - Doses range from 2-16 mg/day
  - Bile salt-sequestering agents and bismuth subsalicylate supported anecdotally
- Serotonin receptor drugs

- 5-HT is a key neurotransmitter in the gut
  - Enteroendocrine cells release 5-HT into the submucosa in response to luminal conditions and state of mucosa
  - Submucosal nerves have receptors for 5-HT which mediate pain and initiate peristaltic reflex
  - Some enteric interneurons also use 5-HT for signaling
- Alterations in 5-HT release or sensitivity of neurons to serotonin are postulated in IBS
- Modulation of 5-HT3 and 5-HT4 receptors is effective in treatment in some patients with IBS
- Tegaserod , serotonin type 4 receptor agonist (5-HT4)
  - Efficacy in constipation-predominant IBS
  - Release of acetylcholine release, prokinetic effects
  - Once approved only for women
  - **Withdrawn in US/Canada – increased CVS, cerebrovascular events in 2007 review of trials
- Alosetron, 5-HT3 antagonist
  - RCT evidence for “adequate” relief of IBS pain after 3 months: 60% (alosetron) vs. 41% (placebo)
  - Meta-analysis (3 studies) for 1.6 RR for global improvement
  - Restricted use – concern for ischemic colitis, severe constipation
  - Indicated for diarrhea-predominant IBS

• Modulation of chloride secretion
  - Chloride secretion by intestinal mucosa is main mechanism of fluid secretion in intestine

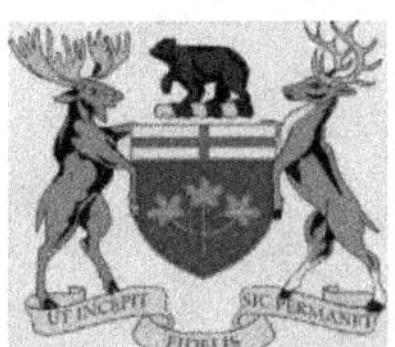

- Mediated by chloride channels in apical membrane of enterocytes that permit exit of chloride from interior of cell to lumen
  - CFTR
  - Chloride C-2 channel
- Na^+ and water follow to maintain electrical and osmotic equilibrium

- Increasing chloride secretion
  - No evidence that chloride secretion is defective in constipation-predominant IBS
  - Lubiprostone
    - Prostaglandin derivative, activates chloride C-2 channels and promotes secretion
    - Approved for treatment of IBS-C in US
    - Global response rates 18% (lubiprostone) vs. 10% placebo
    - Significantly more likely than placebo to improve individual Sx: AP, stool consistency, straining, constipation, QOL
    - ACG IBS Task Force – 8mcg bid more effective than placebo in relieving global IBS Sx in women
    - S/E – Nx (8%), diarrhea (6%)
  - Linaclotide
    - Guanylate cyclase-C receptor agonist, stimulates production of cGMP, which activates CFTR
    - Two Phase 3 RCTs (>1600 pts) found licaclotide superior to placebo for overall and individual Sx of IBS-C
    - S/E: Diarrhea

- Antidepressants
  - TCAs (tricyclic anti-depressants)
    - Meta-analyses have included low-quality studies, report NNT 3-4 for improvement in global well-being
    - Large RCT - Desipramine vs. placebo – in female patients 60% vs. 47% response
    - May be most beneficial in diarrhea-predominant IBS
    - Up to 40% discontinue use because of intolerance
  - SSRIs
    - Fewer side effects, RCTs report more mixed results

- Antibiotics
  - Largest and most rigorously designed studies for IBS are with rifaximin
  - Two Phase 3 RCTs (1260 pts) for non-constipation IBS: rifaximin 550mg tid x 14d improved global Sx and individual Sx (bloating, AP, stool consistency) vs. placebo
    - Benefits persisted up to 3 months – alteration of flora?
    - Side effects: Safe – no C diff
    - Long term prognosis (>10 weeks) unknown

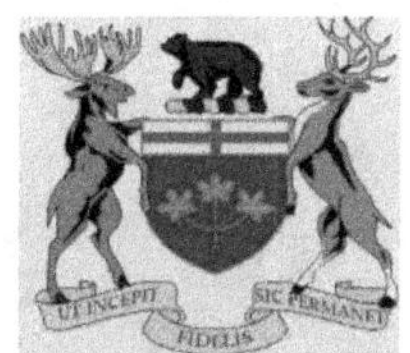

- Complementary Alternative Medicine (CAM)
  - More "educational resources" available to patients
  - 11-53% of IBS patients in N. American and Europe have used at least one type of CAM techniques
  - Review available evidence without bias
  - Prebiotics
    - Non-digestible food ingredients that beneficially affect the host by selectively stimulating the growth/activity of health-promoting bacteria in the colon
    - Few studies
  - Acupuncture
    - May alter visceral sensation and motility by stimulating somatic nervous system and vagus nerve
    - 2006 Cochrane review of 6 RCTs: most of poor quality, inconclusive evidence
    - Subsequent large study showed superiority of acupuncture and sham acupuncture over no treatment
  - Herbal medicines
    - Peppermint oil = cross between water mint and spearmint, active principle being menthol
    - 1998 meta-analysis of 5 RCTs showed significant global improvement of IBS-Sx compared with placebo
    - Recent RCT in Taiwan (110 patients), peppermint oil vs. placebo x 1 month – patients in treatment arm had less abdominal distention, stool frequency, flatulence

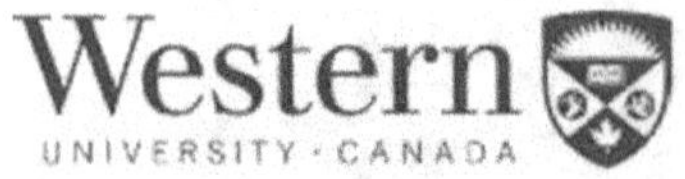

IBS and Call in Residents (Wells et al., 2012)

- Study Objective
  - The aim of this study was to determine whether sleep disruption during overnight call was associated with the presence and severity of IBS in residents.

- Study design
  - 822 Western residents and fellows
  - Survey
  - Exclusion criteria:
    - Residents with pre-existing GI disorders that would preclude a Dx of IBS
    - Inadequate completion of the survey
  - Analysis
    - A priori outcomes
    - Logistic and linear regression

	Resident (n=205)	IBS (n=39)	No IBS (n=166)	p-value
o Age				
Mean ± SD (n)	30.3 ± 3.9 (172)	30.2 ± 5.0 (34)	30.1 ± 3.7 (138)	0.91
o Gender				
Female (n)	52.7% (108)	66.7% (26)	50.3% (83)	0.07
Male (n)	47.3% (97)	33.3% (13)	49.7% (82)	0.07

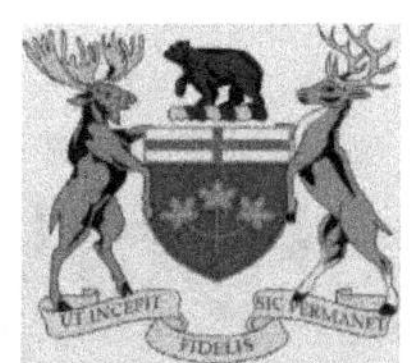

○ Training level	Residents (n=205)	IBS (n=39)	No IBS (n=166)	p-value
R1	31.4% (64)	41.0% (16)	29.1% (48)	0.14
R2	29.9% (61)	30.8% (12)	29.7% (49)	0.88
R3	15.7% (32)	12.8% (5)	16.4% (27)	0.59
R4	11.8% (24)	7.7% (3)	12.7% (21)	0.39
R5	6.9% (14)	5.1% (2)	7.3% (12)	0.64
R6	2.5% (5)	0% (0)	3.0% (5)	0.51
R7	1.5% (3)	2.6% (1)	1.2% (2)	0.53
Other	0.5% (1)	0% (0)	0.6% (1)	

○ Specialty	Residents (n=205)	IBS (n=39)	No IBS (n=166)	p-value
Anatomical Pathology	1.5% (3)	0% (0)	1.8% (3)	0.84
Anesthesiology	5.4% (11)	0% (0)	6.7% (11)	0.23
Diagnostic Radiology	3.0% (6)	7.7% (3)	1.8% (3)	0.07
Emergency Medicine	3.9% (8)	5.1% (2)	3.6% (6)	0.66
Family Medicine	21.6% (44)	17.9% (7)	22.4% (37)	0.55
General Surgery	6.4% (13)	0% (0)	7.9% (13)	0.18
Internal Medicine, including Subspecialties	19.6% (40)	20.5% (8)	19.4% (32)	0.86
Medical Microbiology	0.5% (1)	0% (0)	0.6% (1)	0.84

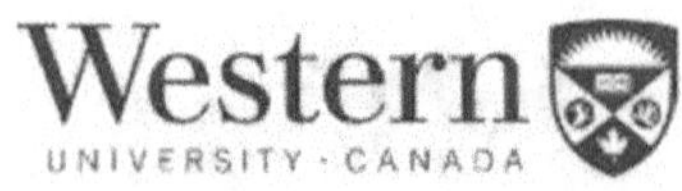

- Specialty

Specialty	Residents (n=205)	IBS (n=39)	No IBS (n=166)	p-value
Neurology	2.0% (4)	5.1% (2)	1.2% (2)	0.14
Neuropathology	1.0% (2)	0% (0)	1.2% (2)	0.14
Neurosurgery	1.0% (2)	2.6% (1)	0.6% (1)	0.30
Nuclear Medicine	2.0% (4)	5.1% (2)	1.2% (2)	0.14
Obstetrics and Gynecology	6.0% (12)	7.7% (3)	5.5% (9)	0.59
Ophthalmology	3.0% (6)	2.6% (1)	3.0% (5)	0.88
Orthopedic Surgery	3.0% (6)	0% (0)	3.6% (6)	0.43
Otolaryngology	2.0% (4)	0% (0)	2.4% (4)	0.60
Pediatrics	4.5% (9)	12.8% (5)	2.4% (4)	**0.01**
Physical Medicine and Rehabitation	2.0% (4)	0% (0)	2.4% (4)	0.60
Plastic Surgery	1.5% (3)	0% (0)	1.8% (3)	0.73
Psychiatry	4.5% (9)	7.7% (3)	3.6% (6)	0.27
Radiation Oncology	1.5% (3)	0% (0)	1.8% (3)	0.73
Urology	1.5% (3)	0% (0)	1.8% (3)	0.73
Other	5.4% (11)	5.1% (2)	5.5% (9)	0.94

- Sleep and Call Characteristics

	IBS (n=39)	*No IBS (n=166)*	Residents (n=205)	p-value
Overnight Call				
Number (Calls / month	5.4 ± 1.4 (39)	5.4 ± 1.7 (166)	5.4 ± 1.6 (205)	1.00
Home Call (%)	53% ± 46% (38)	38% ± 39% (160)	41% ± 41% (198)	0.06

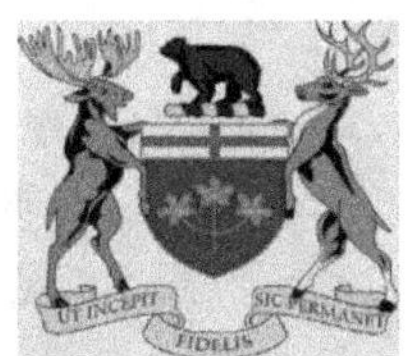

	IBS (n=39)	*No IBS (n=166)*	Residents (n=205)	p-value
Average time leaving the hospital post-call				
Before 8:00am	5.1% (2)	4.3% (7)	4.5% (9)	0.80
8:00 to 10:00am	33.3% (13)	34.8% (56)	34.5% (69)	0.96
10:00am to Noon	46.9% (15)	28.0% (45)	30% (60)	0.16
Noon to 2:00pm	7.7% (3)	5.0% (8)	5.5% (11)	0.48
2:00 to 5:00pm	0.0% (0)	8.1% (13)	6.5% (13)	0.18
After 5:00pm	15.4% (6)	19.9% (32)	19% (38)	0.57
Hours of Sleep				
While on Call	2.9 ± 1.9 (39)	3.6 ± 1.9 (166)	3.5 ± 1.9 (205)	**0.04**
While Not on Call	7.1 ± 0.9 (39)	7.1 ± 1.1 (166)	7.1 ± 1.0 (205)	1.00

- Key Results
  - Sleep disruption was significantly associated with a diagnosis of IBS even when adjusted for age and gender (p= 0.02).
  - For every hour of sleep less while on call, the odds ratio (OR) for a diagnosis of IBS was 1.32
  - Severity of IBS was predicted by:
    - Sleep deprivation while on call (p=0.04)
    - Mean number of calls per block (p=0.01)
    - Specialty program versus family practice (p=0.01)

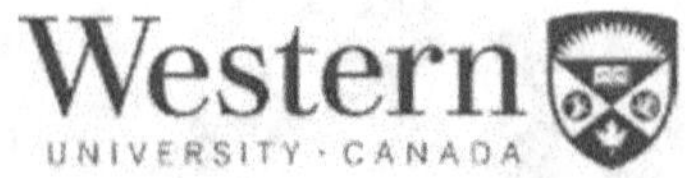

- Conclusions
  - Sleep disruption is an important risk factor for IBS. This study is the first to demonstrate a relationship between overnight call and IBS in residents
  - The sleep deprivation on call, the number of calls per block, and whether the resident was in a family practice vs. specialty program significantly predicted the severity of IBS, as measured by the IBS QOL questionnaire.

- Limitations
  - This survey was completely voluntary which can lead to selection bias.
  - The overall response rate was relatively low (27.5%), which raises concerns about generalizability of our findings.
  - There were a larger number of male participants where IBS has a higher prevalence in females, therefore our study may under-estimate the association in females who are more at risk for IBS.
  - As in any observational study, there may have been unmeasured confounders.

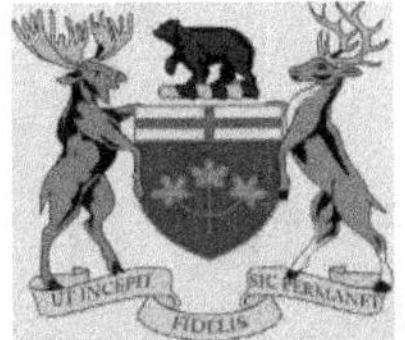

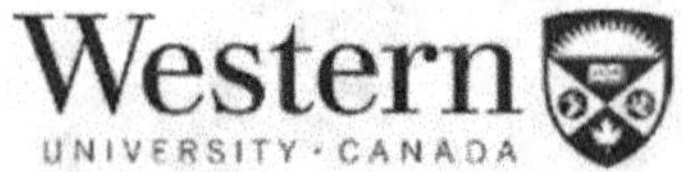
Western
UNIVERSITY · CANADA

LIVER, HEPATOBILIARY TREE AND GALLBLADDER

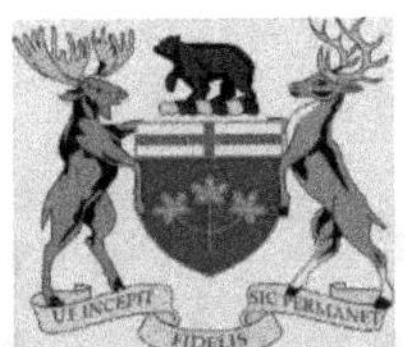

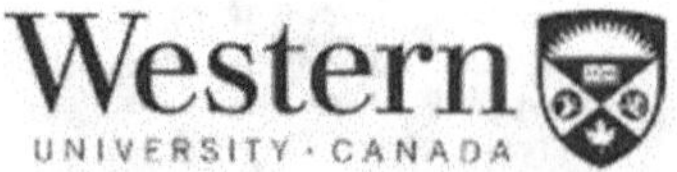

MINI UPDATE

Vascular Diseases of the Liver

Malcolm Wells

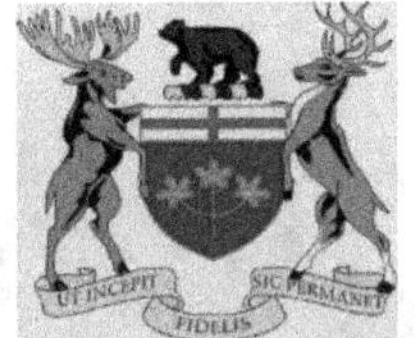

VASCULAR DISEASES OF THE LIVER

➢ Classification

- Classify, and give 6 examples of the vascular diseases of the liver.

  - Disorders of portal venous inflow
    - Acute mesenteric/portal venous thrombosis (PVT)
    - Chronic mesenteric/PVT
  - Disorders of hepatic arterial (HA) inflow
    - HA thrombosis
    - Hepatic arteriovenous fistula
    - Ischemic hepatitis
  - Disorders of hepatic venous outflow
    - Veno-occlusive disease (VOD)
    - Budd-Chiari syndrome (BCS)

Printed with permission: Kamath PS. *Mayo Clinic Gastroenterology and Hepatology Board Review* 2008: pg. 337.

Budd-Chiari Syndrome (BCS)

➢ Definition: obstruction of the hepatic venous outflow anywhere from the right atrium to the small hepatic venules.

  - Classically results from thrombosis of one or more hepatic veins at their opening to the IVC

➢ Causes of Budd-Chiari Syndrome

  - Commonest causes
    - Africa, Asia
      - MOVC (membranous obstruction of the inferior vena cava)

- NA/Europe
  - Thrombosis of hepatic veins, from thrombogenic states, e.g. myeloproliferative disorders (JAK_2 mutations of the gene coding for tyrosine kinase Janus kinase 2)

- Hypercoagulable States
  - Anti-phospholipid syndrome
  - Anti-thrombin deficiency
  - Factor V Leiden mutation
  - Lupus anti-coagulant
  - Methylenetetrahydrofolate reductase mutation TT677
  - Myeloproliferative disorders (including polycythemia vera and essential thrombocytosis)
  - Oral contraeptives
  - Paroxysmal nocturnal hemoglobinuria
  - Postpartum thrombocytopenic purpura
  - Pregnancy
  - Protein C deficiency
  - Protein S deficiency
  - Prothrombin mutation G20210A
  - Sickle cell disease

- Infections
  - Aspergillosis
  - Filariasis
  - Hydrated cysts
  - Liver abscess (amebic or pyogenic)
  - Pelvic cellulitis
  - Schistosomiasis
  - Syphilis
  - Tuberculosis

- Malignancies adrenal carcinoma
  - Bronchogenic carcinoma
  - Hepatocellular carcinoma

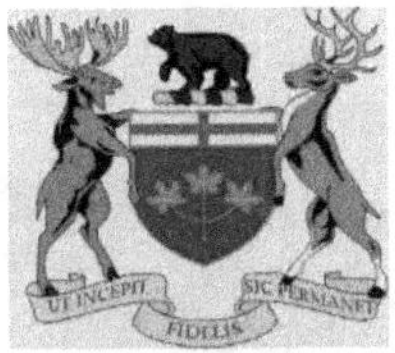

- Leimyosarcoma
- Leukemia
- Renal carcinoma
- Rhabdomyosarcoma
- Miscellaneous
  - Behcet's syndrome
  - Celiac disease
  - Dacarbazine therapy
  - Inflammatory bowel disease
  - Laparoscopic cholecystectomy
  - Membranous obstruction of the vena cava
  - Polycystic liver disease
  - Sarcoidosis
  - Trauma to hepatic veins

➢ Clinical
- Presentation: BCS "….should be considered in patients presenting with decompensated cirrhosis or refractory ascites out of proportion to the magnitude of liver biochemical test abnormalities (Feldman M., et al. Sleisenger and Fordtran's Gastrointestinal and Liver Disease. 9th Edition. Saunders/Elsevier, Philadelphia, 2010, page 1373).

- Give the presentation, etiology, diagnostic imaging and histological changes, as well as management of hepatic vein (HV) occlusion (BCS).

- Presentations
  - Subacute or Chronic Budd-Chiari syndrome
    - Most common
    - Signs and Symptoms occur over 3-6 months
    - Many already have cirrhosis and experience decompensation

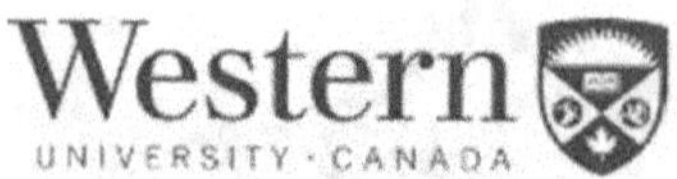

- Signs and Symptoms
  - HSM and ascites usually present
  - Variceal bleeding
  - If IVC obstructed as well:
    - Collaterals over flanks and back
    - Lower limb edema
- Acute BCS
  - Bilirubin typically less than 5
  - AST and ALT typically 2-3X ULN
  - AST and ALT may be non-specifically mildly elevated

- Asymptomatic
  - Occurs in many
  - Especially if thrombosis in only one hepatic vein or if collaterals
  - Elevated liver enzymes may be the only indication

- Acute Budd-Chiari syndrome
  - Common (20-30% of cases)
  - Clinical findings depend on
    - Location of the thrombus
    - Stage and rapidly of evolution
    - Percentage of liver tissue deprived of venous drainage
  - Symptoms and sign develop over 1-2 months
    - Abdominal pain
    - Tender hepatomegaly
    - Ascites
    - Hepatic failure if acute
  - Some patients may have a remitting course

- Fulminant Liver Failure
  - Uncommon
  - Occurs mostly in pregnant women with hypercoagulable disorders

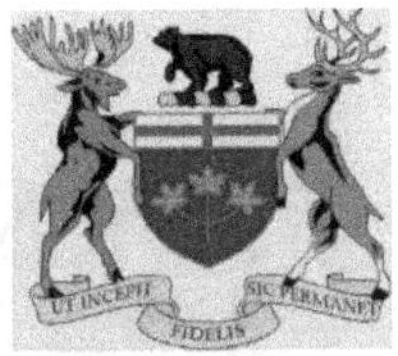

- Presents with:
  - abrupt and severe abdominal pain
  - Vomiting
  - Marked hepatomegaly
  - Jaundice
  - Ascites
  - High hepatocellular enzymes (greater than 1000)
  - Rapid deterioration with HE and renal failure
- Few survive without prompt liver transplantation

➢ Pathology

- Acutely, hepatic histologic features include:
  - Centrilobular congestion
  - Hemorrhage
  - Sinusoidal dilation
  - Non-inflammatory cell necrosis
- Within weeks:
  - Fibrosis in the centrilobular areas more so than in the periportal areas
- Over time:
  - These lesions develop into cirrhosis
  - Large regenerative nodules are common, especially in areas of decreased portal venous perfusion
- Because hepatic vein occlusion is asymetric, the pathology may vary in different parts of the liver
- Massive caudate lobe hypertrophy is common
  - Probably secondary to preservation of drainage directly into the IVC
  - May compress IVC
- Changes (except for cirrhosis) can be reversed with adequate decompression of the sinusoids

- Give the acute and chronic pathological changes of BCS (Budd-Chiari Syndrome).

o Acute centrilobular	– Congestion – Sinusoidal distention – Hemorrhage – Necrosis – Little inflammation
o Chronic	– Patchy, asymmetrical involvement – Perivenular sclerosis – Hepatocellular necrosis – Regenerative nodules – Cirrhosis

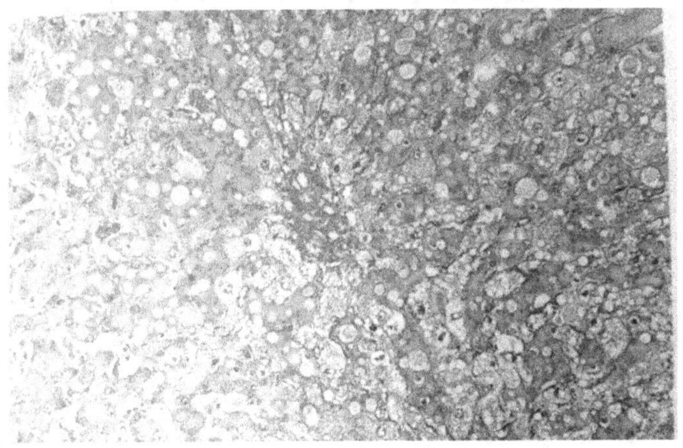

Source: Stevens WE. Sleisenger & Fordtran's gastrointestinal and liver disease: Pathophysiology/ Diagnosis/Management 2006: pg. 1762; and 2010, 1378.

- o The damage occurs mostly in zones 3 and 2
- o Because of ↓total blood flow in the HV, and because the caudate lobe has additional blood flow through the accessory hepatic veins, the caudate lobe may hypertrophy.

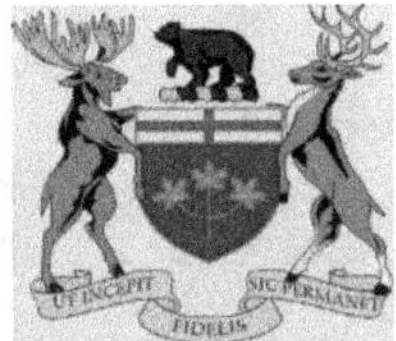

- Laboratory
  - Liver enzymes
    - May be normal or mildly elevated
    - Occasionally >5X ULN with fulminant liver failure or in acute cases
    - Severity of liver disease often out of proportion with the bloodwork

- Diagnostic imaging
  - Doppler U/S
    - SN and SP > 80%
    - Diagnostic procedure of first choice
    - Typical features of Budd Chiari syndrome
      - Lack of visualization of normal hepatic veinous connections to IVC
      - Comma-shaped intrahepatic or subcapsular collateral vessels
      - Absence of flow in the hepatic veins
    - Diagnostic accuracy decreased by large body habitus
    - Operator dependent

  - MRI and CT
    - Also may demonstrate characteristic findings of BCS
    - Usually doesn't add much to the Doppler U/S
    - MRI the preferred second line test:
      - Provides accurate angiographic detail with minimal risk of nephrotoxicity
    - Combination of U/S with MRI or CT should be sufficient to diagnose most cases

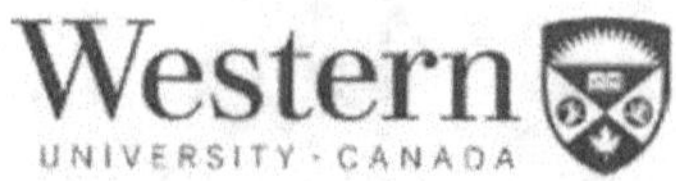

- Venography
  - Was the gold standard, now often not necessary
  - Should be performed when BCS suspected, 1st and 2nd line imaging nondiagnostic and surgery planned
  - Liver biopsy can be performed simultaneously with venography
    - Liver biopsy not essential but may be helpful in planning treatment
  - If a venogram were performed, it might show a "spider web" appearance suggestive of BCS (BCS → ↓ HV flow → ↑ accessary HV flow → spider appearance on venography).
  - Curiosity: a very large candate lobe may compress the IVC (inferior vena cava) and further ↓ HV outflow.

➢ Treatment

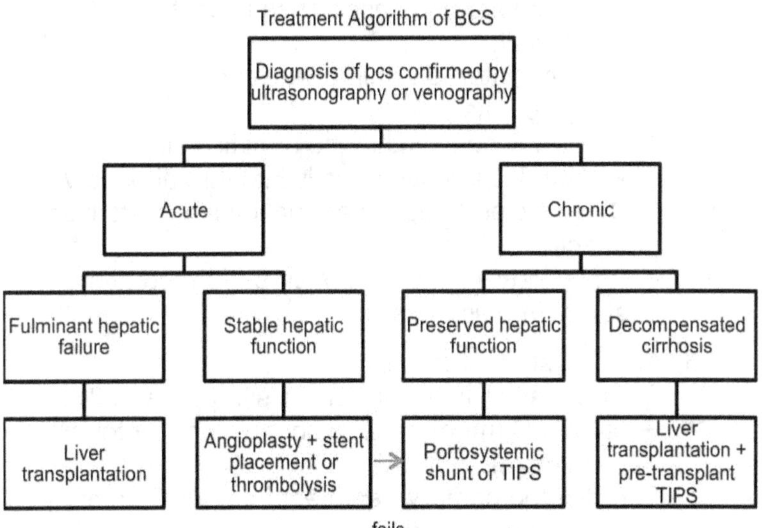

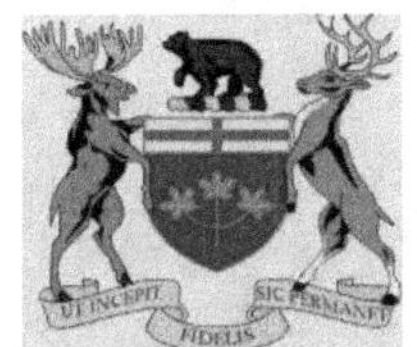

- Depends on etiology, anatomic characteristics and pace of the disease
- Treat precipitating causes
- Collaboration between hepatology, hematology, interventional radiology and surgery
- Medical Treatment alone in only a few patients with milder BCS
  - Control of ascites (lasix, spironolactone, Na restriction, paracentesis)
  - Anticoagulation is recommended
    - Heparin followed by warfarin (target INR 2-3)
  - Treatment considered successful if:
    - Ascites controlled
    - Liver enzymes normalize
    - Symptoms resolve
  - Most patients require further therapy
- Thrombolytic therapy
  - Case reports and case series in acute BCS
  - Effective if:
    - Administered within 3 weeks of onset of symptoms
    - Flow is seen within the hepatic vein
    - Agent is infused directly into thrombosed vein
  - Systemic and hepatic arteria infusions are less effective
  - Angioplaty +/- stenting often performed at the same time as infusion
- Angioplasty and stenting
  - Can restore flow and relieve symptoms in 80% of MOVC (membranous obstruction of inferior vena cava)
    - It's the primary treatment for MOVC in many parts of the world

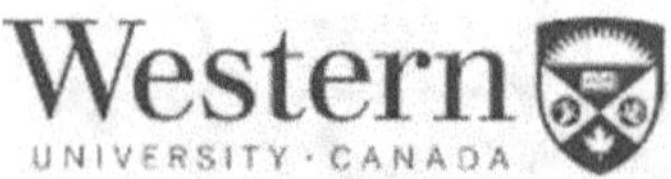

- Rate of restenosis is high and regular doppler U/S are recommended
- Can be combined with creation of portacaval shunt in patients with both IVC and hepatic vein obstruction

- TIPS
  - Gaining popularity
  - Low mortality
  - shunt placement usually successful
  - Useful for:
    - Combined IVC and Hepatic vein obstruction, or
    - Fulminant liver failure awaiting transplant
  - Outcomes:
    - Short-term mortality in 50% of those with fulminant failure undergoing TIPS
    - Can be a longterm treatment in a minority of patients with acute BCS failing thrombolytics and angioplasty
    - TIPS revisions are often required

- Surgical therapy:
  - MOVC
  - Web removal
  - resection
  - Trans-atrial "finger-fracture" of IVC webs

- Portosystemic shunt
  - Relieves portal HTN effectively
    - Relieves hepatic ischemic necrosis,
    - Refractatory ascites,
    - Variceal bleeding
  - When shunt surgery is successful:
    - The portal vein becomes the hepatic outflow tract
    - Hepatomegaly resolves

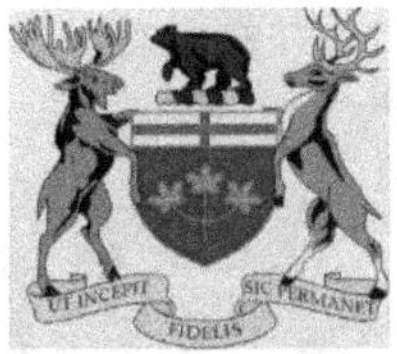

        - Histologic findings resolve and may even normalize
        - Survival is prolonged in >90% of patients
    - Contraindicated if:
        - IVC stenosis present
        - IVC pressure >20mmHg
        - Poracaval pressure <10mmHg
- Surgical therapy: liver tranplantation
    - Appropriate for patients with:
        - Fulminant liver disease
        - Chronic BCS
        - Failed surgical portosystemic shunt
    - Curable for patients with PnC, PnS, and antithrombin deficiencies (although most patients will require lifelong anticoagulation)
    - Myeloproliferative disorders can be managed with hydroxurea and ASA post-transplant
        - There is risk of progression and leukemic transformation
    - Prognosis:
        - Recurrent BCS occurs in 4-10%
        - 5-year survival >85%

- Give the treatment options and indications for the use of 4 different modalities in the patient with Budd-Chiari Syndrome (BCS), and give their advantages and disadvantages.

Treatment	Indication	Advantages	Disadvantages
Thrombolytic therapy	- Acute thrombosis	Reverses hepatic necrosis	Risk of bleeding Limited success
Angioplasty with and without stenting	- IVC webs - IVC stenosis - Focal hepatic vein stenosis	No long-term sequelae Averts need for surgery	High rate of restenosis or shunt occlusion

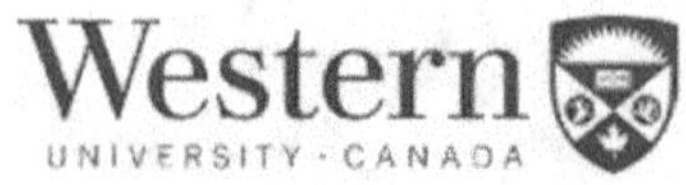

Treatment	Indication	Advantages	Disadvantages
TIPS	- Possible bridge to transplantation in fulminant BCS - Acute BCS	Low mortality Useful even with compression of IVC by caudate lobe	High rate of shunt stenosis Extended stents may interfere with liver transplantation
Surgical shunt	- Subacute BCS if portacaval pressure gradient <10 mm Hg or occluded IVC	Definitive procedure for many patients Low rate of shunt dysfunction with portacaval shunt	Risk of procedure-related death Limited applicability
Liver transplan-tation	- Subacute BCS - Portacaval pressure gradient >10 mm Hg - Fulminant BCS - Presence of cirrhosis - Failure of portosystemic shunt	Reverses liver disease May reverse underlying thrombophilia	Risk of procedure-related death Need for long-term immunosuppression

Abbreviations: IVC, inferior vena cava; TIPS, transjugular intrahepatic portasystemic shunt

Printed with permission: Kamath PS. *Mayo Clinic Gastroenterology and Hepatology Board Review* 2008: pg. 344.

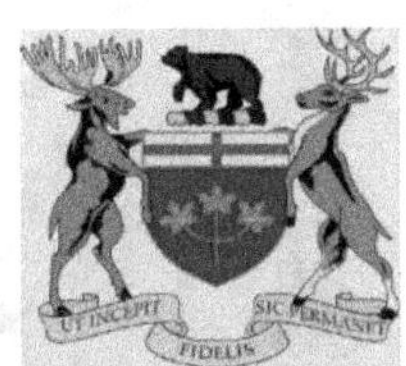

Sinusoidal Obstruction Syndrome (SOS, aka Veno-occlusive Disease [VOD])

- Definition
    - Occlusion of the terminal hepatic venules and hepatic sinusoids
    - Resembles BCS clinically
- Causes / associations
    - Worldwide
        - Ingestion of alkaloids in inadvertently winnowed wheat or "bush tea" is the main cause worldwide
        - Herbal remedy comfrey associated with SOS
        - Rare familial clusters reported in association with immunodeficiency states
    - In the "West"
        - Most commonly post bone marrow (BM) transplant (0-70%)
        - Chemotherapy
            - 6-thioguanine
            - Actinomycin D
            - Azathioprine
            - Cytosine arabinoside
            - Decarbazine
            - Gemtuzumab ozogamicin
            - Mirtramycin
        - Bone marrow transplantation (BMT) occurs
            - Within 2 weeks after BMT
            - In 50% of BMT
            - 70% mortality rate
        - Hepatic irradiation and busulfan/cyclophosphamide associated
        - Longterm immunosuppression with azathioprine and 6-thioguanine

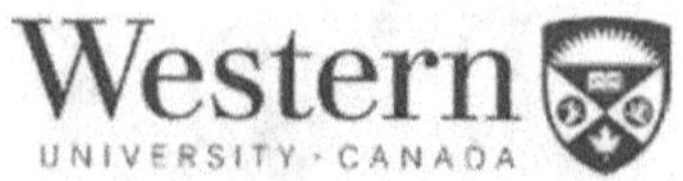

- Older age
- HCV
- C282Y (HH, hereditary hemochromatosis)
- Other pre-existing chronic liver diseases
- Recent bacterial / viral infections

- Pathology
  - Histologic features result from toxic injury to the centrilobular (zone 3) endothelial cells in the hepatic sinusoids and terminal hepatic venules
    - Cellular debris
    - Exfoliated hepatocytes
    - Activated coagulation factors
    - Extravasated red blood cells produce
    - All of which cause progressive occlusion of the sinusoids and venules, sinusoidal dilatation, and severe hepatic congestion
    - Inflammation is noticably absent
  - Progressive venular sclerosis ensues
  - Collagen is deposited into the venuoles
  - Eventually leads to venular obliteration, hepatocellular ischemic necrosis, and widespread fibrosis

- Clinical Features
  - Early: features of portal HTN
  - Classically begins with:
    - Mild hyperbilirubinemia
    - Painful hepatomegaly
    - Weight gain >2%

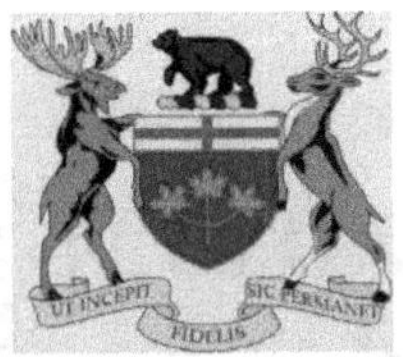

- Later:
  - Jaundice
  - Ascites
  - HE
  - Multi-organ failure
- Occurs within 10-20 days of BM transplantation

➢ Predictors of severity

- Jaundice
- Ascites
- HVPG (hepatic venous pressure gradient) > 20 mm Hg
- Multiorgan failure
- Mortality rate ~25% from multiorgan failure, and not liver failure

Note: be prepared for questions such as: without performing a liver biopsy, distinguish between SOS and GVHD of the liver (easy – see above)

➢ Laboratory

- Serum bilirubin usually peaks at day 17
- Routine blood work not specific
- Serum ALP and aminotransferase elevations may indicate accompanying hepatic ischemic necrosis
- Thrombocytopenia aggravated by portal HTN and splenomegaly
- ↑ conjugated hyperbilirubinemia
- Thrombocytopenia

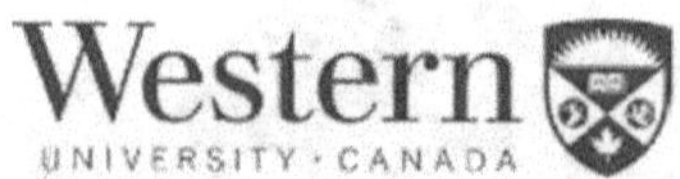

- Diagnostic imaging
  - U/S, CT and MRI are nonspecific early, but are helpful in ruling out other causes. Common findings include:
    - Gall Bladder wall thickening
    - HSM
    - Ascites
    - Portal vein enlargement with sluggish or reversed flow and umbilical vein recanulization
  - U/S can predict disease severity
  - If diagnosis is uncertain:
    - Transjugular liver biopsy and
    - Measurement of the hepatic venous pressure gradient
      - Gradient >10mmHg is predictive of SOS and increased disease severity
  - Bloodwork can be predictive of SOS before it's clinically evident
    - Thrombin are decreased before the onset of SOS
      - PnC, Factor VII
    - Increased before the onset of SOS
      - Plasminogen activator inhibitor type 1
      - TNF-a
      - Procollagen type III are increased

- Give the non-specific changes seen on diagnostic imaging (abdominal ultrasound, CT or MRI) which suggest the diagnosis of SOS (Sinusoidal Obstruction Syndrome).

  - Liver, spleen
    - Hepatosplenomegaly

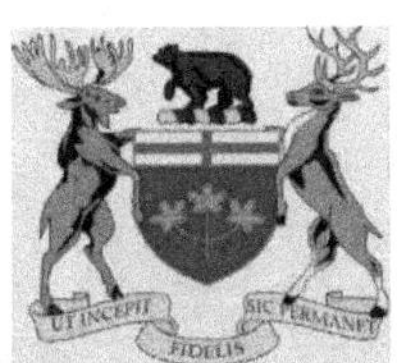

- PV
  - Dilated
  - Flow in PV slow or reversed
- Umbilical vein
  - Recanalization
- Gallbladder thick wall

➢ Diagnosis

- Based on characteristic clinical features and exclusion of other conditions

➢ Differential diagosis:

- SOS develops after BMT on days 10 to 20
- Distinguish from GVHD (graft-versus-host disease) which develops after day 15
- Sepsis and drug toxicity do not usually cause painful hepatomegaly or ascites, as does SOS
  - Hepatic dysfunction via sepsis or drug toxicity
    - Rarely cause painful hepatomegaly and ascites
  - Cholestasis resulting from hemolysis
  - HF (heart failure)

➢ Treatment

- Lack of safe and effective treatment
- Preventative measures
  - Recognizing risk factors and adjusting chemo appropriately
  - Urso, heparin, and LMWH for prevention have yielded inconclusive results

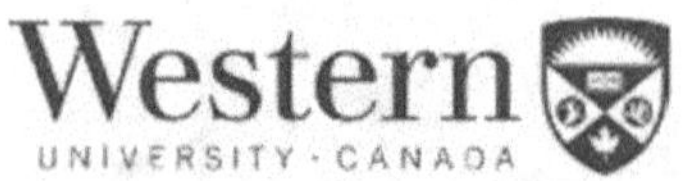

- Mainly supportive (diuresis, analgesia, paracentesis, avoidance of nephro/hepatotoxins
- TPA has response rate of 30% and life-threatening hemorrhage of 20-30%
- Multiple other medications have been ineffective
- Most are unsuitable for liver transplantation due to their malignancy

➢ Prognosis

- SOS evolves over 2-3 weeks
- Overall mortality is 20-50% with
  - Most deaths occuring from multi-organ failure rather than hepatic failure
- Severe SOS progresses rapidly and carries a 100% mortality rate

Portal Vein Thrombosis (PVT)

➢ Pathogenesis

- Thrombosis, constriction or invasion of the portal vein
- Results in
  - Portal hypertension,
  - Portosystemic collaterals, and
  - Esophageal, gastric, jejunal varices
- Fibroblasts transform the clot into a collagenous plus in which venous channels develop (cavernous transformation)
- Mesenteric ischemia can occur if the clot extends into mesenteric vessels

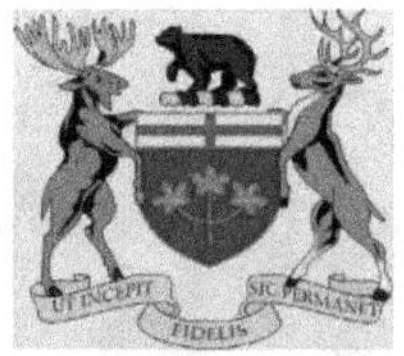

- Ascites, abdominal pain and fever acutely, but wanes, over time with the formation of collaterals

➢ Causes / associations

- Most cases have identifiable causes
  - Hypercoagulable states
  - Inflammation
  - Trauma/surgery
  - Malignancy
- <20% considered idiopathic
- Infection (umbilical vein sepsis) is the main cause in children
- In adults, cirrhosis and abdominal malignancies cause 50% of cases
- Occurs in 10% of patients with cirrhosis (sluggish portal vein flow)

- Classify and give 10 causes of portal vein thrombosis (PVT).

  - Common causes
    - Children
      - Umbilical vein sepsis
    - Adults
      - Cirrhosis
      - Hypercoagulability (e.g. myeloproliferative disorders)
      - Intraabdominal malignancy
        - HCC (hepatocellular cancer)
        - Pancreatic cancer
      - Iatrogenic previous
        - Sclerotherapy of esophageal varices
        - Abdominal surgery
    - Idiopathic

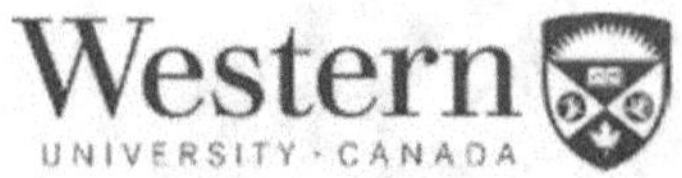

- Hypercoagulable states
  - Antiphospholipid syndrome
  - Antithrombin deficiency
  - Factor V Leiden mutation
  - Methylenetetrahydrofolate reductase mutation TT677
  - Myeloproliferative disorders
  - Nephrotic syndrome
  - Oral contraceptives
  - Paroxysmal nocturnal hemoglobinuria
  - Polycythemia rubra vera
  - Pregnancy
  - Prothrombin mutation G20210A
  - Protein C deficiency
  - Protein S deficiency
  - Sickle cell disease
- Impaired portal vein flow
  - Budd-Chiari syndrome (BCS)
  - Cirrhosis
  - Nodular regenerative hyperplasia (NRH)
  - Sinusoidal obstruction syndrome (SOS)
- Inflammatory diseases
  - Behçet syndrome
  - Inflammatory bowel disease
  - Pancreatitis
- Infections
  - Appendicitis
  - Cholangitis
  - Cholecystitis
  - Diverticulitis
  - Liver abscess
- Cancer
  - Pancreas
  - Bladder cancer
  - Cholangiocarcinoma

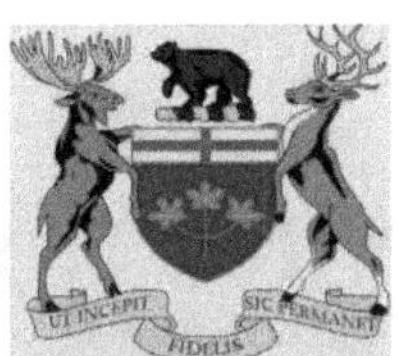

    - HCC

- Intra-abdominal procedures
    - Alcohol injection
    - Colectomy
    - Endoscopic sclerotherapy
    - Fundoplication
    - Gastric banding
    - Hepatic chemoembolization
    - Hepatobiliary surgery
    - Islet cell injection
    - Liver transplantation
    - Peritoneal dialysis
    - Radiofrequency ablation of hepatic tumour (s)
    - Splenectomy
    - TIPS procedure
    - Umbilical vein catheterization

Adapted from: Stevens WE. *Sleisenger & Fordtran's gastrointestinal and liver disease: Pathophysiology/Diagnosis/Management* 2006: pg. 1762; and 2010, 1378.

For more details, please see Feldman M., et al. Sleisenger and Fordtran's Gastrointestinal and Liver Disease. 9th Edition. Saunders/Elsevier, Philadelphia, 2010, Table 83.2, page 1378, for "Causes of Portal Vein Thrombosis".

- Progression over time of obstruction of PV
    - Thrombus
    - Constriction
    - Compression (invasion)

↓

Collagenous plug formed

↓

Cavernous transformation of venous channels

↓

Portal cavernoma

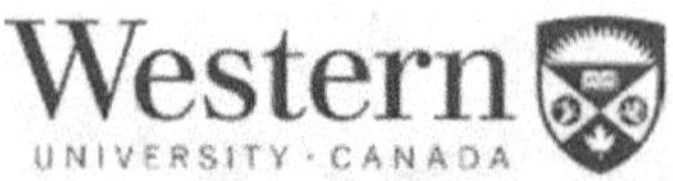

Clinical Alert!

"….long-term anti-coagulation does **not** increase the risk or severity of variceal bleeding and prevents further portal and mesenteric venous thrombotic complications" (Feldman M., et al. Sleisenger and Fordtran's Gastrointestinal and Liver Disease. 9th Edition. Saunders/Elsevier, Philadelphia, 2010, page 1379).

A Little Quiz

- In the context of chronic centrilobular vascular congestion, give the meaning of "reverse lobulation".
    - Reverse lobulation is the formation of bridging necrosis between central veins (CV), (the reverse of bridging necrosis between portal tracts), which is characteristic of cardiac cirrhosis.
    - The bridging necrosis CV ➔ CV in cardiac cirrhosis is different from the bridging necrosis from portal vein to portal vein (PV) as seen in other types of cirrhosis (PV ➔ PV)

Note: Same answer for different question: Give the pathological feature distinguishing portal cirrhosis from cardiac cirrhosis.

- Clinical
    - Found equally in adults and children
    - Initial manifestation almost always variceal bleeding
    - Abdominal pain is unusual unless thrombosis is acute and involves mesenteric vessels
    - Splenomegaly common

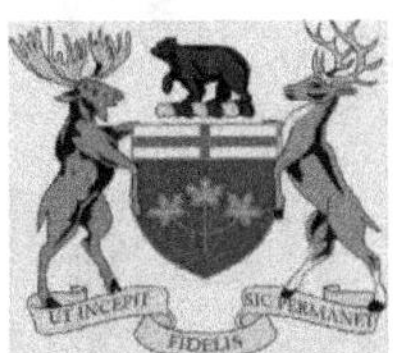

- Ascites unusual, except when acute or when thrombosis complicates cirrhosis

➢ Laboratory

- Liver enzymes usually normal
  - Occasionally bile duct varices can cause obstruction

➢ Diagnostic imaging

- Doppler U/S is highly sensitive
  - Echogenic clot
  - Collaterals
  - Enlarged spleen
  - Occasionally non-visualization of portal vein
- When U/S inconclusive, MRI better than CT
- Portal veinography usually unecessary
- Consultation with hematologist to investigate hypercoaguable risk factors

➢ Treatment

- Varices
  - Repeated Banding or sclerotherpy is first line
  - Prophylactic beta blocker
  - Portosystemic shunt or TIPS (can be technically challenging) if refractatory bleeding
- Anticoagulation
  - Recommended acutely to prevent cavernous transformation and complications of portal HTN
  - Increases rates of recanulization from 20% to 80%
  - Heparin/LMWH followed by warfarin (INR 2-2.5) for 6 months
  - One study has shown this to be safe despite varices
  - Not recommended for chronic PVT

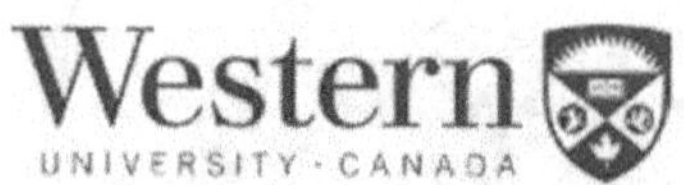

- Antibiotics for cases of pylephlebitis
- Direct thrombolytics in rare cases (effective, but high complication rate)
- Liver transplantation
  - Technically difficult
  - High rates of rethrombosis
  - Overall survival rates not reduced when compared to other indications

➤ Prognosis
- 10 yr survival is 80%
  - In the absence of cirrhosis, cancer, and mesenteric vein thrombosis
- 2% experience fatal variceal bleeding
  - Better outcomes seen than in cirrhosis because of preserved hepatic function & lack of coagulopathy

Ischemic Hepatitis

➤ Definition
- "Hepatitis" is a misnomer because this is not associated with inflammation
- Results from hypoxia of the liver
  - Hypoperfusion from cardiac failure
  - Systemic hypxemia from resp failure
  - Increased O_2 requirements from sepsis

➤ Demography
- Probably the most common form of vascular liver disease

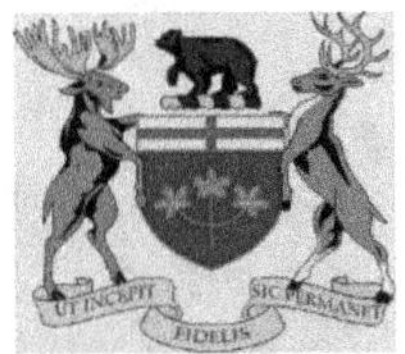

- Give reasons why "Ischemic" or "Hypoxic" hepatitis may not be a satisfactory term.
    - Reduced hepatic blood flow from any cause, such as heart failure, respiratory failure, and systemic hypotension cause the following pathological changes
    - Very little inflammatory infiltrate (i.e. no "hepatitis")
    - Centrilobular necrosis
    - Loss of hepatocytes
    - RBC in sinusoids
    - May progress to centrilobular fibrosis

➢ Pathology

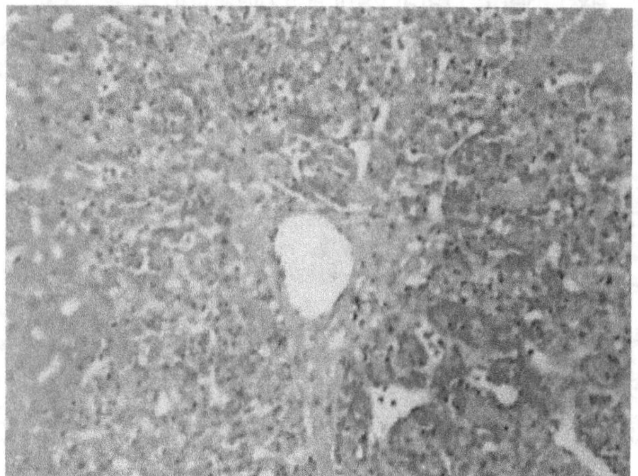

- This low-power photomicrograph
- Centrilobular necrosis
- Loss of hepatocytes
- Sinusoidal congestion with red blood cells
- Only a scant inflammatory infiltration
- Perivenular fibrosis

(Hematoxylin and eosin; courtersy of Dr. Pamela Jensen, Dallas, Tex)

- Causes / associations
  - Cardiovascular disease
    - Most common cause (70% of cases)
    - e.g. Acute MI, severe CHF
    - More than 80% of cases occur in people with pre-existing CHF
  - Respiratory issues/disease
    - Accounts for 10-15% of cases
  - Sepsis
    - Accounts for 10-15% of cases
  - Others account for <5% of cases
    - Acute trauma, acute hemorrhage, burns and heat stroke
  - HoTN seen in >50% of cases but does not have to be present

- Clinical
  - Findings usually dominated by the underlying precipitating medical condition
  - Think of ischemic hepatitis when AST/ALT are markedly elevated in these circumstances
  - Often altered mental status
  - Often patient is in ICU

- Laboratory
  - AST increased markedly
    - Accounts for 50% of all the cases where AST is >3000
    - Aminotransferase levels peak at 1-2 days and return to normal within 7-10 days

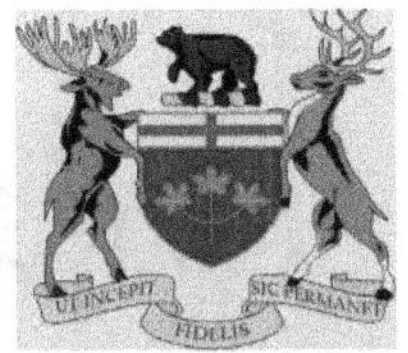

- LDH also profoundly elevated
  - LDH usually greater than ALT
  - Usually ALT-to-LDH ratio of <1.5 is more typical of ischemic hepatitis rather than viral hepatitis
- Prothrombin time usually 2-3
- Serum bilirubin mildly increased
- Cr and BUN often increased due to AKI (potentially ATN)
- Liver Biopsy usually not necessary
  - Reveals bland centrilobular necrosis with preservation of the hepatic architecture

Abbreviations: AKI, acute kidney ischemia; ATN, acute tubular necrosis

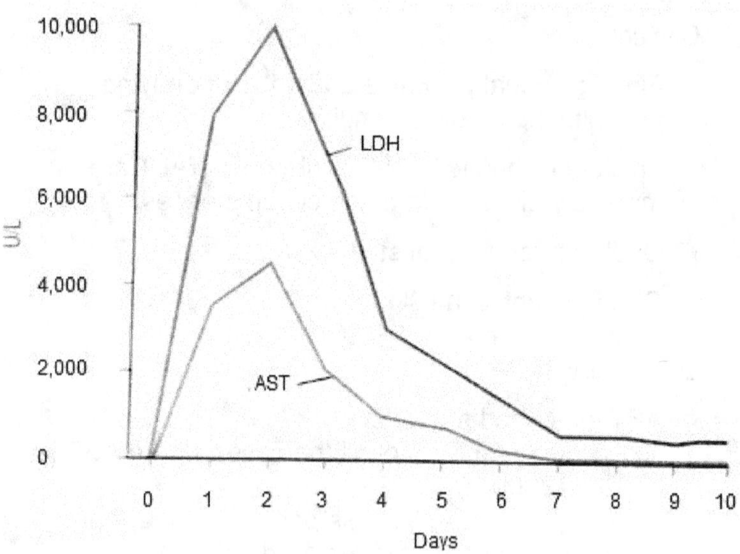

- Give 4 laboratory measurements, which suggest ischemic hepatitis.
    - ↑ AST
    - ↑ LDH
    - ALT-to-LDH ratio of < 1.5
    - Rapid fall of LDH, AST, usually within 4 days
    - In congestive hepatopathy
      – ↑ SAAG
      – ↑ protein in ascites

➤ Differential Diagnosis
- Acute Viral Hepatitis
- Autoimmunity
- Toxins
- Medications

➤ Treatment
- No specific treatment
- Treat underlying condition
- Improve cardiac output and systemic oxygenation

➤ Prognosis
- Usually self-limited (resolves with resolution of the underlying condition)
- Sometimes a manifestation of multiorgan failure and is a signal of poor prognosis

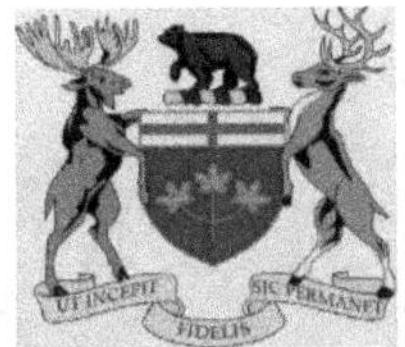

- Fulminant liver disease is uncommon
  - Can occur with chronic CHF or if cirrhosis is also present
- Overall prognosis depends on the severity of the precipitating condition

Congestive Hepatopathy

- Pathogenesis
  - Heart failure effects the liver via:
    - Decreased hepatic blood flow
    - Increased hepatic vein pressure
    - Decreased arterial oxygen saturation
  - RHF
    - Results in transmission of increased CVP from the heart directly to the hepatic sinusoids
    - Results in centrilobular congestionand sinusoidal edema that further decreases oxygen delivery
  - Susceptible to superimposed ischemic hepatitis

Abbreviations: CHF, congestive heart failure; CVP, central venous pressure; RHF, right heart failure

- Pathology
  - Typical features:
    - Atrophy of hepatocytes
    - Sinusoidal distension
    - Centrilobular fibrosis (distribution is variable)
    - Bridging fibrosis typically extends between central veins
  - Often ischemic hepatitis overlaps
    - Centrilobular necrosis

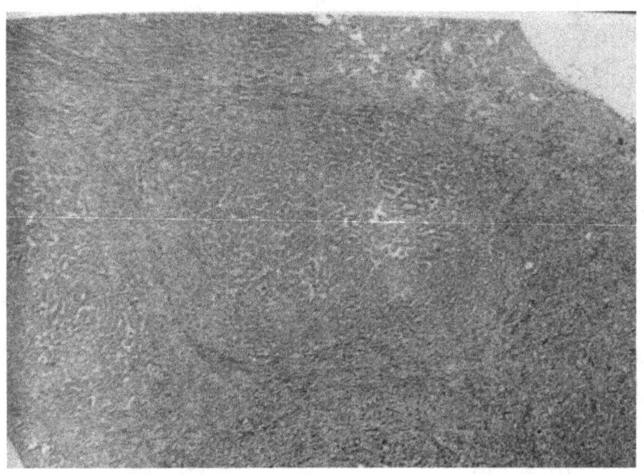

- Portal tract in the center of a regenerative nodule and fibrotic bands bridging central vein
- The size of the scar and the presence of the nodule attest to the long-term course of the fibrotic process
- The bland nature of the cirrhosis is apparent - No inflammatory cells are evident
- The sinusoids are dilated and congested

(Masson trichrome stain; Courtesy of Dr. Edward Lee, Washington, DC)

- Clinical
    - Symptoms and signs of CHF are the predominant features
    - Dull RUQ pain and hepatomegaly are common
    - Liver may be pulsatile if TR present
    - Hepatojugular reflux is often apparent on compression of the liver
    - Spider angioma and varices usually not present

Abbreviations: CHF, congestive heart failure; RUQ, right upper quadrant; TR, tricuspid regurgitation

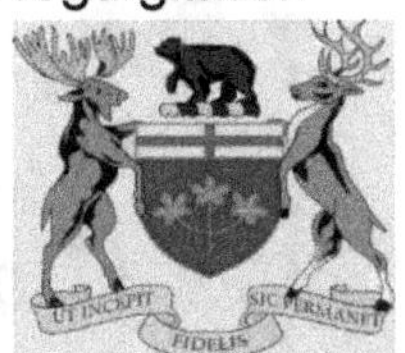

- Laboratory
  - Bloodwork
    - Mild elevation of serum bilirubin
    - Jaundice seen in fewer than 10%, occurring only in the most severe
    - PT is prolonged in more than 75% of cases and is usually resistant to the administration of vitamin K
    - Other liver biochemical tests often normal or mildly elevated
    - Liver tests often improve with treatment of the CHF
- Diagnostic Imaging
  - U/S useful in excluding other Dx
  - CT
    - HSM
    - Ascites
    - Dilation of the IVC and hepatic veins
    - Inhomogenous hepatic enhancement during the portal phase of contrast administration

Abbreviations: HSM, hepatosplenomegaly; IVC, inferior vena cava

- Treatment
  - Paracentesis may be needed if ascites is present
  - Therapy usually aimed at improving cardiac disease
- Prognosis
  - The presence of congestion hepatopathy does not affect the prognosis in patients with CHF
  - Mortality is determined by the severity of liver disease

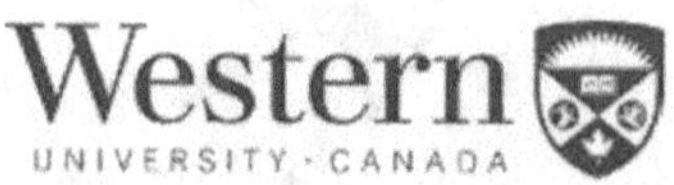

Peliosis Hepatis

- Definition
  - Characterized by the presence of multiple blood-filled cavities distributed randomly throughout the liver
    - Cavities range from few mm to 3cm
  - Seen in association with dilated hepatic sinusoids

- Causes / associations
  - Unknown
  - Leading theories
    - Damage to sinusoidal endothelial cells
    - Outflow obstruction of blood flow at the sinusoidal level
    - Hepatocellular necrosis
  - Associated with drugs, chemical toxins
    - Anabolic steroids
    - OCP
    - Tamoxifen
    - Danazol
    - Vit A
    - Gluccocorticoids
    - 6-Thioguanine
    - Azathioprine
    - Exposure to urethane, vinyl chloride, thorium dioxide
  - Syndrome can regress with discontinuation of offending agent
  - Other associations
    - Myeloproliferative disorders
      - Agnogenic myeloid metaplasia
    - Infections

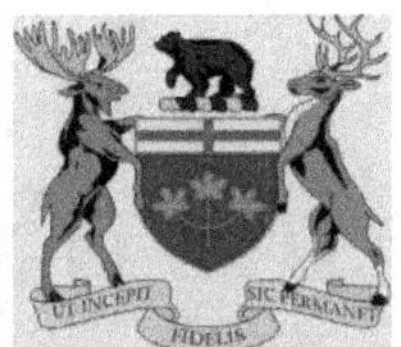

    - *E. coli* pyelonephritis
  - Castleman Disease
    - Giant LN Hyperplasia
- Other associations
  - Myeloproliferative disorders
    - Agnogenic myeloid metaplasia
  - Infections
    - *E. coli* pyelonephritis
  - Castleman Disease
    - Giant LN Hyperplasia
- Seen in 20% of patients post-kidney transplantation
  - Especially after prolonged azathioprine or potentially cyclosporine

- Clinical Features
  - Abnormal liver enzymes

- Pathology
  - Two histologic types:
    - *Parenchymal* type:
      - Blood-filled cavities are lined by hepatocytes
      - Hemorrhagic parenchymal necrosis
      - Congestion
    - *Phlebectatic* type
      - The cavities are lined by endothelial cells
      - Aneurysmal dilation of the central vein
  - Other potential features
    - Fibrosis (may progress)
    - Cirrhosis (portal hypertension)
    - Regenerative nodules
    - Tumours

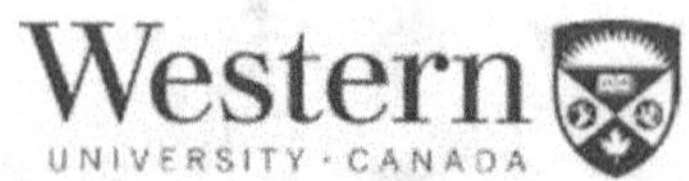

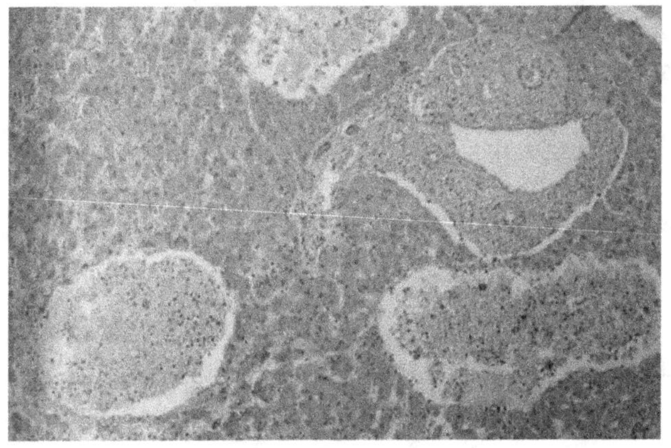

- Blood filled cysts without lining cells and adjacent portal tract
- Sinusoidal dilation

(Courtesy of Dr. Edward Lee, Washington, DC)

Bacillary peliosis

- Causes / associations
  - Caused by *Bartonella*, the bacteria responsible for cat-scratch fever
    - Traumatic exposure to cats is a risk factor
  - Reported in patients with HIV infection, but more commonly with AIDS
- Clinical
  - Anorexia
  - Abdominal pain
  - Fever
  - Lymphadenopathy
  - Cutaneous vascular lesions or nodules
    - Bacillary angiomatosis

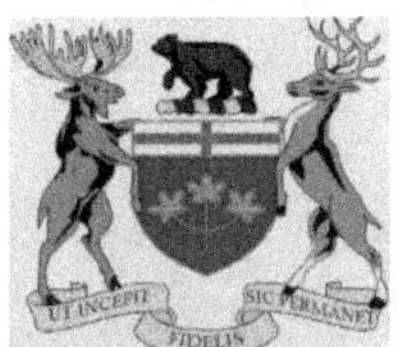

- Liver lesions (Bacillary peliosis)
- Most common:
  - Abnormal liver enzymes in an asymptomatic patient
- Other potential features:
  - Jaundice
  - Painful hepatomegaly
  - Liver failure
  - Fatal hemorrhage

➢ Laboratory

- Anemia
  - Increased ALP
  - Decreased CD4 lymphocyte count <200

➢ Diagnostic imaging

- If the cavities are large enough they can be seen with U/S, CT and MRI

➢ Treatment

- Antibiotics
  - Erythromycin
  - Doxycycline

➢ Prognosis

- Lesions may resolve with stopping azathioprine
- Overall course doesn't change
- Risk of transplant rejection is high

Hepatic Artery Aneurysm

➢ Demography

- Uncommon
- Second leading cause of visceral artery aneurysms (after splenic artery aneurysms)
  - Accounts for >20% of cases

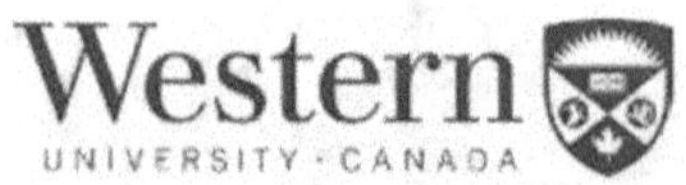

VASCULAR DISEASES OF THE LIVER

- Causes, associations
  - In the past mainly mycotic (infectious)
  - Now:
    - Athersclerosis
    - Mediointimal degeneration
    - Trauma
    - Infection (less commonly)
  - 50% are pseudoaneurysms resulting from injury
    - Liver biopsy
    - Transhepatic biliary drainage
    - Cholecystectomy
    - Hepatectomy
    - Liver transplantation
  - Rare causes:
    - Vasculitidies such as polyarteritis nodosum, systemic lupus erythematosis, Takayasu arteritis, Kawasaki disease
    - CTD (connective tissue diseases): Marfan Syndrome, Ehlers-Danlos syndrome, Osler-Weber-Rendu disease

- Clinical
  - Epigastric or right subchondral pain
  - Most are asymptomatic until rupture
  - Rarely pulsatile RUQ mass or thrill
  - Rupture
    - Into the biliary tree
      - with hemobilia
      - epigastric pain
      - Icterus
    - Into the portal vein
      - Portal HTN
      - Variceal bleeding

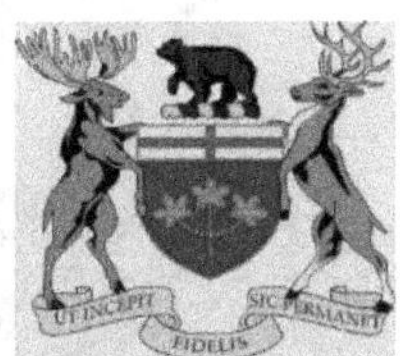

- Into the peritoneal cavity
  - Abdominal pain
  - Shock

➢ Diagnostic imaging

- Doppler U/S and CT demonstrate HAA's
- Angiography is particularly useful for defining lesions, assessing collateral circulation, and planning treatment

➢ Treatment

- Pseudoaneuryms are treated with embolization
- True extrahepatic aneurysms are treated with
  - Embolization
  - Surgical resection

➢ Prognosis

- Mortality from rupture is >30%
- Non-atherosclerotic aneurysms and multiple HAA's carry high risk of rupture, and should be treated
- Risk of rupture is dependent on size
  - Greater than 2 cm in diameter should be treated

Hepatic Artery Atherosclerosis

- Rarely causes liver disease
- Develops later than cardiac atherosclerosis
- Associated with
  - Development of HAA's
  - Ischemic cholangiopathy (as CBD derives its blood supply from the hepatic artery)
- May prevent use of liver for orthoptic transplantation

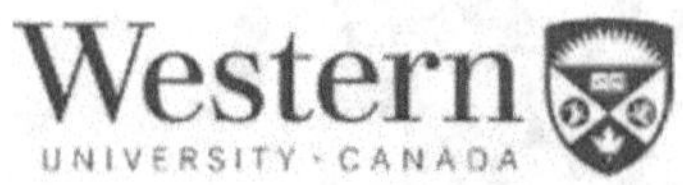

NAFLD and Alcoholic Liver Disease

Melanie Beaton

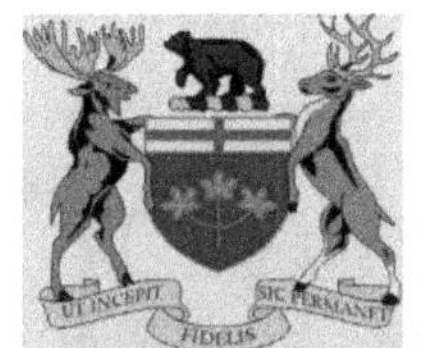

Alcoholic Liver Disease (ALD)

- Demography
  - Alcoholism
    - 15-20 million Americans
    - 100,000 deaths/y
  - Female Gender
    - 2-4X risk than males, at similar intake
  - Responsible for 40% of liver related deaths
  - #3 cause of preventable mortality (cigarettes & obesity, #1 & 2)
  - Alcohol Intake
    - Relative risk (RR) of alcoholic liver disease (ALD) rises at > 30 g/d alcohol
      - Small absolute risk
    - Even at > 60-80 g/d, only 5-15% develop ALD
    - *"Safe"* levels of alcohol ingestion
      - Women 10 g/d, Men 20g/d
      - 1 drink = 12 g alcohol
        - Beer -12 oz, Wine - 6 oz, Liquor - 1 oz

"We are inherently critical as scientists, and inherently kind as physicians."

Grandad

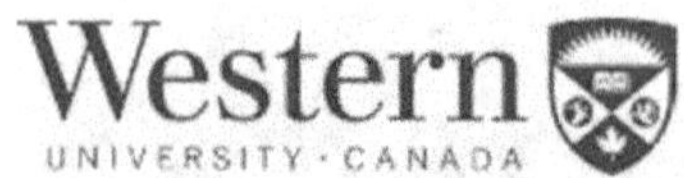

NAFLD AND ALCOHOLIC LIVER DISEASE

➢ Spectrum

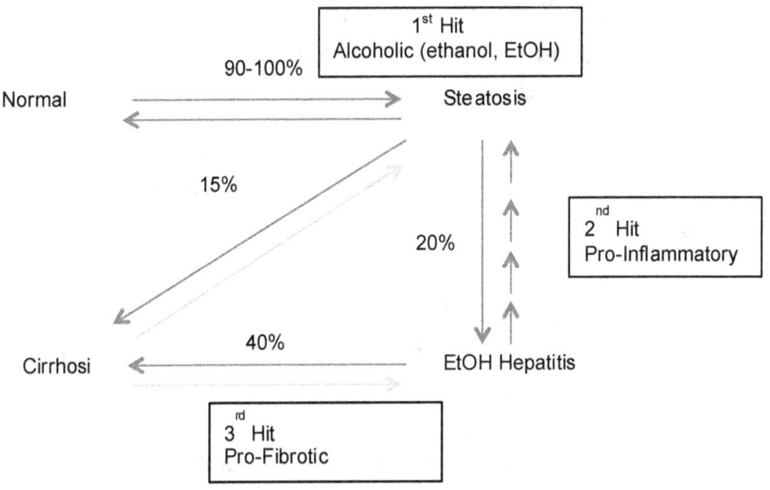

➢ Causes / associations

- Give 5 reasons why only a small % of heavy EtOH drinkers develop ALD.
  - Genetic variation in EtOH metabolizing enzymes
    - Alcohol dehydrogenase (ADH)
  - Genetic variation in response to damage
    - Pro-inflammatory genes (eg. TNF)
    - Autoimmune predisposition
  - Nutritional Status
    - Under- & "Over-" nutrition
  - Co-factors
    - Drugs/Toxins, Iron, α1AT deficiency
    - Hepatotropic viral infection (HBV, HCV, HIV)

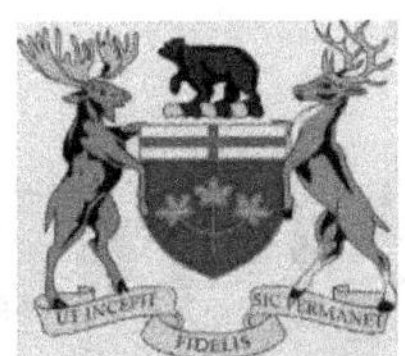

- Pathophysiology
  - Ethanol (EtOH) Absorption
    - Absorbed from Small Intestine & Stomach
    - SIBO aldehyde
    - ↑ gut permeability
    - ↑ bacterial LPS (endotoxin) absorption
  - EtOH metabolism
    - Catabolized by:
      - Cytosol: ADH
        - Metabolism of Acetaldehyde → Acetate is slowed
        - Acetaldehyde accumulates → ↑ acetaldehyde protein adducts (neoantigens)
      - Microsomes: CYP2E1
        - With chronic ingestion, microsomal enzyme oxidation system (MEOS) are induced, and generate O_2 free-radicals (aka reactive oxygen species, ROS)
      - Mitochondria: ↑ NADH, ↓ NAD+, ↑ NADH / NAD
  - ↑ hepatic Fat
    - ↓ FA oxidation → ↓ fat export from liver
    - ↑ peripheral lipolysis & ↑ TG synthesis → ↑ fat accumulates in liver
  - ↑ Kupffer cell activity
    - Production ↑ TNFα, IL-1b, IL-1, IL18
    - Hepatocyte damage

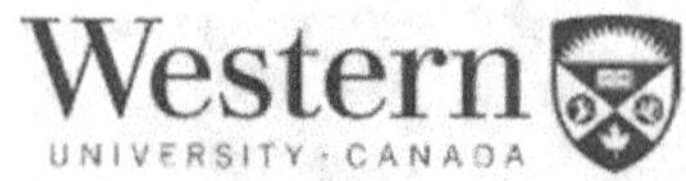

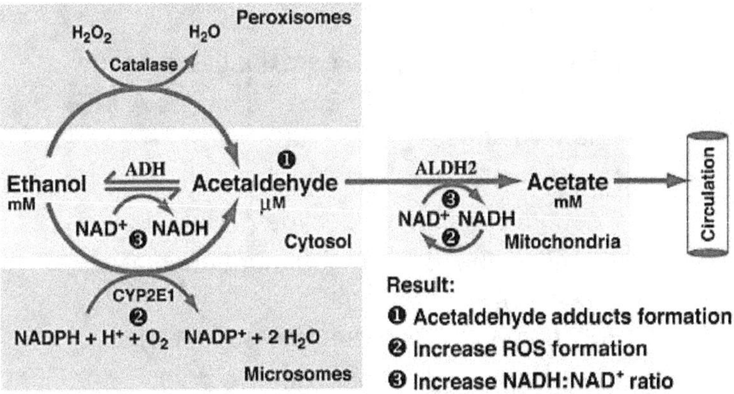

Peroxisomes
H_2O_2 H_2O
Catalase
Ethanol mM
ADH
Acetaldehyde µM ❶
NAD^+ ❸ NADH
Cytosol
ALDH2
Acetate mM
❸ NAD^+ NADH ❷
Mitochondria
Circulation
CYP2E1 ❷
$NADPH + H^+ + O_2$ $NADP^+ + 2\ H_2O$
Microsomes

Result:
❶ Acetaldehyde adducts formation
❷ Increase ROS formation
❸ Increase NADH:NAD⁺ ratio

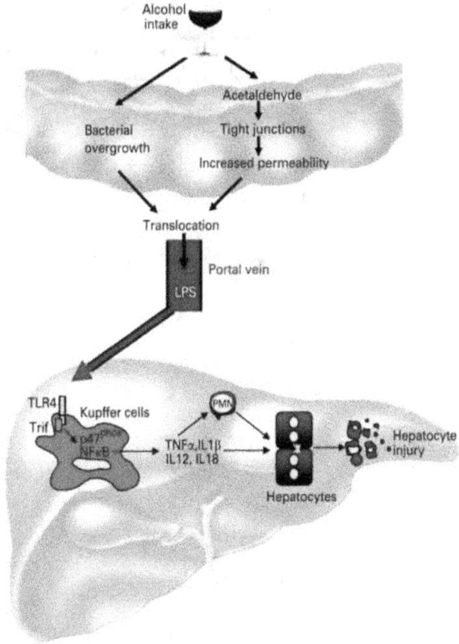

- Gut endotoxins
  - ADH → ↑ TJ leakiness →
    - ↑ Gut permeability of LPS
    - ↑ bacterial overgrowth (SIBO)

Alcohol intake
Acetaldehyde
Tight junctions
Increased permeability
Bacterial overgrowth
Translocation
Portal vein
LPS
TLR4
Trif
Kupffer cells
p47phox
NFκB
TNFα, IL1β, IL12, IL18
PMN
Hepatocytes
Hepatocyte injury

- ↑ Kupffer cell activity
  - ↑ TNFα

Abbreviation: LPS, lipopolysaccharides; SIBO, small intestinal bacterial overgrowth; TNFα, tumor necrosis factor alpha

Source: Wheeler M. Alcohol Res Health. 2003; 27(4) 300-6; Zakhari S et al. Alcohol Res Health. 2006; 29 (4) 245-54.

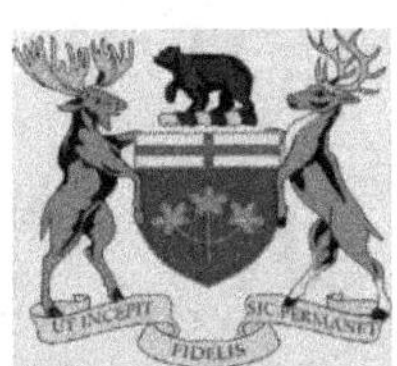

- Oxidative Damage
  - ↑ Free radicals → lipid peroxidative damage
  - ↓ Antioxidants (Glutathione, Vit amins A & E) → oxidative stress
  - ↑ oxidative stress
  - ↑ neoantigens (acetaldehyde-protein adducts)
    - Antibodies to APA → immune-mediated damage
  - Polymorphonuclear leukocytes (PMNs)
    - Attracted by lipid peroxidative damage & neoantigens
    - PMN release proinflammatory cytokines, leukotrienes, prostagladins
- Proliferation of stellate cells → transformation into myofibroblasts → collagen deposition, fibrosis → cirrhosis

➢ Progression to Cirrhosis

	5yr Mortality	
	Abstinent	Drinking
○ All alcoholics	35%	60%
○ No complications	10%	30%
○ Complications	40%	70%

- The worse prognosis in ALD is the presence of alcoholic hepatitis and continued drinking

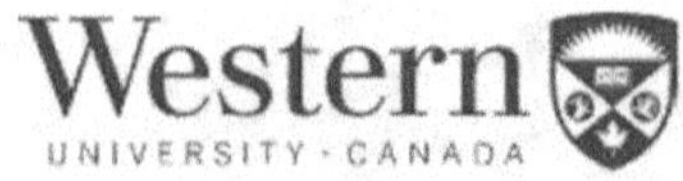

- Treatment
  - Manage the associated
    - Alcoholism
    - Psychosocial issues
    - Nutrition
    - Hepatic complications
      - Alcoholic hepatitis
      - Cirrhosis

Alcoholic Hepatitis (AH)

- Laboratory
  - AST: ALT > 2
    - Reduced ALT activity
    - Alcohol-induced depletion of hepatic pyridoxal 5'-phosphate
    - Increased hepatic mitochondrial aspartate
  - ↑ WBC (PMN)
  - ↑ Bilirubin
  - ↑ INR

"We know what we are, but know not what we may be."

William Shakespeare

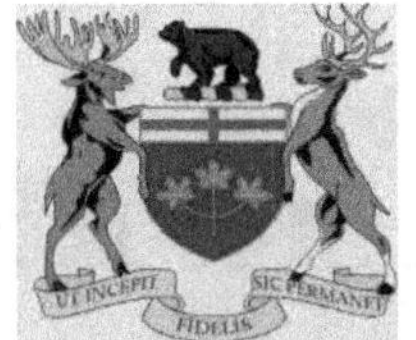

- Pathology

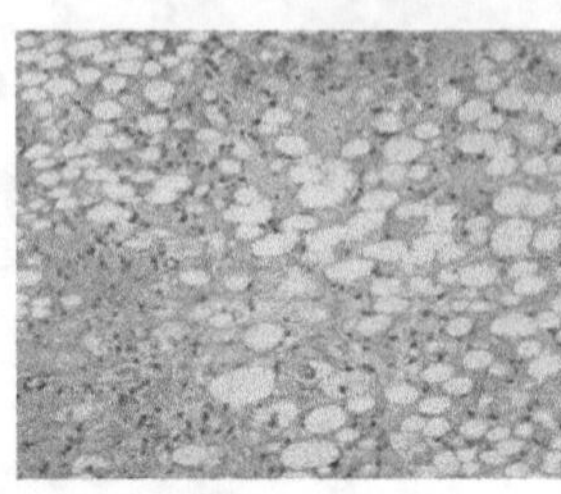

-Steatosis (Macro & Microvesicular)
-Mallory Bodies
-PMN infiltration zone
-Perivenular (3) Inflammation

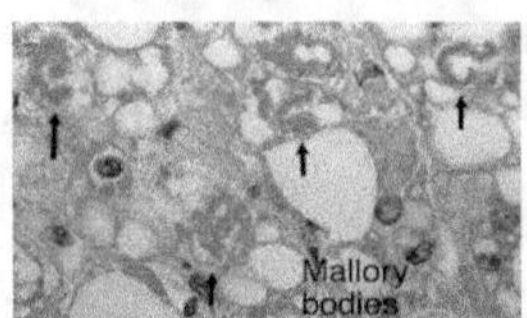

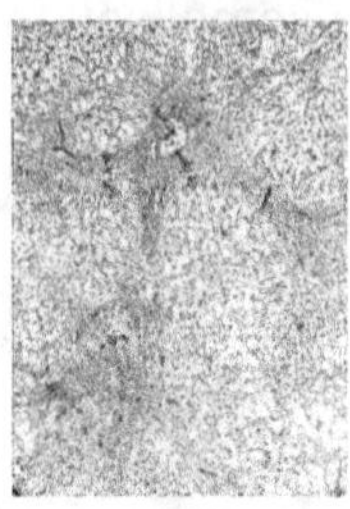

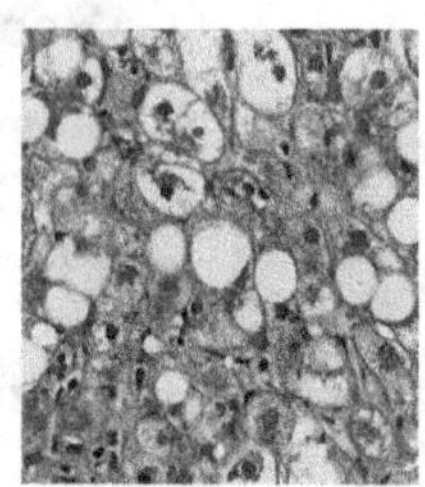

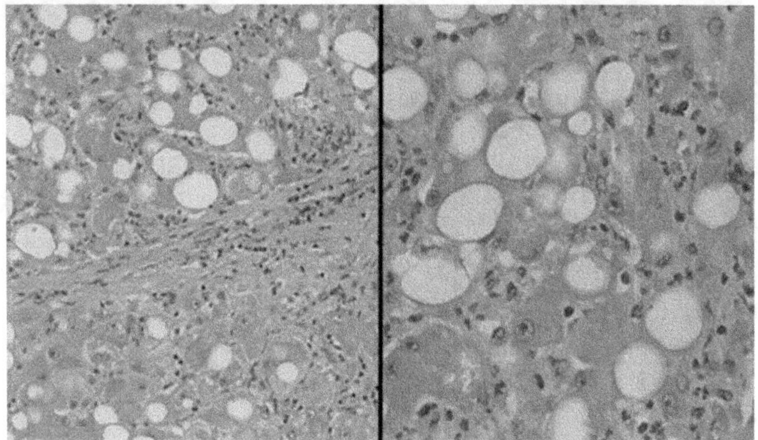

- Risk Stratification (Prognosis Scores)
  - Maddrey Discriminant Function (DF)
    - DF>32 high short-term mortality (50% at 1mo)
    - Used to determine need for CS Rx
    - DF = 4.6(PT- Control PT) + Total Bili/17
  - Presence of Ascites & Bili > 176

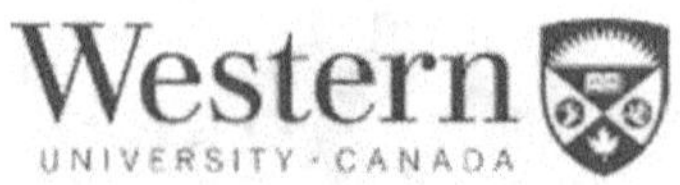

- ↑ Creatinine
  - Ominous
  - Often portends onset of HRS (hepatorenal syndrome)
- MELD Score
  - Designed to predict risk of dying while waiting for liver transplantation
  - Predict 30 & 90 d mortality rate
  - MELD Score = 10 * ((0.957 * ln (Creatinine)) + (0.378 * ln(Bilirubin)) + (1.12 * ln(INR))) + 6.43
  - www.mayoclinic.org/meld/mayomodel7.html
- Other scores
  - Glasgow AH Score, Lille Score, ABIC Scores, Child-Pugh (C-P) Score

Source: Srikureja, Hepatol 2005; Dunn, Hepatol 2005; Sheth, BMC Gastro 2002

- Treatment
  - Monitor for and treat acute ethanol withdrawal
  - Search for possible infection
    - *AH as a cause of fever is a diagnosis of exclusion!*
  - Nutrition
    - Thiamine, Folate, B6, Phosphate, Mg, vitamin K
    - Enteral preferred
    - Do not routinely restrict protein
    - BCAA may be helpful if HE develops during feeding
  - Corticosteroids
    - Multiple trials, mixed results

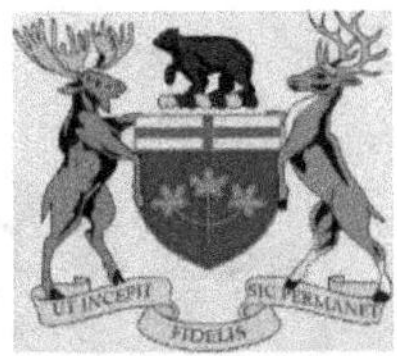

- 3 Meta-analyses:
  - Short-term mortality reduced if encephalopathy is also present (Source: Imperiale, Annals IM, 1990 & Reynolds, Gastro Intl 1989)
  - Studies too heterogenous, No significant effect on mortality (Source: Cochrane Review, Rambaldi, APT 2008)

- Pentoxifylline (PTX)
  - Inhibitor of TNF synthesis
  - Alternative to Prednisolone for severe AH
    - Especially if Prednisolone contraindicated
  - 400 mg po tid x 4wk
  - Meta-analysis (5 trials, N=336)
    - *"A possible benefit [of pentoxifylline] on mortality and HRS and a possible increase in serious and non-serious adverse events"*

- Other Drugs Investigated (+, helpful; -, not helpful)
  - Etanercept (-), Infliximab (-), PTU (+/-), SaME, Insulin + Glucagon (+/-), Silymarin (Milk Thistle) (-), Colchicine (-), Insulin (+), PTK, glucagon (+/-), Etanercept, SAM

- Guidelines

AASLD & ACG Consensus Statement 2009

- Mild/Mod AH (DF<32) w/o HE + Improvement in Bilirubin or decline in DF during 1st wk
  - Nutritional support & abstinence

- Severe AH (DF ≥32) +/- HE & no contraindications to steroids
  - Prednisolone 40mg/d x 4wk, then d/c or taper over 2-4 wk

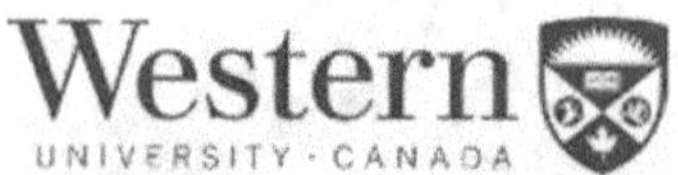

Liver Transplantation

- Survival similar to non-EtOH indications
- Recidivism
  - 1y 10-15%
  - 5y 25-50-%
- Strategies to reduce recidivism
  - Family Supports
  - New Social Circle
  - Social worker / Psychologist
  - Addiction Rehabitation Program (e.g. AA)
  - No other substance abuse
  - Treat psychiatric problems (depression)
  - Develop supportive MD-Patient relationship
- Aware of the HUGE role addiction plays in the alcoholic's life
- As physicians we must acknowledge that for many of these patients, the addiction will 'win' but if we are able to develop a trusting, non-judgmental relationship with patients and their families the chance of success in abstaining is greater
- State clearly and honestly that ongoing use is harmful to their health as well as family/social/professional relationships
- Listen effectively, picking up on non-verbal cues)
- Elicite& synthesizerelevant information & perspectives from the patient, their family & other professionals (i.e. Social Work, Support Groups, Church/Cultural groups)
- Requires far more from us than simply telling them that they need to quit drinking

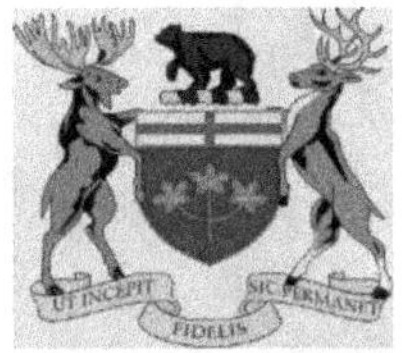

NAFLD (NON-ALCOHOLIC FATTY LIVER DISEASE)

- Demography (General US Adult Population)
  - NHANES III (N=15,700)
    - Assessed NAFLD with aminotransferases
    - *General prevalence of NAFLD 5.5%*
  - Dallas Heart Study (N=2,200)
    - Assessed with liver imaging
    - *General prevalence of fatty liver ~31%*
    - Most (79%) do not exhibit aminotransferase elevations
    - Responsible for ≈90% asymptomatic ↑LFTs when other causes excluded

NAFLD Prevalence
5.5-31%

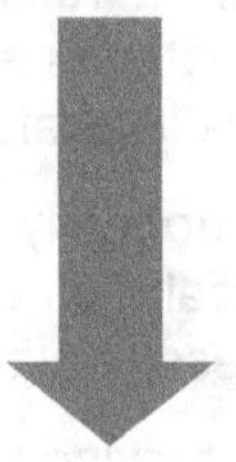

3-10X more prevalent than HCV (1.8% population)

- Pathology
  - NAFLD: Spectrum of Disease

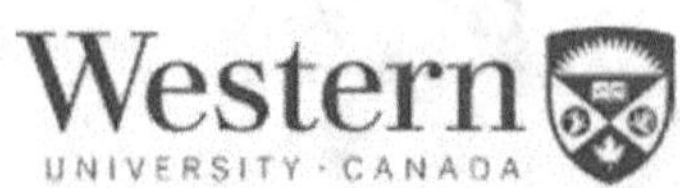

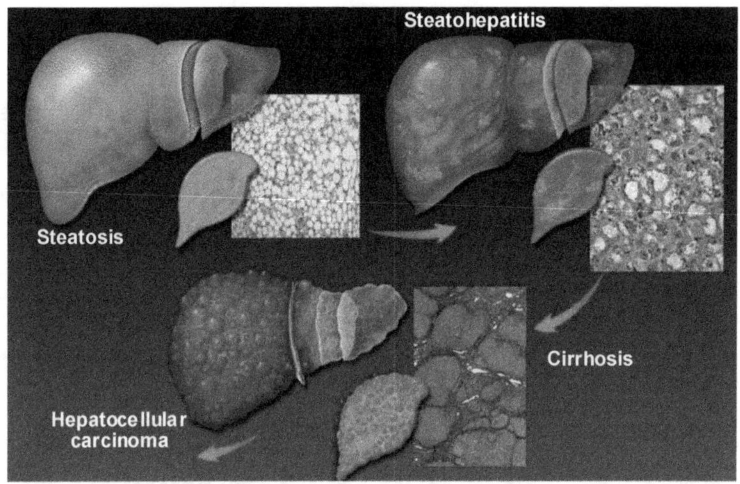

Source: American Gastroenterological Association

- Natural History of NAFLD / NASH

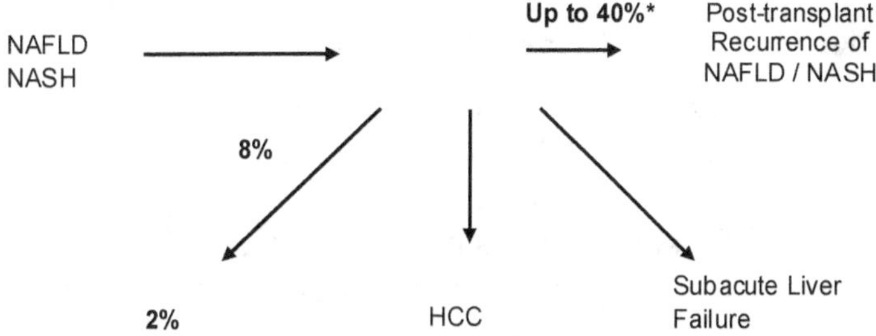

  - NASH shows more consistent and rapid progression to cirrhosis than NAFLD

Source: *Dureja P, et al. Transplantation 2011 ;91(6):684-9; Matteoni C, et al. Gastroenterology 1999; 116:1413-9; McCullough AJ. Clin Liver Dis 2004;8:521-33.

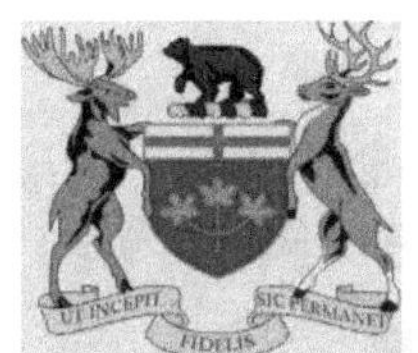

➢ Causes, associations (comorbidities)

Established conditions	Emerging conditions
o Obesity	– Obstructive sleep apnea
o Types 2 diabetes glucose intolerance	– Hypothyroidism
o Dyslipidemia	– Obstructive sleep apnea
o Metabolic syndrome	– Hypopituitarism
	– Polycystic ovary syndrome

Source: Vuppalanchi R and Chalasani N. Hepatology 2009;49:306-17.

➢ Special consideration

- **NAFLD & Cardiovascular Disease**
  - o Association with CV Risk Factors
    - – Obesity, DM, Metabolic syndrome
    - – ↓ Plasma Adiponectin*
    - – ↑ Plasma markers of lipid peroxidation*
    - – ↓ Hepatic synthesis of apolipoprotein B-100*
  - o Association with CV Disease
    - – ↑ carotid artery intima-media thickness
    - – ↑ carotid atherosclerotic plaques
    - – ↑ rate of coronary, cerebrovascular and peripheral vascular disease

*Independent of metabolic syndrome

Source: Targher G. Diabetic Med 2007;24(1):1-6.

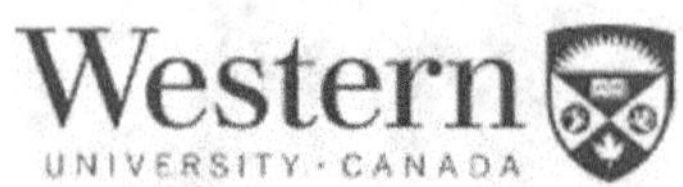

- NAFLD and Type 2 DM

Prevalence of NAFLD is high
- ~50% on U/S
- 70% on biopsy

NASH
- 10-20%
- *Extensive fibrosis/cirrhosis not uncommon*

Source: Gupte P, et al. J Gastroenterol Hepatol. 2004;19(8):854-8; Tolman KG, et al. Ann Intern Med 2004;141(12):946-56.

- **HCV and Insulin Resistance**
  - Host-Related
    - BMI >25
    - Diet
    - Race
    - Age
    - Family history of diabetes
    - Sedentary Lifestyle
  - Viral-related
    - Genotype 3
    - ↑ inflammatory cytokines
    - ↑ Oxidative stress
    - ↑ fatty acid synthesis
    - ↓ PPARα expression
- NAFLD and HCV Genotype 3
  - Greater degrees of steatosis
    - Direct pathogenicity of virus vs. combination of viral & host factors
    - High viral overload related to severity of steatosis

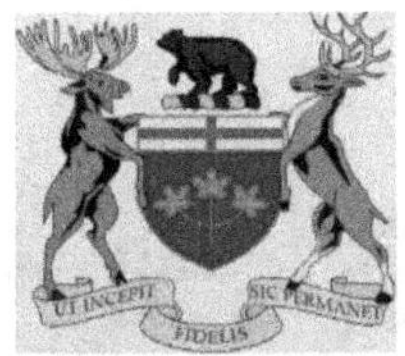

- Also worse prognosis with HIV or HIV plus HCV infection
- Steatosis & Insulin resistance (IR) are each linked to fibrosis progression
- BMI, waist circumference, IR & steatosis:
  - All independently associated with disease progression and lower SVR
- Poorer response to therapy

- If SVR (sustained viral response) achieved, steatosis often reversible

Source: Adinolfi LE, al. Hepatology. 2001;33(6):1358-64.

- NAFLD and other commonly associated diseases
  - TPN
    - NAFLD can occur rapidly
    - Typically reversible
  - Intestinal Surgery
    - J-I Bypass, Gastroplasty, Extensive SB resection
    - Small intestinal bacterial overgrowth (SIBO)
  - Metabolic Disorders
    - Metabolic Syndrome
    - Abetalipoprotenemia
    - Wilson Disease
    - Glycogen storage disease

Source: Svegliati-Baroni G, et al. Gut 2007;56(9):1296-301; Poynard T, et al. J Hepatol. 2003;38(4):518-20; Castera L, et al. Gut 2003 ;52(10):1531

- Treatment
  - Modify treatable risk factors
    - Insulin resistance
    - Hyperlipidemia
    - At-risk lifestyle

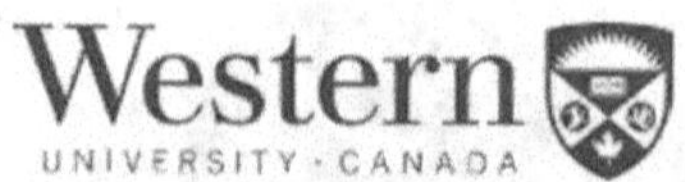

- Stop hepatotoxic drugs & those associated with steatosis, e.g.
  - EtOH, MTX, Steroids, Tamoxifen, TPN, Amiodarone, Valproate
- Lifestyle Modification
  - First line therapy
    - ↑ Insulin sensitivity
    - ↓ Adipose tissue inflammation
    - ↓ Hepatic supply of free fatty acids
  - Modest (10%) ↓ weight improves LFTs & liver histology
- Pharmacologic agents studied in NASH
  - Insulin sensitizers
    - Troglitazone
    - Pioglitazone
    - Rosiglitazone
    - Metformin
  - Antioxidants
    - Vitamin E
    - Vitamin C
    - Betaine
  - Cytoprotective agents
    - Ursodeoxycholic acid (UDCA)
    - Taurine
    - Lecithin
    - Silymarin
      - Carotene
    - Metadoxine

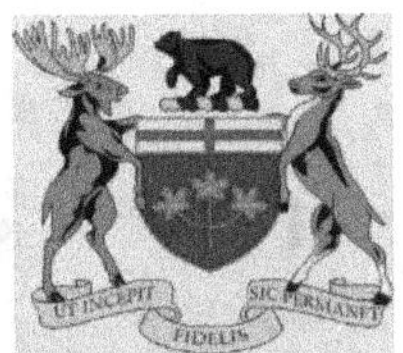

- Antihyperlipidemic agents
  - Clofibrate
  - Gemfibrozil
  - Atorvastatin
  - Pravastatin
  - Probucol
  - Omega-3 fatty acids
- Antiobesity drugs
  - Orlistat
  - Sibutramine
- Novel treatments
  - Losartan
  - Probiotics
  - Lactulose
  - Pentoxifylline
  - Oligofructose
  - Nateglinide

- Insulin sensitizing agents (metformin, TZD, Gliptins)
- Lipid lowering drugs (statins, fibrates)

Insulin Sensitizers

- Metformin
  - Small studies, short duration, many with incomplete histologic follow-up
  - Improved LFTs, steatosis & inflammation in most studies
    - Benefit on fibrosis in only one trial
  - Benefit in DM patients with NAFLD not known
    - *Potential significant as DM is a major risk factor for NAFLD & its progression to NASH!*

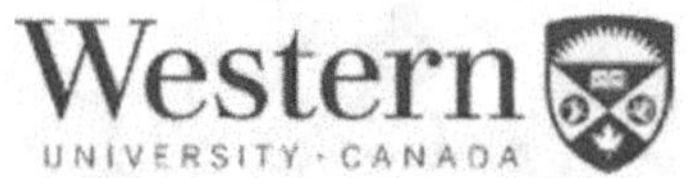

- Glitizones
    - ↑ Fatty acid oxidation & decrease its synthesis in hepatocytes
    - ↑ insulin sensitivity
    - ↑ Circulating adiponectin levels
    - Problems
        - Weight gain
        - Hepatotoxicity
        - Possible
        - Indefinite therapy needed (relapse after withdrawal)

Vitamin E

- 247 Non-diabetic NASH patients
- Pioglitazone 30 mg vs. Vit E 800 IU vs. Placebo for 96 wk
- Pioglitazone and vitamin E vs. placebo
    - ↓ ALT, ↓ AST, ↓ IR
- Large systematic review of antioxidant trials showed ↑ risk of death
    - Doses of vitamin E >400 IU ↑all cause of mortality
    - Likely ↑ risk of prostate cancer

Source: Sarnyal AJ, et al. N Engl J Med. 2010;362(18):1675-85.

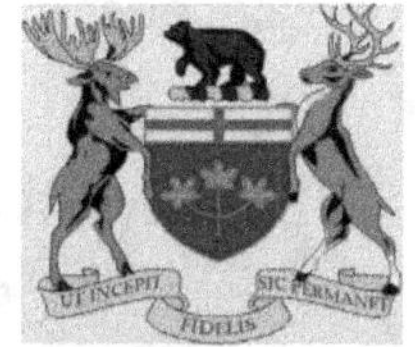

Bariatric Surgery

- Difficult to achieve sustained weight loss via lifestyle modification
- Surgery increasingly popular with patients
- Newer techniques demonstrate benefit on liver histology of NAFLD NASH

Source: Mattar SG, et al. Ann Surg 2005; ;242(4):610-7; Clark JM, et al. Obes Res 2005;13(7):1180-6.

- Suggested management based on risk stratification
  - Those with mild elevations in liver enzymes, normal liver function tests, no signs of portal hypertension, normal FibroScan, mild histology (NAS < 4, no Fibrosis)
  - Diet & Lifestyle
  - Compassionate physician support
  - BMI <35, NAS ≥4, any Fibrosis
    - No DM: Vit E (800 IU/d)
    - DM: Vit E or Pioglitazone (need to assess risk/benefit ratio of pioglitazone in each patient)
  - BMI >35, DM, NAS ≥ 4, fibrosis, plus comorbidities
    - OSA (obstructive sleep apnea)
    - CAD (coronary artery disease)
    - Dyslipidemia
    - Consider Bariatric surgery on case-by-case basis
  - NASH Cirrhosis
    - Diet & lifestyle
    - No evidence to support any drug therapy
    - Monitor for complications of cirrhosis

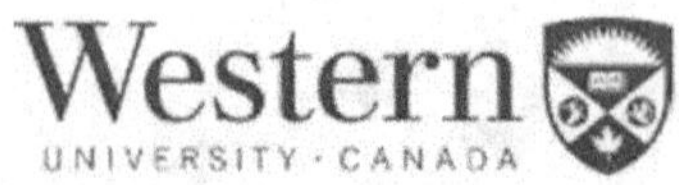

- Follow annually with
  - History and physical examination
  - Laboratory testing
    - Liver enzyme / function tests
  - FibroScan
  - Diabetic tests
  - Fasting lipid profile
- Continued encouragement re weight loss, exercise
- Careful monitoring for & treatment of hypertension, diabetes and dyslipidemia
- As these patients are often followed by a number of health care providers (yourself, GP, Endocrinologist, Dietician +/- Cardiologist), clear and accurate delivery of information to these individuals, as well as to the patient's family helps to facilitate better care, and better outcomes.
- Good communication is one of the most important factors in fostering patient satisfaction (*and as an added bonus, physician satisfaction!)*

"With the new day comes new strength and new thoughts."

Eleanor Roosevelt

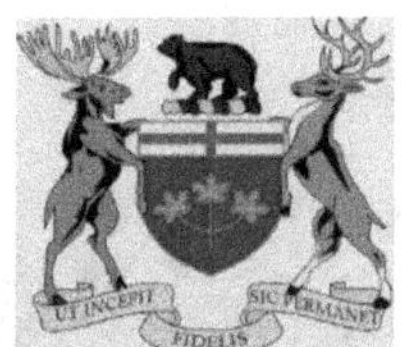

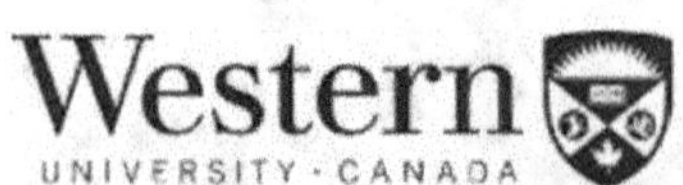

MINI UPDATE

Complications of Portal Hypertension

Mohammed Aljawad

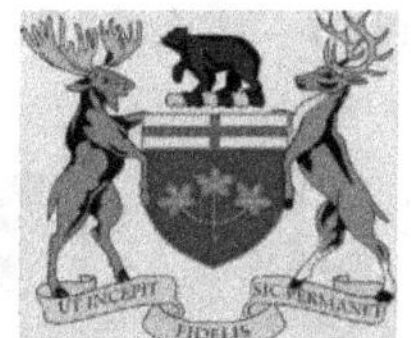

Stigmata of Chronic Liver Disease

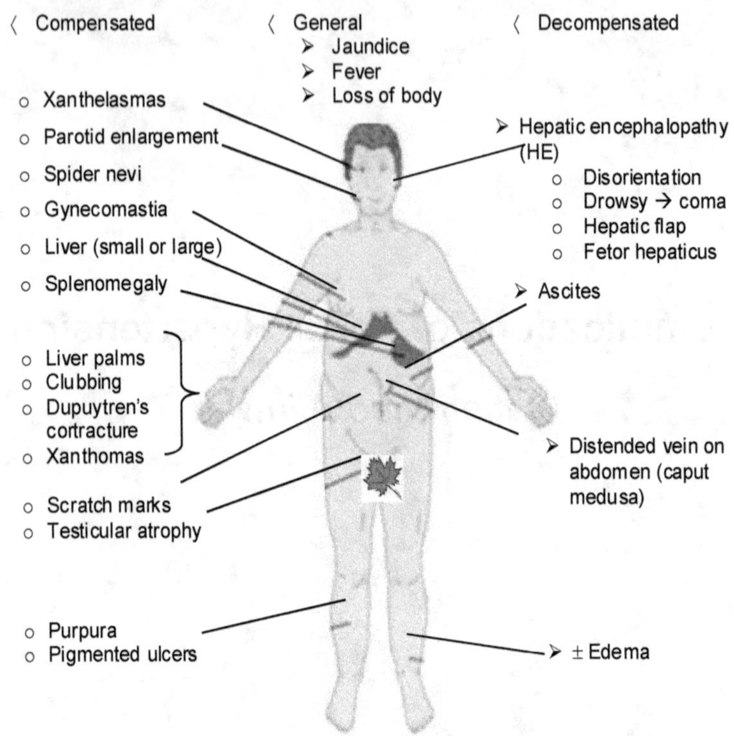
〈 Compensated
〈 General
➢ Jaundice
➢ Fever
➢ Loss of body
〈 Decompensated
o Xanthelasmas
o Parotid enlargement
o Spider nevi
o Gynecomastia
o Liver (small or large)
o Splenomegaly
o Liver palms
o Clubbing
o Dupuytren's cortracture
o Xanthomas
o Scratch marks
o Testicular atrophy
o Purpura
o Pigmented ulcers
➢ Hepatic encephalopathy (HE)
o Disorientation
o Drowsy → coma
o Hepatic flap
o Fetor hepaticus
➢ Ascites
➢ Distended vein on abdomen (caput medusa)
➢ ± Edema

Refractory Ascites

- Definition
  - No response to Na^+- restriction and high-dose diuretics (no weight loss)

- Demography
  - Occur in < 10 % of ascites patients
  - Compliance :
    - 24 hr urine Na^+ > 78 mmol /d
    - Spot urine Na^+/K^+ ratio > 1

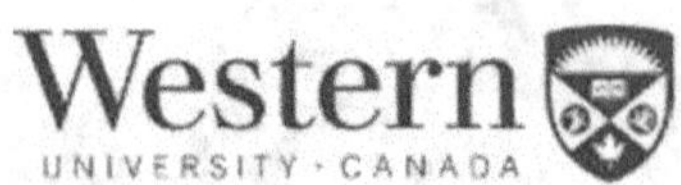
Western
UNIVERSITY · CANADA

Ascites

- Definition
  - Accumulation of free fluid in the peritoneal cavity
  - Ascites is the most common complication of cirrhosis

- Pathogenesis
  - Portal HTN : portal pressure >12 mm Hg is required for fluid retention in the peritoneal cavity
  - Vasodilation and hyperdynamic circulation
    - ↑ synthesis of systemic prostacyclin
    - Nitric oxide (NO)
    - ↑ Na^+ & water retention from activation of
      - renin
      - angiotensin
      - ADH
    - Renal vasoconstriction
  - Hypoalbuminemia
  - Imbalance in formation and removal of lymphatic fluid

Abbreviation: ADH, anti-diuretic hormone (vasopressin); HTN, hypertension

- Clinical
  - Ascites
    - Bulging, distention
    - Physical examination

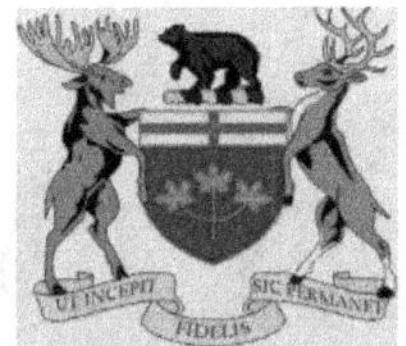

Performance characteristics of physical examination for ascites

Physical sign	Sensitivity	Specificity	PLR	NLR
○ Bulging flanks	0.81	0.59	2.0	0.3
○ Flank dullness	0.84	0.59	2.0	0.3
○ Shifting dullness	0.77	0.72	2.7	0.3
○ Fluid wave	0.62	0.9	6.0	0.4

Abbreviations: NLR, negative likelihood ratio; PLR, positive likelihood ratio
Note: only the presence of a fluid wave has a PLR >3; the puddle sign is not recommended because of patient discomfort, and a PLR <2.

Adapted from: Williams, J W Jr. Simel, D L.. *JAMA*, 1992;267(19):2645-2648

➢ Laboratory

Routine	Optional	Unusual	Unhelpful
○ Cell count	- Amylase	- Bilirubin	- Cholesterol
○ Albumin	- Culture in blood culture bottles	- Cytology	- Fibronectin
○ Total protein	- Glucose	- TB smear, culture, and PCR test	- Lactate
	- Gram stain - LDH	- Triglycerides	- pH

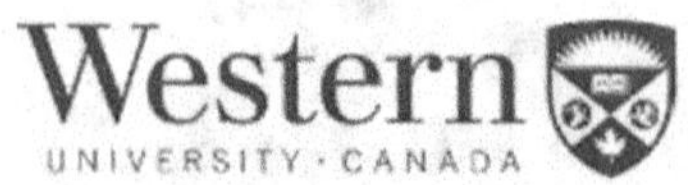

COMPLICATIONS OF PORTAL HYPERTENSION

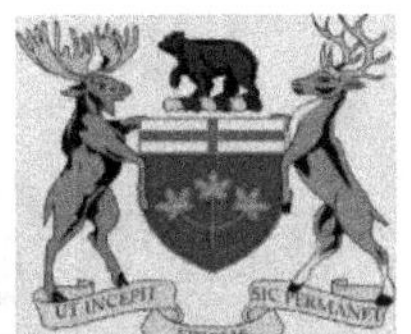

Causes of ascites by SAAG

High SAAG gradient ≥1.1 g/dL (11 g/L)	Low gradient <1.1 g/dL (11 g/L)
○ Alcoholic hepatitis	○ Biliary ascites
○ Budd-Chiari syndrome	○ Bowel obstruction or infarction
○ Cardiac ascites	○ Nephrotic syndrome
○ Cirrhosis	○ Pancreatic ascites
○ Fatty liver of pregnancy	○ Peritoneal carcinomatosis
○ Fulminant hepatic failure	○ Postoperative lymphatic leak
○ Massive liver metastases "Mixed" ascites Myxedema	○ Serositis in connective tissue diseases ○ Tuberculous peritonitis
○ Portal vein thrombosis	
○ Sinusoidal obstruction syndrome	

Abbreviation: SAAG, serum albumin-ascites gradient

Data from: Runyon, BA, Montano, AA, Akriviadis, EA, et al. Ann Intern Med 1992; 117:215

- Complications of ascites
  - Refractory ascites
  - Ascitic Fluid Infection
  - Hepatorenal syndrome (HRS)
  - Cellulitis
  - Tense Ascites
  - Pleural effusion
  - Abdominal Hernias

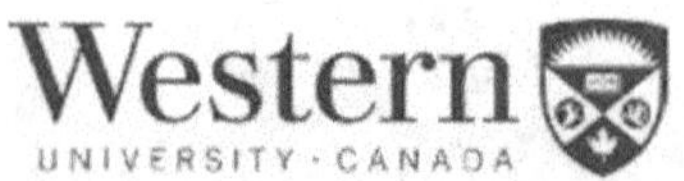

➢ An approach to ascites, based on paracente

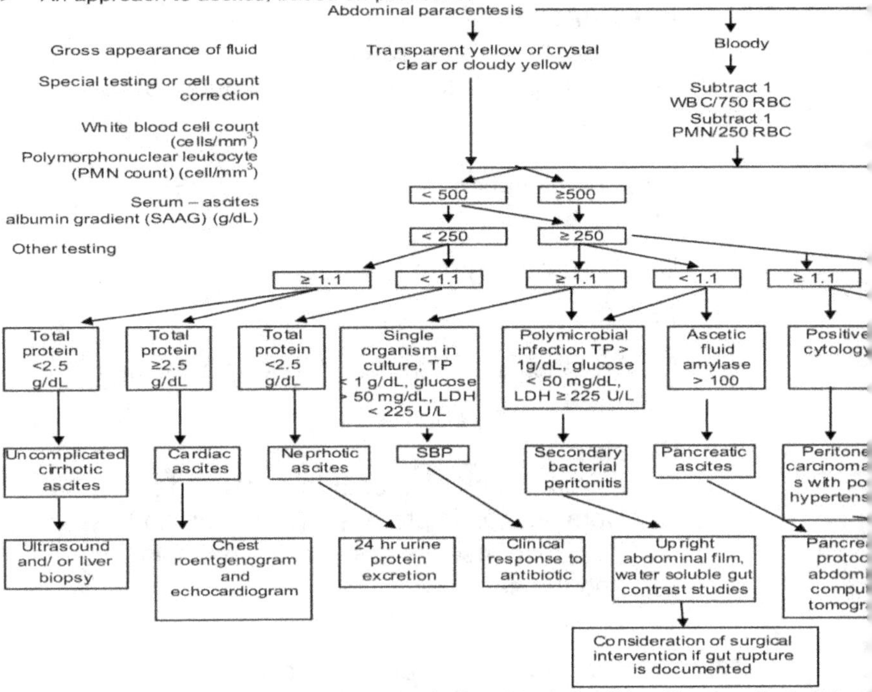

Abdominal paracentesis

Gross appearance of fluid: Transparent yellow or crystal clear or cloudy yellow | Bloody

Special testing or cell count correction: Subtract 1 WBC/750 RBC; Subtract 1 PMN/250 RBC

White blood cell count (cells/mm^3): < 500 | ≥500

Polymorphonuclear leukocyte (PMN count) (cell/mm^3): < 250 | ≥ 250

Serum – ascites albumin gradient (SAAG) (g/dL): ≥ 1.1 | < 1.1 | ≥ 1.1 | < 1.1 | ≥ 1.1

Other testing:

- Total protein <2.5 g/dL → Uncomplicated cirrhotic ascites → Ultrasound and/ or liver biopsy
- Total protein ≥2.5 g/dL → Cardiac ascites → Chest roentgenogram and echocardiogram
- Total protein <2.5 g/dL → Neprhotic ascites → 24 hr urine protein excretion
- Single organism in culture, TP < 1 g/dL, glucose > 50 mg/dL, LDH < 225 U/L → SBP → Clinical response to antibiotic
- Polymicrobial infection TP > 1g/dL, glucose < 50 mg/dL, LDH ≥ 225 U/L → Secondary bacterial peritonitis → Upright abdominal film, water soluble gut contrast studies → Consideration of surgical intervention if gut rupture is documented
- Ascetic fluid amylase > 100 → Pancreatic ascites → Pancrea protoc abdomi compu tomogr
- Positive cytology → Peritone carcinoma s with po hypertens

Modified with permission from: Sleisenger & fordtran's Gastrointestinal and Liver Disease: pathophysiology Feldman, M, Scharschmidt, BF, Sleisenger, MH (Eds), WB Saunders Company 2002. P.1522. Copyright ©

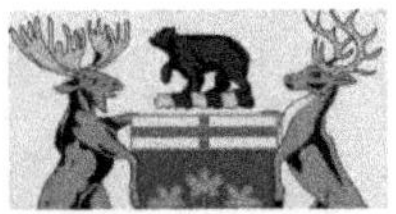

- Treatment
  - Low SAAG
    - Treat underlying cause
    - No response to Na^+ restriction or diuretics
  - High SAAG
  - Treat precipitating factors (e.g. Avoid NSAIDs, ACEI)
  - Diet: ↓ Na : < 2 gm /day
  - Protein restriction : not recommended [3]
  - Fluid restriction : No recommended unless serum Na < 120
  - Diuretics
    - spironolactone superior to furosemide
    - Combination is preferred (100/40 ratio)
    - If no response, increase both spironolactone and furosemide
    - IV diuretics
  - Therapeutic large volume paracentesis (LVP)
    - Single or serial
    - 1st line for tense ascites
    - avoid serial LVP in patients with diuretic-sensitive ascites
  - Albumin replacement paracentesis
    - Albumin not needed for taps < 5 L
    - Albumin is optional for taps > 5 L
    - Dose: 6-8 of albumin per 1 L removed
  - Other options
    - TIPS
    - Peritoneovenous Shunt
    - Liver Transplantation
  - Treatment of complications of ascites

Spontaneous Bacterial Peritonitis (SBP)

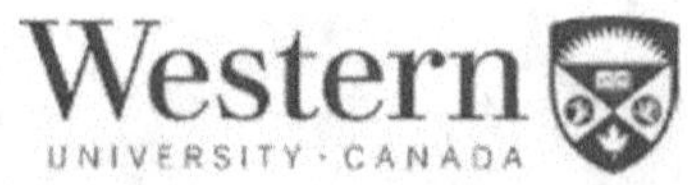

Suggested pathophysiology of SBP and SNNA

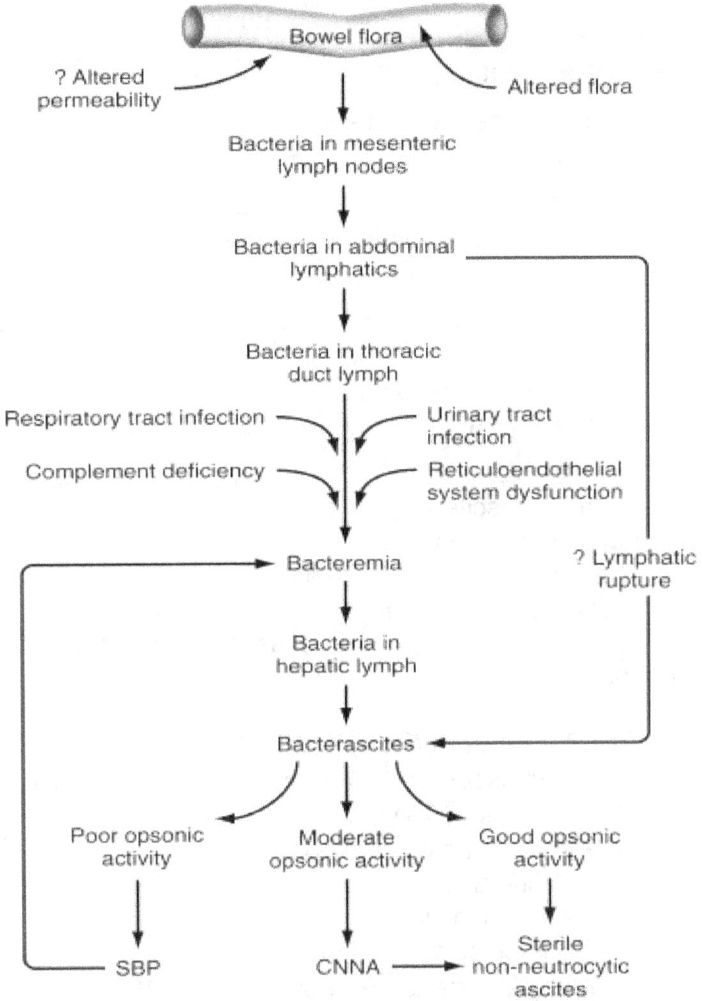

Bowel flora
? Altered permeability
Altered flora
Bacteria in mesenteric lymph nodes
Bacteria in abdominal lymphatics
Bacteria in thoracic duct lymph
Respiratory tract infection
Urinary tract infection
Complement deficiency
Reticuloendothelial system dysfunction
Bacteremia
? Lymphatic rupture
Bacteria in hepatic lymph
Bacterascites
Poor opsonic activity
Moderate opsonic activity
Good opsonic activity
SBP
CNNA
Sterile non-neutrocytic ascites

Abbreviation: SNNA, sterile non-neutrocytic ascites

Source: Sleisenger and Fordtran's. Gastroenterology and Liver Disease 9th Edition, Fig 91-4

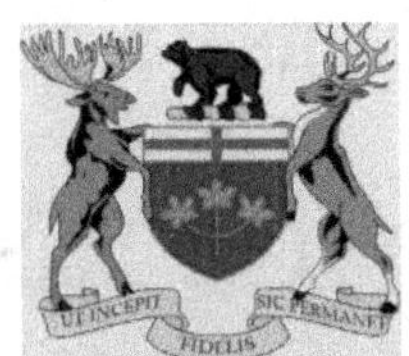

- Ascitic fluid infection variants

Variant	Ascetic fluid culture	Absolute PMN per mm³*
o Surgery not required		
- Spontaneous bacterial peritonitis (SBP)	+	≥ 250
- Culture negative neutrocytic ascites (CNNA)	No growth	≥ 250
- Monomicrobial non-neutrocytic bacterascites (single organism)	+	< 250
- Polymicrobial bacterascites	+	< 250

- Surgery required
  - Secondary bacterial peritonitis with PMN >> 250 PMN per mm³, and a positive polymicrobial culture, is the fifth form of ascetic fluid infection.

*cell count

Secondary Bacterial Peritonitis (SBP)

- ↑ WBC in ascetic fluid tap (> 250 PMN per mm³)
- Other causes of ↑ WBC
  - Peritoneal carcinomatosis
  - Pancreatitis
  - Hemorrhage
  - Tuberculosis
- Aggressive diuresis → may ↑ WBC > 1000
  - Lymphocytes predominate
  - No symptoms
- Bloody tap → falsely high PMN
  - Subtract 1 PMN for each 250 RBCs

Frequency

(%)*

Organism	SBP	Monomicrobial Non-Neutrocytic Bacterascites	Secondary Bacterial Peritonitis
➢ Monomicrobial			
○ *Escherichia coli*	37	27	20
○ *Klebsiella pneumoniae*	17	11	7
○ *Streptococcus pneumoniae*	12	9	0
○ *Streptococcus viridans*	9	2	0
○ *Staphylococcus aureus*	0	7	13
○ Miscellaneous gram-negative	10	14	7
○ Miscellaneous gram-positive	14	30	0
➢ Polymicrobial	1	0	53

Abbreviations: SBP, spontaneous bacterial peritonitis

- Causes, association
  - Risk factors
    - Ascitic fluid total protein < 1 g/dL (<10 g/L)
    - Prior episode of SBP
    - Variceal hemorrhage
    - Total bilirubin > 2.5 mg/dL (42.5 mmol/l)
    - Possibly malnutrition
    - Use of proton pump inhibitors (PPIs)

- Clinical
  - Fever 69 %
  - Abdominal pain 59 %
  - Altered mental status 54 %
  - Abdominal tenderness 49 %

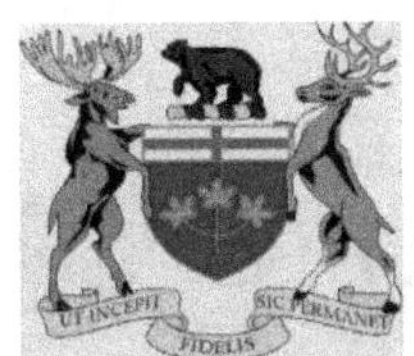

- Diarrhea 32 %
- Paralytic ileus 30 %
- Hypotension 21 %

- Hypothermia 17 %
- No signs or symptoms 13 %
- Associated risk factors

➢ Treatment
- 3rd generation Cephalosporin
  - E.g. Cefotaxime 2 g IV 98 h for 5 days (5 days as good as 10 days)
- Quinolones : if Penciliin allergy
- Oral vs parenteral
  - Similar outcome : Ofloxacin 400 mg twice daily vs parenteral Cefotaxime
- IV albumin plus antibiotic (recommended by AASLD)
- When
  - Serum creatinine >1 mg/dL (77 mmol/l)
  - Total bilirubin >4 mg/dL (68 mmol/l)
- Why
  - 1/3 of persons with SBP develop renal failure (RF)
  - Treating SBP ↑ survival
- Dose :
  - 1.5 g/kg at diagnosis of SBP, on Day 1
  - 1 g/kg on day 3

Abbreviation: AASLD, American Association for the Study of the Liver

➢ Prophylaxis
- Previous SBP
  - long-term prophylaxis with daily norfloxacin or Septra

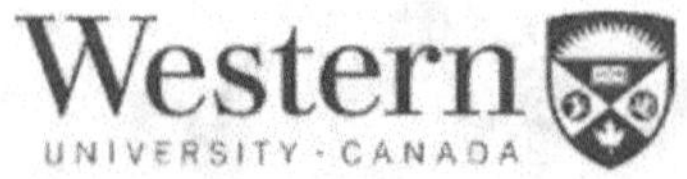

- Cirrhosis, ascites, plus GI bleeding
  - 7 days of ABX
- Cirrhosis and ascites but no GI bleeding, long-term prophylaxis can be justified if
  - the ascitic fluid protein <15 g/L, and at least one of the following is present:
    - serum creatinine ≥1.2 mg/dL (92 mmol/L)
    - serum sodium ≤130 mEq/L,
    - Child-Pugh ≥9 points with bilirubin ≥3 mg/dL (51 mmol/l)
- Note
  - Intermittent dosing of antibiotics to prevent bacterial infections may be inferior to daily dosing

Hepatorenal syndrome (HRS)

- Definition
  - Cirrhosis with ascites plus serum creatinine concentration ≥ 1.5 mg/dL (133 mmol/L)
    - No or insufficient improvement in serum creatinine level after 48 hr of diuretic withdrawal, and adequate volume expansion with intravenous albumin
    - Absence of shock
    - No recent nephrotoxic agents (e.g., NSAIDs)
    - No intrinsic renal disease, ie
      - proteinuria < 500 mg/day,
      - microhematuria < 50 red blood cells/high power field)
      - normal renal ultrasound
  - Develops in ~ 25% per year

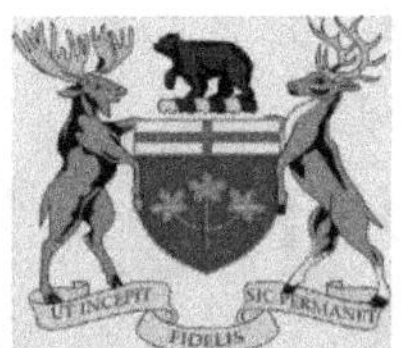

- Demography
  - Incidence, % per year
    - overall, ~25%
    - 10%, ascites, requiring serial large-volume paracentesis
    - 25%, severe alcoholic hepatitis
    - 30%, SBP or other infection
    - 8% to 40% overall

- Pathogenesis
  - Splanchnic arterial vasodilatation
  - ↑ production/ activity of vasodilators :
    - NO
    - Carbon monoxide
    - Glucagon
    - Prostacyclin
  - ↓ effective circulating blood volume
    - ↓ systemic blood pressure ↑ cardiac out put
  - ↑ RAAS/ SNS activity, ↑ plasma ADH
  - Na^+/ H_2O retention, hyponatremia, ascites
  - Renal arterial vasoconstriction/ ↓ GFR
    - NSAIDs
    - ACEIs
    - ARBs

- Types
  - Type 1 :
    - rapidly progressive
    - creatinine level doubles to a value higher than 2.5 mg/dL in a period of two weeks or less
    - triggers :
      - severe bacterial infections
      - gastrointestinal bleeding

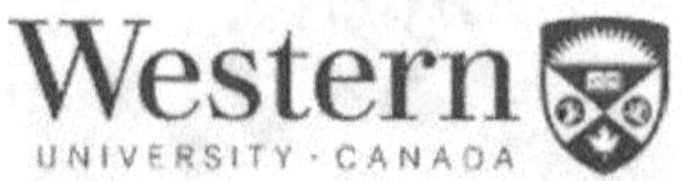

        - surgical procedures
        - acute liver injury

  - Type 2
    - slowly progressive
    - Severe ascites (diuretic resistant) serum
    - creatinine levels lower than 2.5 mg/dL
    - median survival of only six months

- Treatment
  - Prevention
  - Avoid intravascular volume depletion
  - Avoid nephrotoxins
  - Prophylaxis
    - SBP
    - Variceal bleeding
  - Treatment
    - IV albumin
      - 20 -60 g /d
    - Albumin plus
      - Norepinephrine
      - Terlipressin (selective vasopressin 1 agonist)
    - Midodrine and octreotide
      - midodrine (systemic vasoconstrictor), 7.5-12.5 mg po tid
      - octreotide (an inhibitor of endogenous vasodilator release), 100 -200 mic sc tid
    - TIPS
      - Improve hemodynamics and renal function
      - No survival benefits
    - Liver Transplantation
      - Three-year survival rate is approximately 60%

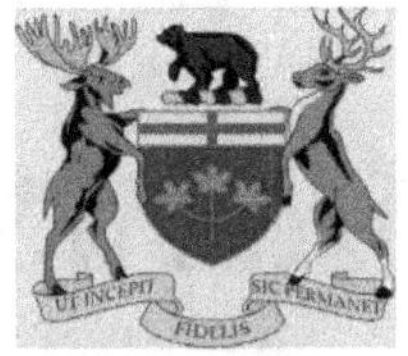

Hepatic Encephalopathy (HE)

- Definition: Transient and reversibly impaired intellectual and neuromuscular function, usually found in patients with chronic liver disease and portal hypertension, but also seen in patients with acute liver failure

- Demography
  - Prevalence - 50% to 70% of patients with cirrhosis
  - Survival after appearance of HE
    - 1 yr, 42%
    - 3 yr, 23%

- Pathophysiology
  - Gut
    - ↑ production from ↑ NH_3 load ↓ metabolism
    - ↑ permeation of gut tight junctions (TJs)
  - Liver
    - ↓ metabolism (loss of normal hepatocytes function)
    - ↑ shunting
  - Skeletal muscle
    - ↓ metabolism of $NH_3 \rightarrow NH_4$
  - Kidney
    - ↓ metabolism of $NH_3 \rightarrow NH_4$ (alkalosis)
  - Brain
    - ↑ blood – brain barrier (BBM) from NH_3
    - ↑ neurotoxins (GABA)
    - ↑ brain edema
    - Altered neurotransmission
    - ↓ metabolism of glucose

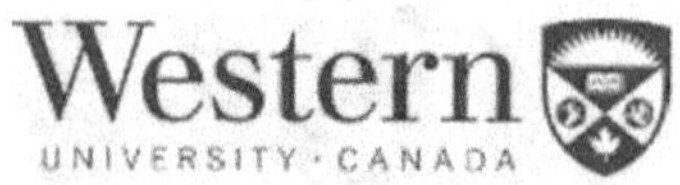

- Clinical
    - Grades of HE

Grade	Impairment Intellectual function	Neuromuscular function
0	- Normal	▪ Normal
Minimal, subclinical	- Normal examination findings. Subtle changes in work or driving	▪ Minor abnormalities of visual perception or on psychometric or number tests
1	- Personality changes, attention deficits, irritability, depressed state	▪ Tremor and incoordination
2	- Changes in sleep-wake cycle, lethargy, mood and behavioral changes, cognitive dysfunction	▪ Asterixis, ataxic gait, speech abnormalities (slow and slurred)
3	- Altered level of consciousness (somnolence), confusion, disorientation, and amnesia	▪ Muscular rigidity, nystagmus, clonus, Babinski sign, hyporeflexia
4	- Stupor and coma	▪ Oculocephalic reflex, unresponsiveness to noxious stimuli

- Causes / precipitants
    - Gut
        - Gastrointestinal bleeding
        - Constipation

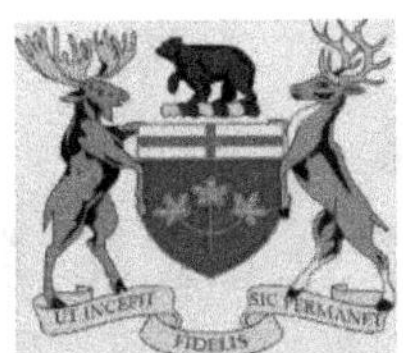

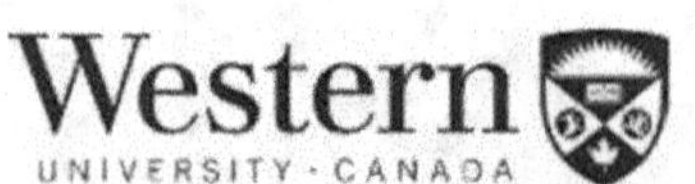
Western
UNIVERSITY · CANADA

- Liver
  - Increase protein intake
  - Vascular occlusion
  - Primary HCC
- Muscle
  - Wasting malnutrition
- Kidney
  - Hypovolemia
  - Hypokalemia and/or metabolic alkalosis
  - Hypoxia
- CNS
  - Hypoglycaemia
  - Infection (including SBP)
  - Sedatives or tranquilizers

➢ Diagnosis

- Clinical suspicion
- EEG – supportive of presence of encephalopathy, but not specific to HE
- ↑ Ammonia concentration
  - In acute liver failure ↑ arterial level may predict presence of brain edema and herniation
    - Supportive of clinical diagnosis
    - Wide differential of ↑ NH_3 levels
- Differential diagnosis of hyperammonemia
  - GI
    - Gastrointestinal bleeding
    - Parenteral nutrition
  - Liver
    - Reye syndrome
    - Certain inborn errors of metabolism (eg. urea cycle defects and organic academia)

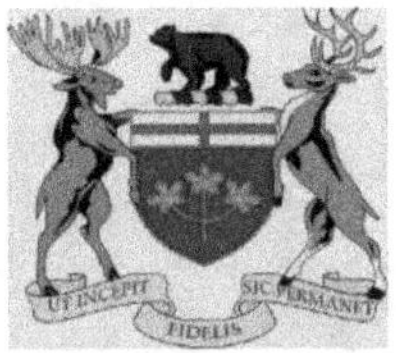

        - Any cause of porto-systemic shunting of blood
    - Muscle
        - Severe muscle exertion/ heavy exercise
    - Kidney
        - Renal disease
        - Urinary tract infection with a urease-producing organism (eg Proteus mirabilis)
        - Ureterosigmoidostomy
    - CNS
        - Drugs such as:
            - Alcohols
            - Barbiturates
            - Diuretics
            - Narcotics
            - Valproic acid
        - Salicylate intoxication
    - Miscellaneous
        - High-dose chemotherapy
        - Shock
        - Cigarette smoking
        - Transient hyperammonimia in newborns

- Treatment
    - Correct precipitating causes
    - Reduction in ammoniagenic substrates
        - Diet restriction: low protein diet (not recommended
        - Lactulose orally or rectally
            - Modification of colonic flora
            - ↑ bacterial utilization of NH_3 incorporation of ammonia by bacteria for synthesis of nitrogenous compounds
            - ↓ pH in colon - ↑ conversion of $NH_3 \rightarrow NH_4$ (non-absorbable)
            - Cathartic effects of a hyperosmolar load

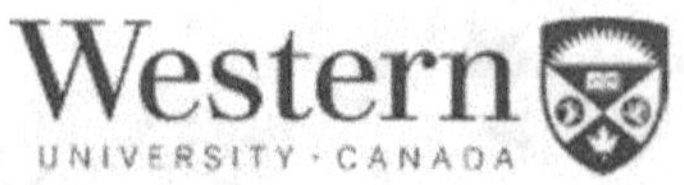

        - increase in stool volume >>>> Increased fecal nitrogen excretion
        - ↓ formation of potentially toxic short-chain fatty acids
- ↓ intestinal NH_3 production and absorption (modification of colonic flora)
    - Oral antibiotics:
        - Rifaximin ,Metronidazole, Neomycin
    - probiotics and prebiotics
    - Acarbose
- ↑ ammonia metabolism
    - Sodium benzoate
- ↓ neurotoxic GABA
    - Benzodiazepine ($GABA_A$ receptor) antagonist
    - Flumazenil

Hepatopulmonary Syndrome

- Definition: Impaired pulmonary function in the patient with chronic liver disease

- Demographics
    - Found in up to 30% of patients evaluated for liver transplantation
    - Associated with increased mortality

- Pathogenesis
    - GI tract
        - Inflammation
        - Bacterial translocation
        - ↑ vasoactive mediators
    - Liver
        - Hepatocyte/ cholangiocyte injury
        - ↑ TNF – α endotoxemia
        - ↑ TGF - β → ↑ ET1

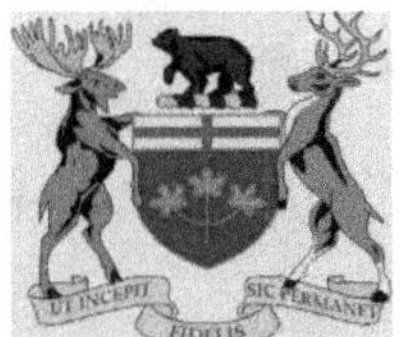

- Lung vessels
  - ↑ eNOS
  - ↑ VEGF
  - Monocyte adhesion/ activation
    - ↑ iNOS
    - ↑ HO-1
  - Vasodilatation
  - Angiogenesis
  - Hypoxemia

Abbreviations: eNOS, endothelial nitric oxide synthetase; ET1, endothelin-1; GI, gastrointestinal; HO-1, heme oxygenase-1; iNOS, induced nitric oxide synthetase; TGF, transforming growth factor; TNF, tumor necrosis factor; VEGF, vascular endothelial growth factor;

➢ Diagnosis :based on the triad of :

- Portal HTN
- Impaired oxygenation
- Intrapulmonary vascular shunt
- ↓ oxygenation
  - AaO_2 gradient
    > 15 on room air
    > 20 mm Hg in patients > 64 years
- ↑ Intrapulmonary shunting
  - Contrast-enhanced "bubble" echocardiography
  - ^{99m}Tc-labeled macroaggregated albumin scan
  - Pulmonary Angiogram
- No intrinsic cardiopulmonary disease
  - CT chest

➢ Clinical

- Liver
  - Signs and symptoms of chronic liver disease, portal hypertension

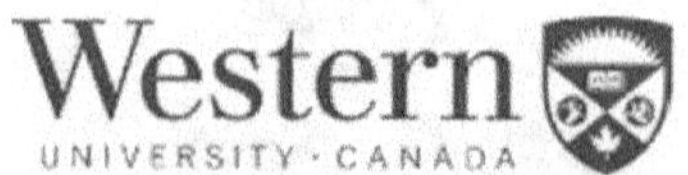

- Lung
    - platypnea (dyspnea worsened by an erect position and improved by a supine position)
    - orthodeoxia (exacerbation of hypoxia and hypoxemia in an upright position)
    - slow progression of dyspnea
    - clubbing
    - distal cyanosis

➢ Treatment

- No established medical therapy
- Pulmonary symptoms - O_2 supplement
- TIPS - not recommended in absence of other indications
- Liver transplant
    - Reverses HPS in 80% of patients
    - Might take more than one year to resolve

CLINICAL REMINDER

What is Portopulmonary Hypertension:

- Pulmonary arterial hypertension in the presence of portal hypertension after excluding all causes of pulmonary HTN
- Characterized hemodynamically by :
    - Mean pulmonary artery pressure (mPAP) >25 mmHg at rest
    - Pulmonary capillary wedge pressure (PCWP) <15 mmHg

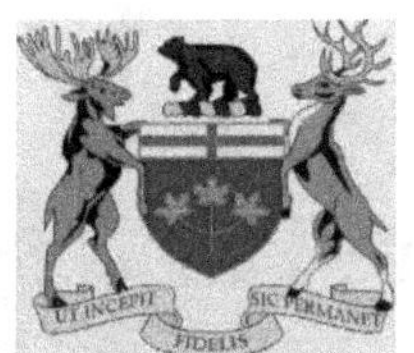

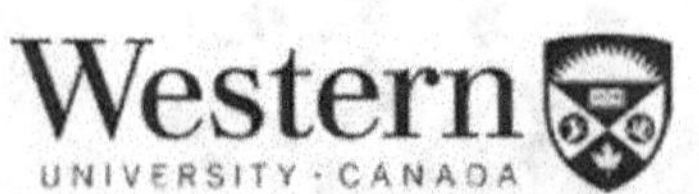
Western
UNIVERSITY · CANADA

Viral Hepatitis B (HBV) and C (HCV) Infections

Keith McIntosh and Jeff So

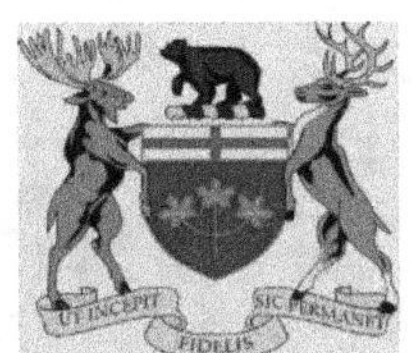

HEPATITIS B VIRUS (HBV)

- Demography
  - 400 million HBV carriers worldwide; one million die annually from HBV-related liver disease
    - 75% reside in Asia and the Western Pacific
  - Major cause of cirrhosis & HCC worldwide
  - USA - incidence of acute hepatitis B < 2 / 10^5 per year
  - Worldwide chronic hepatitis B prevalence

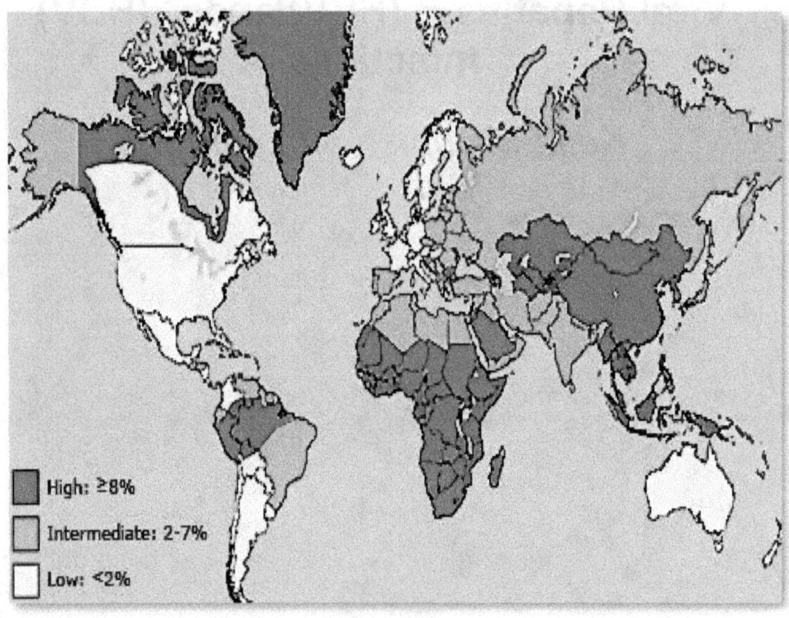

http://wwwnc.cdc.gov/travel/yellowbook/2010/chapter-2/hepatitis-b.aspx

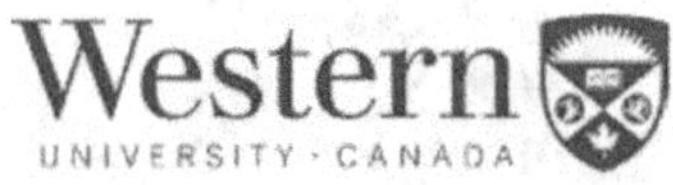

HBV AND HCV INFECTION

➤ Incidence in the United States

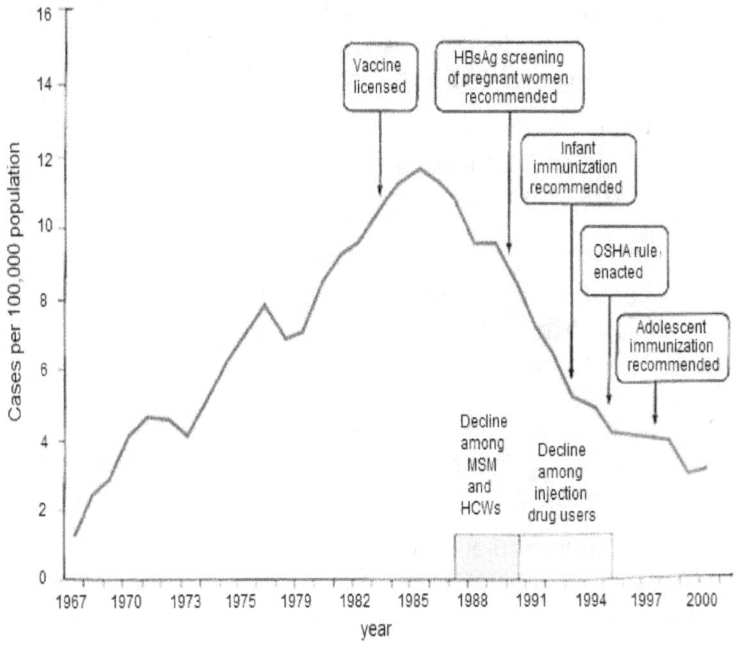

➤ Microbiology

- Modes of Transmission
  - Perinatal
    - Mother HbEAg+ : 60-90% transmission rate
    - Mother anti-HBe+ : 15-20% transmission rate
    - Neonatal vaccination very effective
    - Screening done at first maternal visit
  - Breastfeeding – no increased risk of transmission, provided infant received appropriate immunoprophylaxis

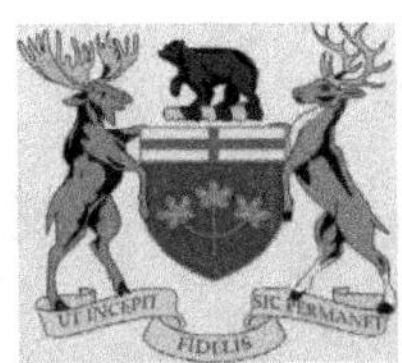

- Horizontal transmission – close household contacts via breaks in the skin/mucous membranes
  - HBV DNA has been detected by PCR testing in most body fluids, except for stool not contaminated with blood
- Transfusion
  - 1-4 per 1 million units in North America
  - Routine screening in 1970's
- Sexual
- Percutaneous
  - IV drug use
  - Tattoos
  - Piercing
  - Acupuncture
  - Sharing razors/toothbrushes
  - Needle stick injury
- Organ transplantation

• Virology
  - dsDNA virus belonging to Hepadnaviridae family
  - Four viral genes
    - Core
    - Surface
    - X
    - Polymerase
  - Replication occurs through RNA intermediate, requiring viral reverse transcriptase/polymerase enzyme
  - Mutation rate higher for HBV than for other DNA viruses (10^{10} to 10^{11} point mutations per day)

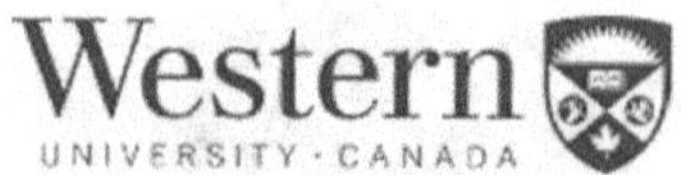

- Life cycle

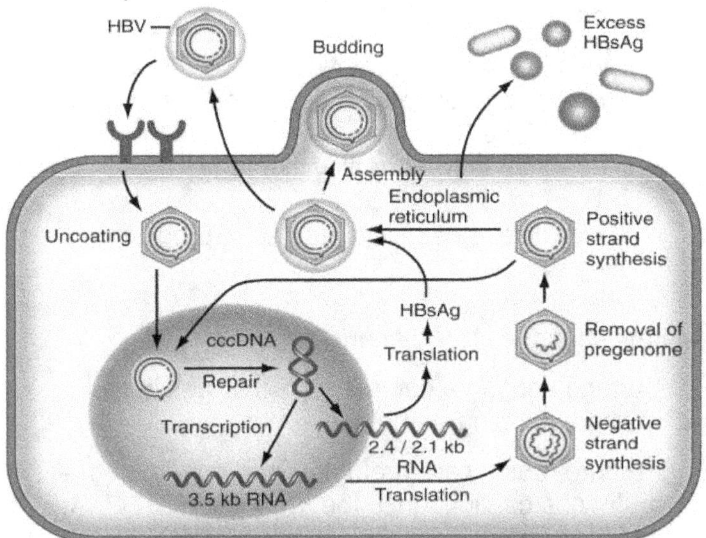

Source: Feldman M, Friedman L, Brandt L. Sleisenger and Fordtran's Gastointestinal and Liver Disease 8th edition. Saunders Elsevier: Philadelphia, PA. 2006.

- HBV Genotypes
    - Geographic Distributions
        - Northwestern Europe, North America, Central Africa
        - Southeast Asia, including China, Japan, and Taiwan (prevalence is increasing in North America)
        - Southeast Asia (prevalence is increasing in North America)
        - Southern Europe, Middle East, India
        - West Africa
        - Central and South America, United States (Native Americans), Polynesia

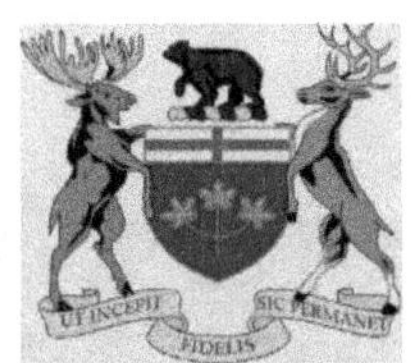

- United States, France
- Central and South America

- Proposed Clinical Associations
  - HBeAg seroconversion occurs earlier in type B than in type C
  - Response to treatment with interferon-α: type A > B ≥ C > D
  - Liver disease activity and risk of progression: type C > B

- Mutations in the HBV Genome
  - Surface antigen – can result in changes in the antibody-binding domain
  - Precore, basal core promoter, and core genes – mutations can influence the production of HBeAg, increase risk of HCC, influence immunologic response to HBV, and possibly affect rate of response to interferon
  - DNA polymerase – mutations can lead to resistance against nucleoside analogs

➢ Pathogenesis

- Severity related to the intensity of the host immunologic response to the virus rather than cytotoxic liver injury
- Cellular immune response primarily involved in pathogenesis of disease
- $CD8^+$ CTLs contribute to the disease process in the liver and result in apoptosis of infected hepatocytes

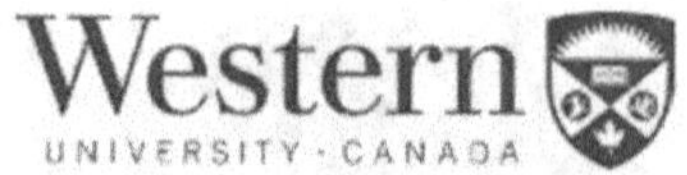

Acute HBV Infection

- Clinical
  - Serum sickness–like prodrome in 10-20% (fever, arthralgia, and rash) before manifestations of liver disease
  - Incubation period from weeks to 6 months (average 60-90 days) after exposure
  - Symptoms
    - Nausea / vomiting
    - Constitutional symptoms
    - Abdominal pain
    - Pruritus
  - Only 30% develop jaundice
  - Symptoms usually resolve within 1-3 months.

- Prognosis
  - Adults:
    - Usually causes clinical acute episode
    - 1 – 5% go on to chronic infection
  - Neonates
    - 95% become chronic HBV carriers
  - Fulminant Hepatitis < 1% of cases
    - Mortality rate approaches
      - 80% without transplant
      - 40% with transplant
    - Thought to be related to massive immune-mediated lysis of infected hepatocytes

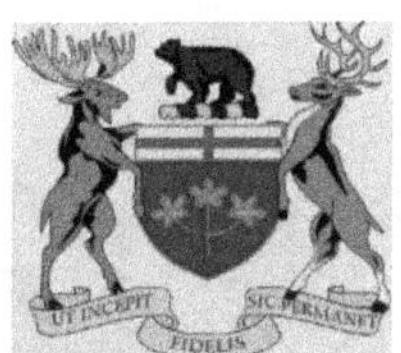

➢ Pathology of HBV

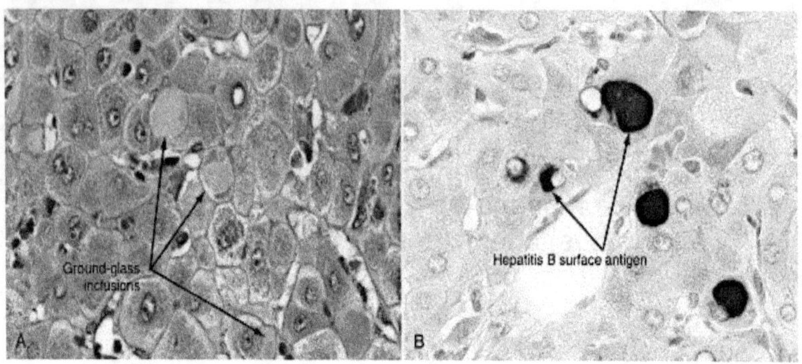

➢ Laboratory

- Liver enzymes / function tests
  - Transaminase levels and serum HBsAg titers tend to decline and then to disappear together
  - Bilirubin rise often lags behind ALT
  - No correlation between ALT peak and prognosis
  - INR is a prognostic indicator
  - After clinical recovery and HBsAg seroconversion, HBV DNA often remains detectable
  - HBsAg persistence beyond 6 months implies chronic infection
  - ALT > AST, and levels often > 1000

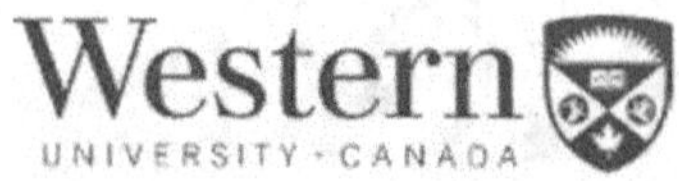

- Serology

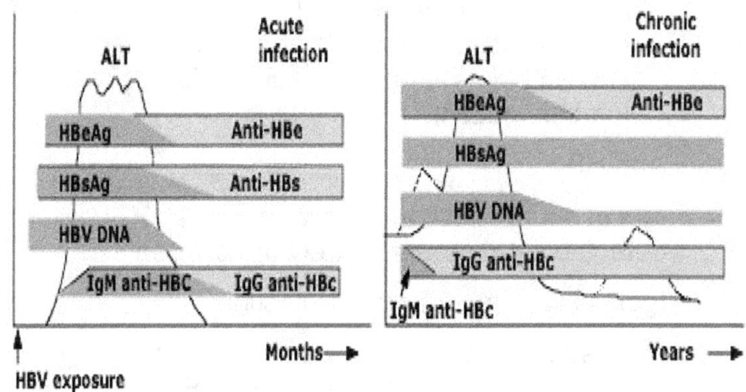

Source: Lok A, Serologic Diagnosis of Hepatitis B infection virus infection. UpToDate.com, 2013.

- HBsAg
  - Positive for 2-10 weeks after exposure, and before onset of symptoms or transaminase elevation.
  - If self-limited hepatitis, undetectable after 4-6 mon.
  - HBsAg persistence > 6 m implies progression to chronic HBV.
- Anti-HBs
  - Develops a few weeks after HBSAg disappears
  - Usually persists for life and provides long-term immunity.
  - May not be detectable during a *window period* of several weeks to months after the disappearance of HBsAg
  - Acute HBV infection is diagnosed by detection of IgM anti-HBc .

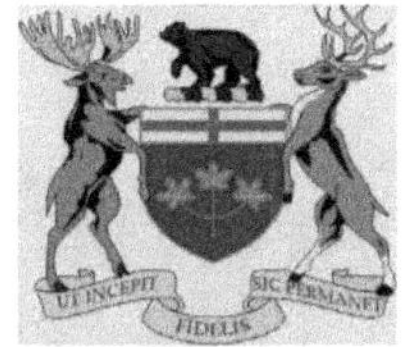

- Coexistence of HBsAg and anti-HBs
  - Anti-HBs usually low level, non-neutralizing, and heterotypic , i.e. directed against a subtype of HBsAg different from the subtype present in the infected patient.
- Anti-HBc
- IgM in acute infection or flare of chronic HBV; detectable 4-6 months (rarely up to 2 years)
- IgG in recovery or chronic infection
- Isolated reactivity for anti-HBc may be caused by:
  - Window period of acute hepatitis B
  - Many years after recovery from acute hepatitis B, when anti-HBs undetectable
  - False-positive
  - After many years of chronic HBV infection, when the HBsAg titer has undetectable
  - Coinfection with HCV
  - Rarely, poor sensitivity of HBsAg assays
- HBeAg - soluble viral protein, found early during acute HBV infection
  - In acute HBV, reactivity usually disappears at or soon after peak aminotransferase levels
  - Persistence >3 months after onset of illness indicates high likelihood of chronic HBV infection.
  - Indicates greater infectivity, a high level of viral replication, and the need for antiviral therapy.
- Most HBeAg-positive patients have active liver disease
  - Exceptions: HBeAg-positive children and young adults with perinatally acquired HBV infection

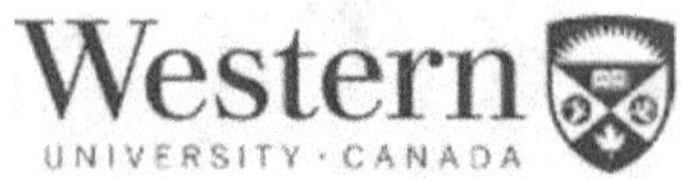

- Used to assess suitability for antiviral therapy and monitor during treatment
  - High pretreatment levels less
    - Likely to respond to interferon
  - Less predictive of response to other antivirals
  - Sensitive quantitative assays (such as real time PCR assays
  - With lower limit of detection of <10 IU/mL [<50 copies/mL] will
    - Identify suboptimal response that may benefit from additional therapy
    - Detect virologic breakthrough

Chronic HBV Infection

- Clinical
  - Often no clear history of symptomatic acute infection; fatigue tends to be predominant symptom
  - Physical findings may be normal, or hepatosplenomegaly may be found
  - Progression to cirrhosis should be suspected with
    - Hypersplenism
    - Hypoalbuminemia
    - ↑ INR
  - In decompensated cirrhosis
    - Spider angiomata
    - Jaundice
    - Ascites
    - Peripheral edema

HBV Cirrhosis

- Demography
  - 2 to 5 per 100 person-years
  - Higher in HBeAg - than in HBeAg + patients.

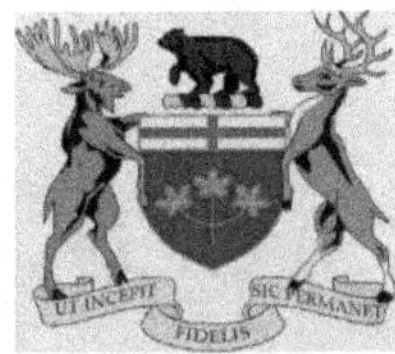

HBV AND HCV INFECTION

- Risk factors include
  - Older age
  - Stage of fibrosis at presentation
  - Ongoing HBV replication
  - Co-infection with
    - HDV
    - HCV
    - HIV
  - Concomitant alcohol abuse

- Clinical
  - Hepatic decompensation
    - 5 year frequency of 16%
  - HCC
    - 5 year frequency of 14%
    - Risk factors: male, age > 45 years, first-degree relative with HCC, cirrhosis, HBeAg +
    - HCC can still develop in HBsAg + persons with none of the identified risk factors
    - Screening is recommended in all patients with cirrhosis and HBsAg carriers older than age 40 years with AFP & US

- Laboratory
  - Usually completely normal during inactive HBV carrier state
  - During exacerbation "flares"
    - Serum ALT levels may be as high as 1000 U/L or more
    - Clinically / labs indistinguishable from acute hepatitis B (including presence of IgM anti-HBc)
  - AST > ALT in patients with advanced cirrhosis

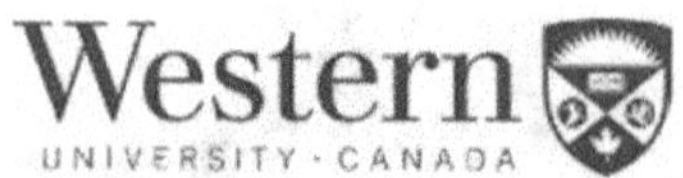

- Triggers for Acute Flares

Cause of Flares	Comment
o Spontaneous	Factors that precipitate antecedent viral replication are unclear
o Superinfection with other hepatitis viruses	May be associated with suppression of HBV replication
o Antiviral therapy for HBV	
– Interferon	Flares are often observed during the second to third month; may herald virologic response
– Lamivudine	
o During treatment	Flares are no more common than with placebo
– YMDD mutant	Can have severe consequences in patients with advanced liver disease
o On withdrawal	Flares are caused by rapid re-emergence of wild-type HBV; can have severe consequences in patients with advanced liver disease
– Immunosuppressive therapy	Flares are often observed during withdrawal; requires preemptive antiviral therapy
– HIV treatment	Flares can occur with HAART or with immune reconstitution; in addition, HBV increases the risk of antiretroviral drug hepatotoxicity

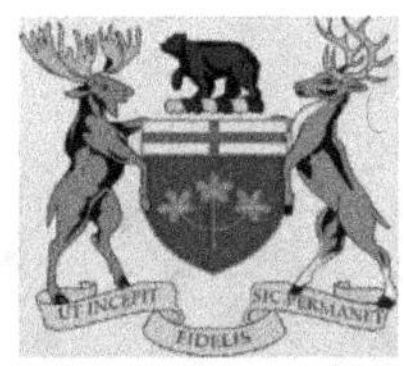

Cause of Flares	Comment
o Genotypic variation	
o Precore and core promoter mutants	Fluctuations in serum ALT levels are common with precore mutants

Source: Feldman M, Friedman L, Brandt L. Sleisenger and Fordtran's Gastointestinal and Liver Disease 8th edition. Saunders Elsevier: Philadelphia, PA. 2006.

HEPATITIS C INFECTION

➢ Demography

- o 170 million people affected worldwide; prevalence ranges from 1.5% in US to 15% in Egypt
- o Prevalence higher in 40-49 year olds, males, and African Americans
- o 55-85% of those infected develop chronic infection
- o Leading indication for transplant in North America and Europe

➢ Risk Factors

- o IV drug use
  - 65% seroprevalence in those injecting < 1 year
- o Blood transfusion before 1992
  - Current risk < 1 in 1 million per unit
- o > 50 lifetime sexual partners
  - Sexual transmission thought to be low risk
- o Incarceration
- o Low family income

- Perinatal (~ 5% risk); breastfeeding thought to be low risk
- Contaminated equipment (medical, tatoo, piercing)

➢ Virology

- Structure
    - Enveloped RNA virus belonging to Flaviviridae family
    - E1 and E2 envelope proteins assemble into tetramers; anchored to host cell–derived lipid bilayer envelope membrane surrounding nucleocapsid.
    - Nucleocapsid composed of multiple copies of the core protein that encapsulates HCV RNA.
    - Circulates in various forms in infected host, including
        - Virions bound to VLDL and LDL and appear to represent the infectious fraction
        - Virions bound to immunoglobulins
        - Free virions

- Replication
    - Hepatocytes are major site of viral replication
    - Envelope proteins E1 and E2 attach to cell surface molecules. CD81 is essential for HCV entry into hepatocytes
    - Once the HCV virus attaches to the cell, endocytosis occurs
    - Viral particle formation is initiated by the interaction of the core protein with genomic RNA in the endoplasmic reticulum

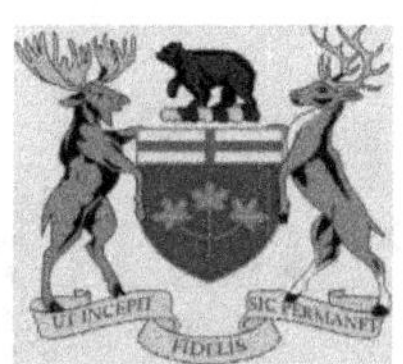

- The large polyprotein generated by translation of the HCV genome is cleaved by cellular and viral proteases to form structural and nonstructural proteins
- Following release, viral particles may infect adjacent hepatocytes or enter the circulation, where they are available for infection of another cell or host

- Heterogeneity
    - HCV RNA polymerase lacks proofreading ability - unable to correct copying errors made during viral replication.
    - Viral heterogeneity results from:
        - Distinct genotypes (6 types). Sequence homology <80%. Does not change with time
        - Quasispecies are families of highly similar strains that develop within an infected host over time. Nucleotide sequence homology is greater than 95 percent.

- Genotypes
    - Genotype 1 is most common (60 to 70 percent of isolates) in the United States and Europe; genotypes 2 and 3 are less common in these areas and 4, 5, and 6 are rare.
    - Genotype 3 is most common in India, the Far East, and Australia
    - Genotype 4 is most common in Africa and the Middle East; Genotype 5 is most common in South Africa
    - Genotype 6 is most common in Hong Kong, Vietnam, and Australia

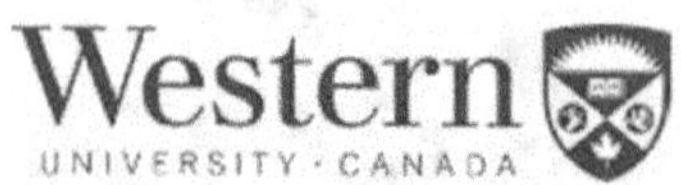

- HCV Polyprotein

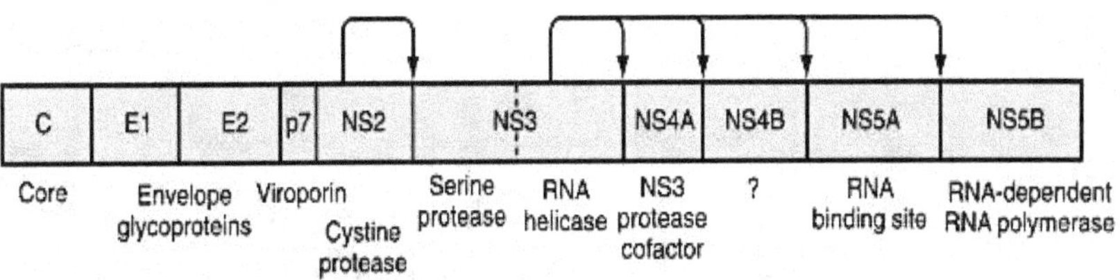

➢ Pathogenesis

- 55% to 85% of acute HCV infections → inability to clear virus despite the development of antibodies against several viral proteins
- In patients in whom acute HCV resolves → early and multispecific $CD4^+$ T-cell proliferative response occurs, with predominance of $CD4^+$ Th1 cells in the peripheral blood, producing interferon-α
- In those without viral clearance, hepatic cell destruction and fibrosis is likely a result of immune mediated liver injury and viral mechanisms
- Likely a direct cytopathic effect of the virus
  - Immune compromised patients with minimal liver inflammation can demonstrate severe liver disease
  - May induce steatosis (30-70%)
- Immune mediated mechanisms
  - CD8+ T cells predominate and may be significant perpetrators of hepatocellular injury
  - Also a humorally directed response

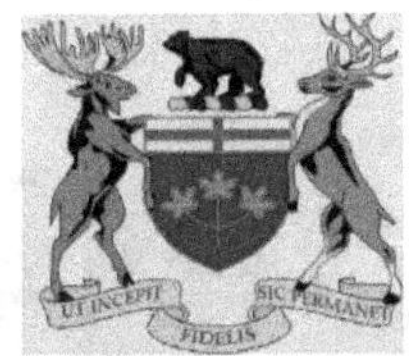

➢ Natural history

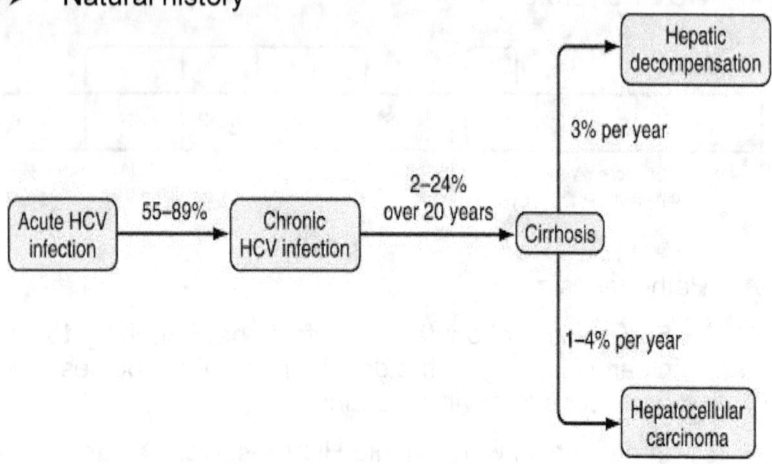

Acute HCV Infection

➢ Clinical
- o Often asymptomatic

➢ Laboratory
- o When symptomatic
  - Jaundice - 10% of patients, usually resolving within 1 month
  - Fatigue, nausea / vomiting - 20% to 30%
  - May be more apparent and severe when acute HCV infection occurs in patients with EtOH, or HBV/HIV coinfection
- o In patients whom infection resolves spontaneously, loss of HCV RNA from serum occurs 3-4 m after onset of disease

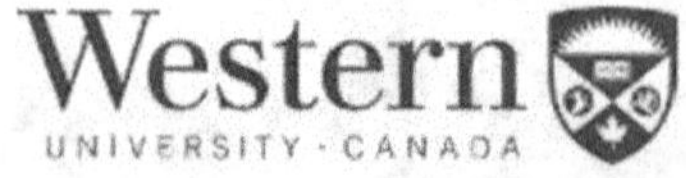

Chronic HCV Infection

- Risk
  - Patients who did not become jaundiced
  - Older patients
  - Males
  - Also possibly influenced by
    - Size of inoculum
    - Immune status of host, and
    - Race
  - ALT often elevated but can fluctuate in given patient

- Clinical
  - Usually asymptomatic before onset of advanced fibrosis
  - Symptoms include
    - Fatigue
    - Depression
    - Arthralgias
    - Parethesias
    - Myalgias
    - Sicca syndrome
    - Nausea
    - Anorexia
    - Difficulty concentrating
  - Symptom severity is not necessarily correlated with severity of underlying liver disease

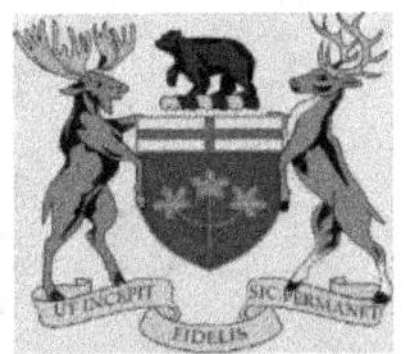

HCV Cirrhosis

- Clinical
  - Manifestations of liver failure
    - Ascites
    - Gastrointestinal bleeding
    - Hepatic encephalopathy
    - Hepatorenal syndrome
    - Synthetic dysfunction
  - Liver failure (decompensatation) develop in 3% per year
  - HCC develops in 1% to 4% per year
  - Extrahepatic Manifestations

	Proven Associations:	Possible Associations
Skin	▪ Lichen planus ▪ Porphyria cutanea tarda	- Sicca syndrome - Vitiligo
Endocrine	▪ Diabetes mellitus ▪ Autoimmune thyroiditis	- Thyroid cancer
Hematology	▪ Mixed cryoglobulinemia ▪ Monoclonal gammopathies	
Cancer	▪ B-cell non-Hodgkin's lymphoma	- Thyroid cancer

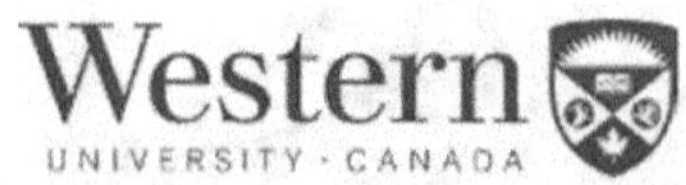

	Proven Associations:	Possible Associations
– Kidney		– Renal cell carcinoma – Non-cryoglobulinemic nephropathies
– Lung		– Idiopathic pulmonary fibrosis
– MSK		– Chronic polyarthritis

➢ Risk Factors for Progression of Fibrosis in Chronic HCV

Established	Possible	Not Associated
○ Age >40 years	– White race	▪ Viral genotype
○ Male gender	– Smoking	▪ Viral load
○ Hepatitis B / HIV coinfection	– Serum ALT level	
○ Immuno-suppressed state	– NASH/Obesity/ DM	
○ Alcohol intake	– Fe Overload	
○ Severe hepatic necro-inflammation		

➢ Pathology

- Reasons to consider performing liver biopsy
  - Assessment of the need for surveillance for HCC
  - Evaluation for concomitant liver diseases

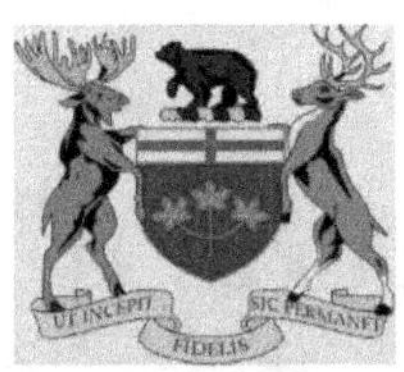

    - Guidance for decisions regarding treatment of hepatitis C
    - Staging of fibrosis
  - Limitations
    - Complications
      - Pain up to 30%
      - Bleeding or bile leak, up to 0.3%, and mortality, $30/10^5$
    - Cost
    - Poor patient acceptance
    - Intraobserver and interobserver variability in interpretation of findings (85-90% concordance for staging fibrosis)
    - Sampling error (up to 33% difference in one stage of fibrosis, 2.4% difference in two stages of fibrosis)
  - Recommendations
    - Initial assessment of genotype 1 or 4, when examination of liver histology will influence treatment plans
    - Genotype 2 or 3 who wish to defer treatment
    - Not required when cirrhosis is already suggested by clinical findings or imaging
    - Not indicated following successful antiviral therapy, although histology generally improves significantly over time following eradication of HCV
- Laboratory
  - Presence of anti-HCV in blood indicates exposure to the virus but does not differentiate among acute, chronic, and resolved infection

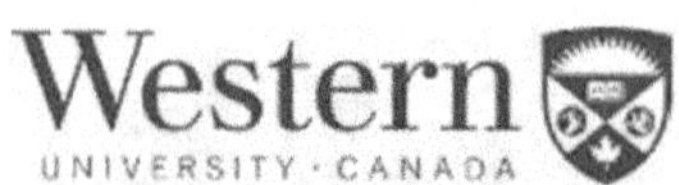

- EIAs detect antibodies against HCV core, NS3, NS4, and NS5 antigens 7 to 8 weeks after infection, with sensitivity and specificity rates of 99%
- Qualitative HCV RNA tests – for screening only (e.g. blood donor)
- Quantitative HCV RNA tests - essential for monitoring the response to antiviral therapy
  - Lower limit of detection 10-15 IU/mL
  - Can't compare using different assays
- Patients suspected of having acute or chronic HCV infection should first be tested for anti-HCV.
- HCV RNA testing should be performed:
  - In patients with a positive anti-HCV test
  - Patients for whom antiviral treatment is being considered (using a sensitive quantitative assay)
  - Patients with unexplained liver disease whose anti-HCV test is negative and who are immunocompromised or suspected of having acute HCV infection.
- HCV genotyping should be performed in all HCV-infected persons before interferon-based treatment

"Those tool were given to you by your parents,

your grandparents, each generation receiving from the previous,

building and refining....It is your obligation

to strive hard to unfold the gifts given to you."

Robert Barney

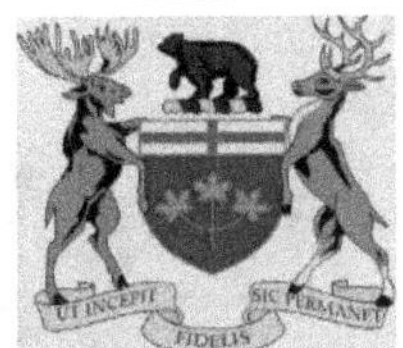

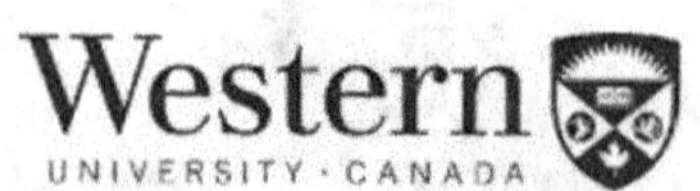
Western
UNIVERSITY · CANADA

Post-Transplantation HCV Infection

Malcolm Wells

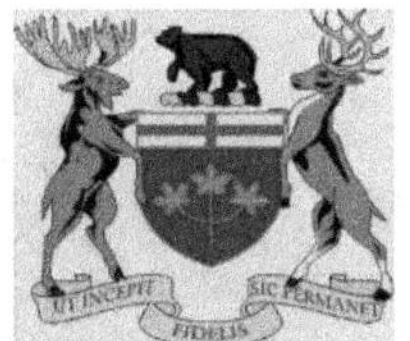

POST-TRANSPLANTATION HCV INFECTION

- Definition
  - Recurrent HCV infection is defined by the presence of HCV RNA in serum and/or liver alone
  - Diagnosis of recurrent disease requires histological confirmation
  - Reinfection of liver allografts is universal and occurs at reperfusion in patient with HCV (recurrent HCV Infection)
  - HCV RNA levels
    - During the anhepatic phase, HCV RNA levels decline to be undetectable
    - After only a few hours, HCV RNA increase rapidly
    - HCV RNA peaks by the 4th postoperative month
    - At 1 year, HCV RNA levels are 1 to 2 log higher than before liver transplant (LT)

- Pathology
  - Histologic features of liver injury can be demonstrated as soon as 9 days post-LT
  - Most typically develop after 3 months
  - Resemble those seen in the non-transplanted graft

- Clinical
  - Analysis of 901 fibrosis measurements in 401 patients showed that

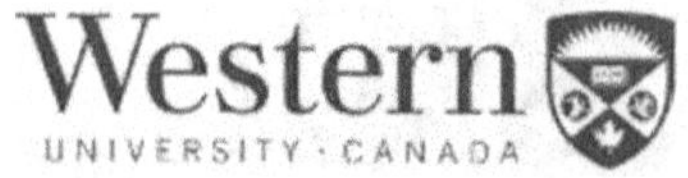

- There is a decreasing risk of progression as time in a given stage increases
- A longer time to reach that stage does not predict a lower risk of further progressing to a higher stage

(Bacchetti P, et al. Non-Markov multistate modelling using time-varying covariates, with application to progression of liver fibrosis due to hepatitis C following liver transplantation. Int J Biostatistics 2010;6(1):7)

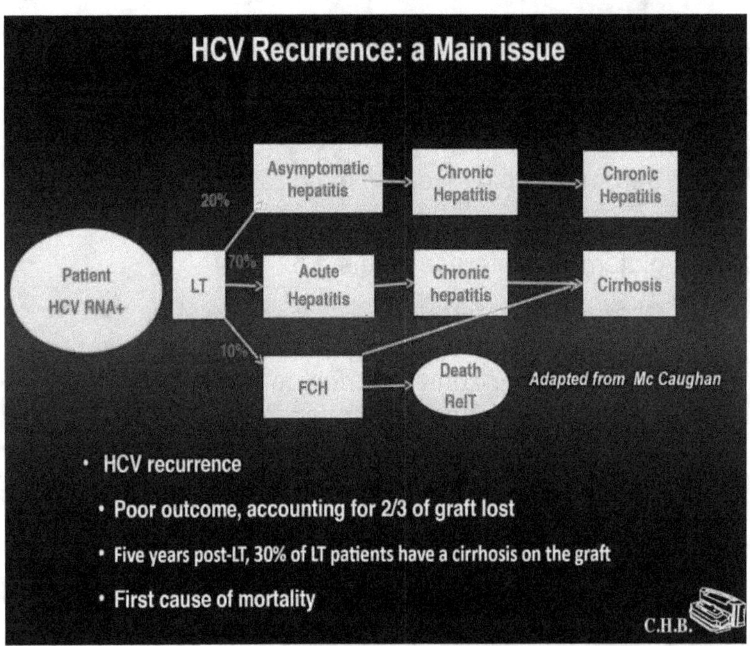

Source:http://www.aphc.info/pdf/2014/pleniere_13012014/1430/Didier_SAMUEL.pdf

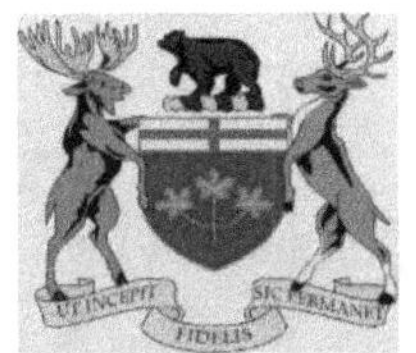

Fibrosing Cholestatic Hepatitis (FCH)

- Clinical
  - Less common presentation (< 10%) of post-LT HCV but severe presentation
    - Possibly a direct cytopathic mechanism
    - Has extremely high viral burdens and reduced immune response
  - Graft failure occurs in 50% within a few months of onset

- Diagnosis (all of the following criteria)
  - Longer than 1 month posttransplantation (usually ≤ 6 months)
  - Serum bilirubin level > 6 mg/dL
  - Serum alkaline phosphatase and g-glutamyltransferase levels > 5x ULN
  - Characteristic histology
    - Ballooning of hepatocytes predominantly in the perivenular zone (not necrosis or fallout)
    - Paucity of inflammation, and
    - Variable degrees of cholangiolar proliferation without bile duct loss
  - Very high serum HCV RNA levels
    - Absence of surgical biliary complications (normal cholangiogram)
    - Absence of evidence for hepatic artery thrombosis
  - Note: many studies of FCH do not commonly use this definition

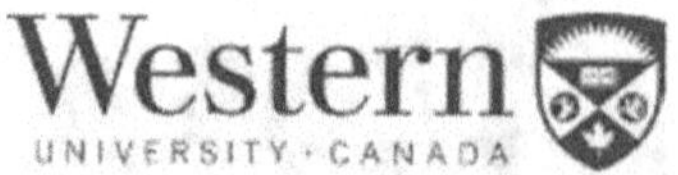

- Treatment
  - The response to antiviral therapy is poor
  - No clear recommendations regarding the duration of therapy in responding patients

(Wiesner RH, et al. Report of the first international liver transplant society consensus conference on liver transplantation and hepatitis C. Liver Transpl 2003;9: S1-9)

- Natural history
  - Progression of fibrosis
    - Fibrosis scope > 2 (Scheuer score) within 10 yr
  - Fibrosis stage achieved in first year post-OLT

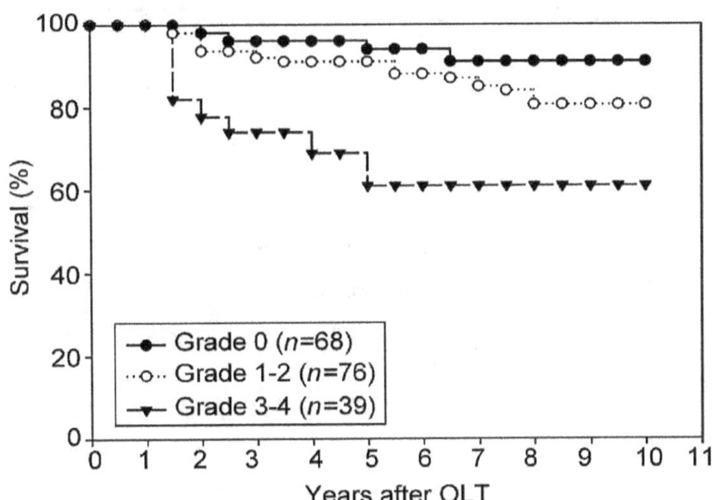

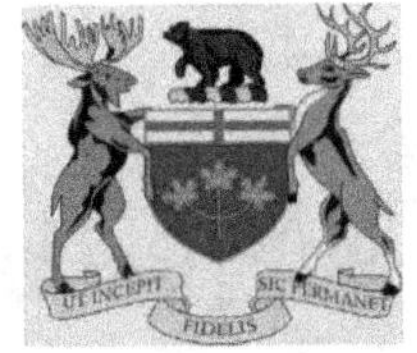

- Cirrhosis or death

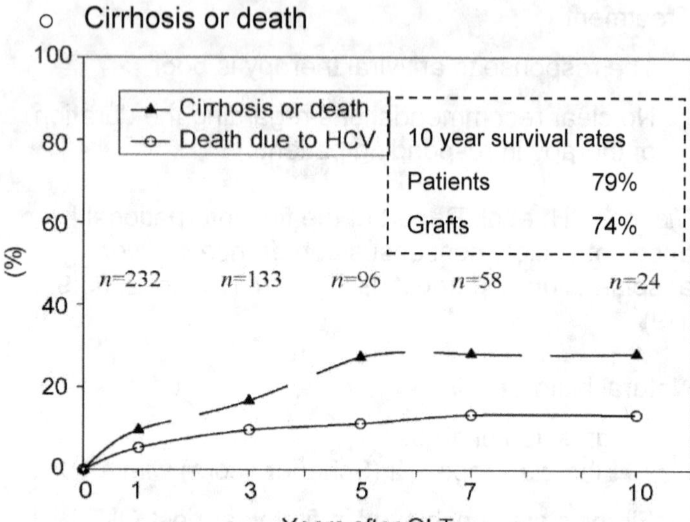

Importance of Sustained Virology Response Post-LT

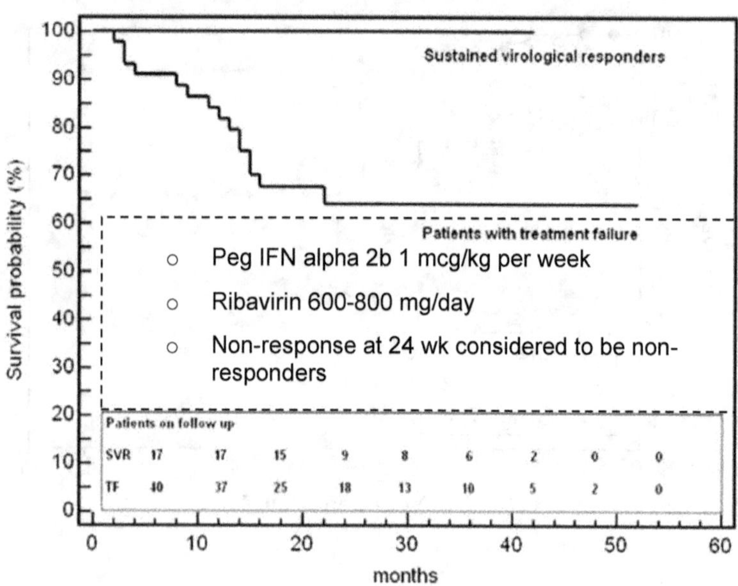

- Peg IFN alpha 2b 1 mcg/kg per week
- Ribavirin 600-800 mg/day
- Non-response at 24 wk considered to be non-responders

$X^2 = 6.9$ $P < 0.01$

Printed with permission: Picciotto FP, et al. / Journal of Hepatology 46 (2007) 459-465)

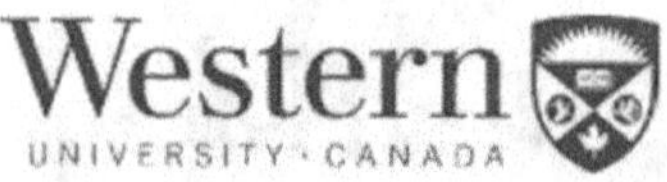

Post Transplantation HCV Infection

Efficacy of antiviral therapy on hepatitis C recurrence after liver transplantation: effect on EVR, BR, SVR and HVPG

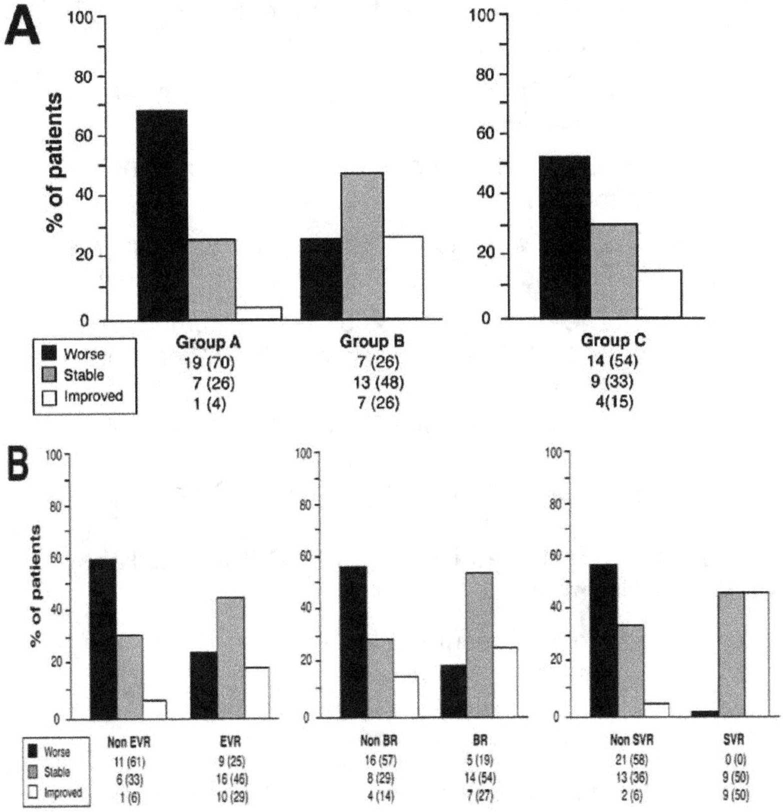

A

% of patients

	Group A	Group B	Group C
Worse	19 (70)	7 (26)	14 (54)
Stable	7 (26)	13 (48)	9 (33)
Improved	1 (4)	7 (26)	4(15)

B

% of patients

	Non EVR	EVR	Non BR	BR	Non SVR	SVR
Worse	11 (61)	9 (25)	16 (57)	5 (19)	21 (58)	0 (0)
Stable	6 (33)	16 (46)	8 (29)	14 (54)	13 (36)	9 (50)
Improved	1 (6)	10 (29)	4 (14)	7 (27)	2 (6)	9 (50)

- Group A: Mild hepatitis (F0-F2), no treatment
- Group B: Mild hepatitis (F0-F2), PEG/riba
- Group C: severe recurrence (F3-F4 or FCH), PEG/riba

Printed with permission: Carrión JA, et al. Gastroenterology. 2007; 132(5): 1746-56.

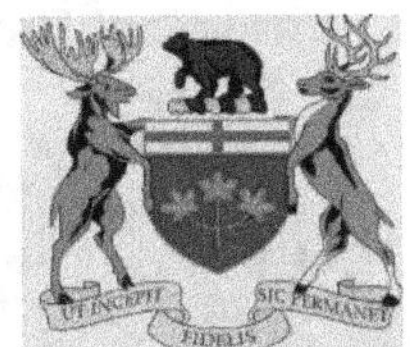

Hepatic Venous Pressure Gradient (HVPG)

- HVPG increased (6.5 to 13 mm Hg, $P < .01$) in patients in whom fibrosis worsened
- HVPG decreased (5 to 3.5 mm Hg, $P = 0.017$) in those with fibrosis improvement
- HVPG remained unchanged in those where fibrosis was stable
- PEG-IFN alfa-2a plus ribavirin in recurrent HCV after OLT.
- Therapy was started with lower fibrosis scores (≤F3) and extended until 72 weeks, if possible
- Between November 2001 and December 2010
  - 279 OLTs were performed in 262 patients at their hospital
  - 81 (31%) for HCV-related cirrhosis
  - 19 patients died in the first 6 months
  - 28 of 62 patients treated for HCV post-LT

Benefit of Early and Extended PEG-IFN plus Ribavirin Dual Treatment

- 28 post-LT recurrent HCV
  - F1, 19 patients (68%)
  - F2, 4 patients (14%)
  - F3, 45 patients (18%).
- Mean time to recurrence was 23 months (3-90 months)
- Adverse effects
  - Leukopenia in 82%
  - Anemia in 79%
  - Four patients (14%) were withdrawn due to SAE
- Efficacy
  - EVR in 19/28 (68%)
  - SVR was 54% (15 of 28 patients)
  - 5 patients died (18%)

(Garcia-Pajares C et al. Transplant Proc 2012;44:1571-3)

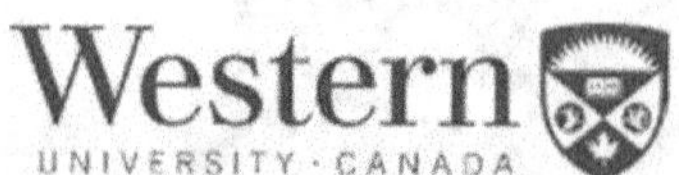

- Extended IFN plus ribavirin from 48 to 72 wk increased SVR in post-LT HCV, using analysis by a logistic regression model

(Wells MM, et al. Saudi J Gastroenterol. 2013;19(5):223-9)

- 76 patients (64 male, mean age 57±6years), treated for G1 HCV recurrence with either BOC (n=41) or TVR (n=35), NS3/4A protease inhibitors
- In BOC group cyclosporine dose reduction was 2.2±1.0 fold, and 8.6±2.4 fold with tacrolimus.
- In TVR group, dose reduction was 3.0±1.4 and 12±5.7 fold with cyclosporine and tacrolimus, respectively.

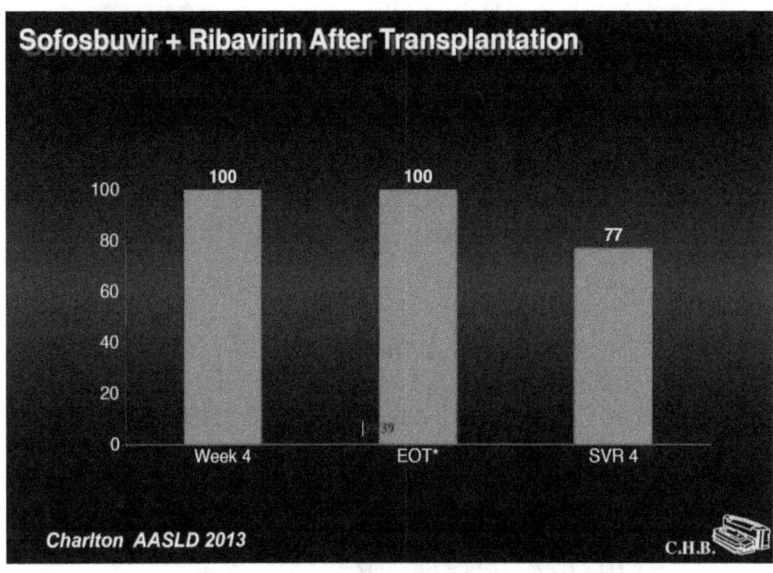

Forn X, et al. Sofosbuvir Compassionate Use Program For Patients With Severe Recurrent Hepatitis C Including Fibrosing Cholestatic Hepatitis Following Liver Transplantation, Abstract, EASL April 9-13, 2014

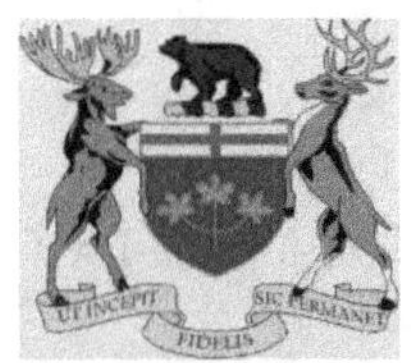

- Methods
  - Patients who had exhausted all treatment options and had poor clinical prognoses received SOF as compassionate use for severe recurrent hepatitis C following LT
  - The regimen included:
    - SOF 400 mg/day and RBV for up to 48 weeks
    - PEG-IFN at the physician's discretion

- Patient Characteristics
  - 87 patients received a SOF-containing regimen by January 1, 2014
    - 57 SOF + RBV
    - 30 SOF + RBV + PEG
  - Genotypes
    - 72 had HCV GT1
    - 2 GT2
    - 6 GT3
    - 3 GT4
    - 4 mixed GTs;

- Results
  - Preliminary SVR12 rates
    - 54% for patients treated with SOF+RBV
    - 44% for those treated with SOF+RBV+PEG
  - Among 76 patients whose outcomes have been reported
    - 53 (70%) have improved on treatment
    - 10 (13%) have stabilized
    - 13 (17%) died, with all deaths attributed to progression of liver disease or associated complications
  - A total of 29 (33%) subjects reported SAEs, none attributable to study drug

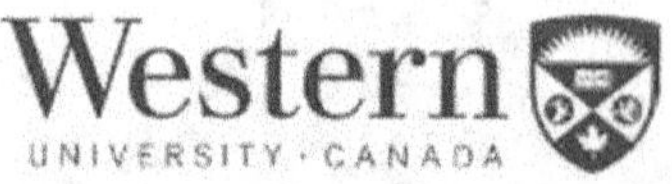

- Conclusions
  - In patients with severe HCV recurrence, a compassionate-use regimen containing SOF+RBV (with or without PEG) was well-tolerated and demonstrated potent antiviral activity, with many patients achieving SVR and clinical improvement.

Kwo P, et al. Result of phase 2 study M12-999: Interferon-free regimen of ABT-450/r/ABT-267 +ABT-333 + Ribavirin in Liver Transplant recipients with recurrent HCV genotype 1 infection. EASL April 9-13, 2014.

- Background
  - ABT-450 Is a potent NS3/4A protease inhibitor
  - Ombitasvir is a potent NSSA inhibitor
  - Dasabuvir is a non-nucleoside NSSB polymerase inhibitor

- Result

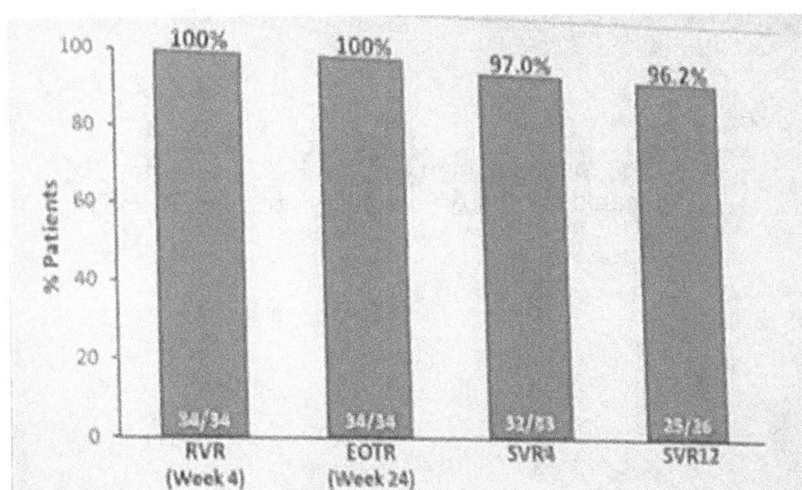

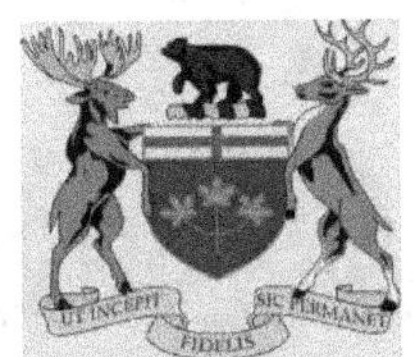

- No patients had breakthrough
- One patient had relapse (post-treatment [day 3])

- Case reports have reported successful therapy for post-LT
  - Recurrent cholestatic HCV[1]
    - Daclatasvir, peg-IFN plus ribavirin
  - Severe recurrent cholestatic HCV[2]
    - Daclatasvir plus sofosbuvir

[1]Fontana RJ, et al. Liver Transplant 2012; 18; 18: 1053-1059

[2]Fontana RJ, et al. Amer J Transplant 2013; 13: 1601-1605

- Abstract publication
  - Pre-LT sofosbuvir + Ribavirin until LT[3]
    - Post-LT virological response 93%

[3]Curry AASLD 2013, Washington, DC, Oral #213

➢ Summary

- The promise of high SVR for HCV may extend to patients treated pre- or post-liver transplantation

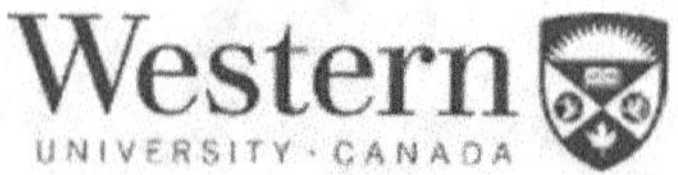

What to Expect When You're Expecting: Liver Disease in Pregnancy

Aze Wilson

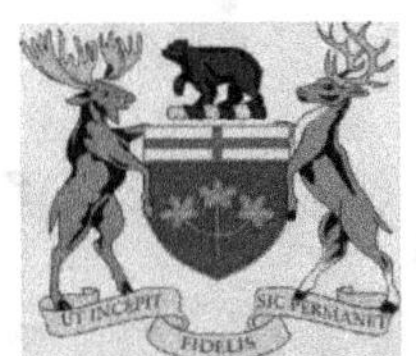

LIVER DISEASE IN PREGNANCY

Normal Changes in Pregnancy

- CVS
  - ↑ intravascular volume
  - Peripheral vascular resistance ↓
  - ↓ systemic pressure
  - ↑ Heart rate, ↑ stroke volume, ↑ cardiac output
  - ↑ Hyperdynamic circulation
- Skin
  - Telangiectasia
  - Spider angiomas
  - Palmar erythema
- Laboratory
  - ↑ alkaline phosphatase
  - ↓ serum albumin
  - ↑ cholesterol
  - ↑ alpha-fetoprotein
  - Note: no change in
    - ALT / AST
    - GGT
    - Bilirubin
    - INR

Pregnancy-related Liver Diseases

- Hyperemesis Gravidarum (HG)
- Intrahepatic cholestasis of pregnancy (ICP)
- Pre-eclampsia and eclampsia
- HELLP syndrome
- Acute fatty liver of pregnancy (AFLP)

Abbreviation: HELLP, hemolysis elevelated liver enzymes low platelets

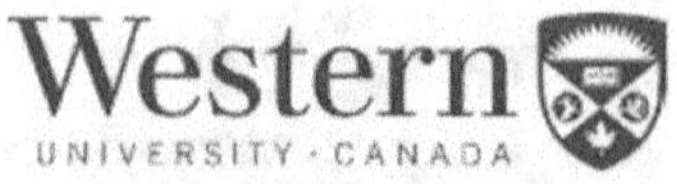

Trimester of Liver diseases in pregnancy

Disease category	Specific disease	Trimester of pregnancy
Pregnancy-related liver disease	- Hyperemesis gravidarum - Intrahepatic cholestasis of pregnancy - Preeclampsia - HELLP syndrome	1 2-3 3, late 2 3, late 2, postpartum 3
Liver disease coincidental with pregnancy	- Acute viral hepatitis - Budd-Chiari syndrome - Gallstones - Drug-induced hepatitis	1-3 1-3, postpartum 1-3 1-3
Chronic liver disease	- Chronic viral hepatitis - Autoimmune hepatitis - Liver disease - Wilson disease	1-3 1-3 1-3 1-3

Kondrackiene J and Kupcinskas L. Medicina 2008;44(5):337-45.

- % of pregnant women with
  - Abnormal liver tests ~3%
  - Liver disease ~1%

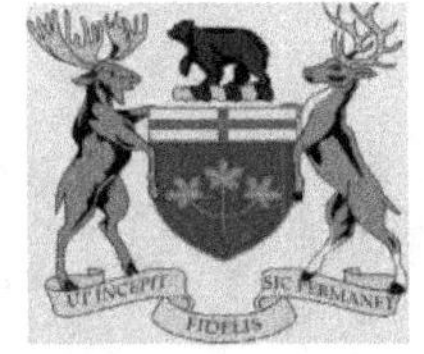

Hyperemesis Gravidarum

- Definition
  - Intractable vomiting, resulting in dehydration, ketosis, and weight loss of ≥ 5% (Fairweather DVI. Am J Obstet Gynecol 1968;102:135-75)
  - May resultin nutritional deficiency requiring hospitalization
  - 10% resolve with delivery

- Demography
  - 0.3-2% of all live births; occur in T1 (4-10 weeks)
  - Resolves by 20 weeks in 90% (Lee NM and Brady CW.World J Gastroenterol 2009;15(8):897-906)
  - Risk factors (Lee NM and Brady CW.World J Gastroenterol 2009;15(8):897-906)
    - Molar pregnancy
    - Multiple pregnancies
    - Pre-existing diabetes mellitus
    - Psychiatric illness
    - ↑ BMI

Abbreviation: T, trimester; BMI, body mass index

- Pathophysiology
  - Poorly understood
  - None of the proposed etiologies are consistently associated or highly predictive of disease

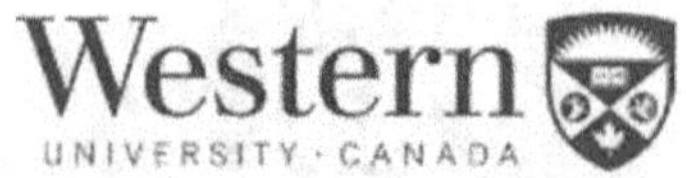

- Possible combination of the following:
  - Hormonal
    - ↑ β-HCG stimulates secretory processes in the UGIT (Verberg MF et al. Hum Reprod Update 2005;11(5):527-39.)
    - ↑ estrogen, decreases in prolactin result in overactivity of the HPA-axis (Kaplan PB et al. Fertil Steril 2003 ;79(3):498-502)
    - Pathway mediated through TNF-α, IgG, IgM, C3, C4 (Leylek OA et al Gynecol Obstet Invest 1999 1999;47(4):229-34.
  - Immunologic
  - Genetic factors
    - ↑ secretion in UGIT
    - ↓ motility

- Pathology
  - Liver involvement in 50% of cases
    - ↑ AST/ALT (> 400 AST and > 1000 ALT have been reported)
    - Mild ↑ bilirubinemia and jaundice
  - Histology
    - Typically normal
    - Can see mild
      - Steatosis
      - Cholestasis
      - Occasional necrotic hepatocytes
  - No mechanisms of liver damage are described

(Kondrackiene Jand Kupcinskas L. Medicina 2008;44(5):337-45)

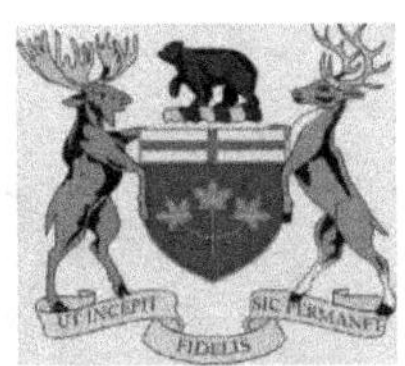

- Prognosis
  - Maternal morbidity is well-documented
  - Recurrence is common
  - Fetal outcomes are less clear:
    - No significant difference in peri-natal mortality
    - Some studies show no difference btw HG and non-HG mothers with respect to fetus outcome (Hepburn IS and Schade RR. Dig Dis Sci. 2008;53(9):2334-58)
    - One large cohort study showed that HG fetuses may have
      - ↓ birth weights
      - ↑ rates of being small for gestational age

- Treatment
  - Mainly supportive
    - IV rehydration
    - Antiemetics
    - Vitamin supplementation (thiamine)
    - Electrolyte replacement
    - Avoid triggers
    - Enteral nutrition in the setting of weight loss

(Jewell D and Young G. Cochrane Database Syst Rev. 2003;(4):CD000145)

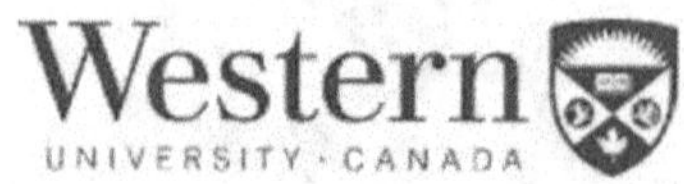

Intrahepatic cholestasis of pregnancy

- Definition
    - Pruritus with ↑ serum bile acids occurring in the second half of pregnancy, which resolves after delivery

- Demography
    - Most common liver disease unique to pregnancy (T2 and T3)
    - 1/1000-1/10,000 pregnancies (Reyes H and Sjövall J. Ann Med 2000;32(2):94-106)
    - Occurs in the late 2nd or 3rd trimester
    - More common in South Asia, South America and Scandinavian countries Lee NM and Brady CW. World J Gastroenterol. 2009;15(8):897-906)
    - Risk factors
        - Advanced age
        - Multiparous women
        - Cholestasis and OCP

Abbreviations: OCP, oral contraceptive pill; T, trimester

- Pathophysiology
    - Unknown, multifactorial
    - Possibly
        - Genetic
        - Hormonal
        - Environmental
    - Abnormalities in the metabolism and disposition of sex hormones and/or bile acids

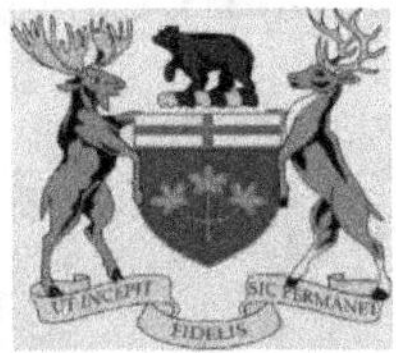

- Defective hepatic canalicular bile salt export pump (BSEP)
- Multidrug resistant protein 3 (MDR3) → ↑ retention of bile acids / pruritis jaundice
- Myometrial contractions → preterm labor and fetal distress

(Kondrackiene J and Kupcinskas L. Medicina 2008;44(5):337-45)

➢ Pathology

- Centrilobular cholestasis without inflammation
- Bile plugs in hepatocytes and canuliculi in zone 3

(Lammert F et al. J Hepatol. 2000;33(6):1012-21)

➢ Clinical

- Usually disappears within 48 hr of delivery
- Maternal complications
  - Pruritus of palms, soles
  - Jaundice in 10-25%
  - Fatigue
- Hyperbilirubinemia (up to 100 micromols/L)
- 60% have mild ↑ AST/ALT (> 2-x10 ULN)
- ↑ ALP
- Fetal complication
  - May occur within the first 1st 4 weeks of the onset of pruritus
  - Worse at night
  - Most often good prognosis
  - Placental insufficiency and fetal distress
  - IU death
  - Pre-term labour

Abbreviations: IU, intrauterine; ULN, upper limit of normal

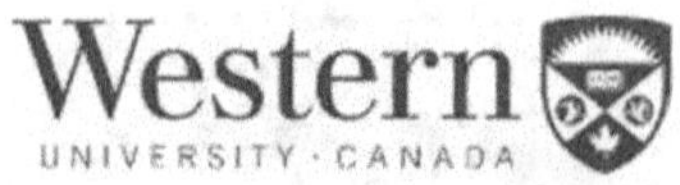

- Treatment
  - Ursodeoxycholic acid
    - Helps target and insert key transporter proteins (such as MDR3 or BSEP into canulicular membranes and ↑ expression of placental bile acid transporters → improved bile salt transfer
    - ↑ bile flow → ↓ pruritus, improves biochemical tests (PBC)
    - Meta-analysis of 9 RCTs/454 pts: URSO pts' outcomes (pruritus, liver chemistry, preterm labour) better than placebo, dex, cholestyramine
    - No adverse effects on mother or fetal

Pre-eclampsia/Eclampsia

- Definition
  - Pre-eclampsia:
    - Triad of HTN (>140/90 on 2 occasions) + edema + proteinuria (>300mg in 24 hrs or 2+protein on dipstick >6hrs apart) (SOGC guidelines JOCC 2008)
  - Eclampsia
    - Triad above plus
      - Neurologic symptoms
      - Visual disturbance
      - Coma

- Demography
  - 5-10% of pregnant woman are affected
    - 2nd/3rd trimester (Lee NM and Brady CW.World J Gastroenterol 2009;15(8):897-906)

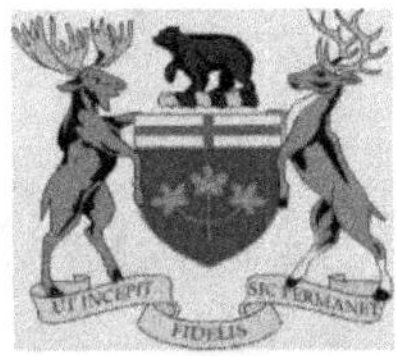

- Pathogenesis
  - Utero-placental ischemia
    → procoagulation and proinflammatory states
    → activation of the endothelium → ↑ vascular tone
    → ↑ SBP
    →↑ vascular permeability
    → proteinuria
    → SIRS → multiorgan damage

- Laboratory
  - AST/ALT 10-20 x > ULN
  - Mild ↑ ALP, Bili

- Pathology
  - Hepatic sinusoidal deposition of fibrin
  - Periportal hemorrhage
  - Hepatocyte necrosis
  - May see microvesicular steatosis
  - Possible overlap with acute fatty liver of pregnancy (AFLP)

- Treatment (Lee NM and Brady CW.World J Gastroenterol 2009;15(8):897-906)
  - Tight control of blood pressure is essential
  - Liver involvement
    - Suggests severe disease → delivery is necessary

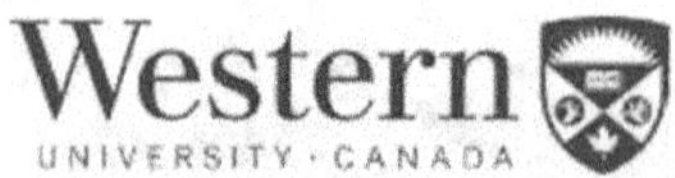

- Prognosis
  - Maternal mortality is 15-20% in developed countries (Thadhani R and Solomon CG. N Engl J Med. 2008 Aug 21;359(8):858-60)
    - CVA
    - Pulmonary edema
    - Fetal growth retardation (FGR)
  - Fetal mortality is 1-2% (Lee NM and Brady CW.World J Gastroenterol 2009;15(8):897-906)
    - Abruption
    - Preterm delivery
  - Liver biochemical profile usually normalizes within 2 weeks of delivery

HELLP Syndrome

- Definition: triad
  - Hemolysis
  - Elevate liver enzymes
  - Low platelets
- Demography
  - 70% occur antenatally
  - Majority of cases in T3
  - 30% of cases within 48 hrs of delivery, but can be seen for up to 7 days post-partum
  - Occurs in 1/1,000 pregnancies

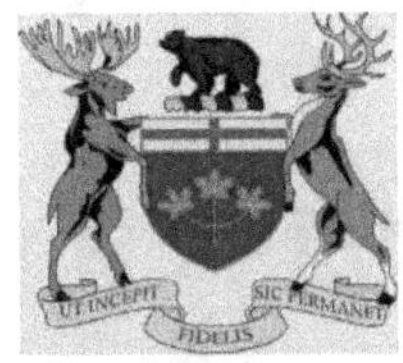

- Pathogenesis
  - Alterations in platelet activation → ↑ pro-inflammatory cytokines
  - Segmental vasospasm → vascular endothelial damage

    ↓
  - Intravascular fibrin deposition and sinusoidal obstruction

    ↓
  - Hepatic hemorrhage and infarction

- Risk factors
  - ↑ maternal age
  - Multiparity
  - White ethnic origin

- Pathology (Barton JR, et al. Am J Obstet Gynecol. 1992;167(6):1538-43)
  - Periportal hemorrhage
  - Fibrin deposition
  - Focal hepatocyte necrosis

- Clinical
  - GI
    - Asymptomatic
    - RUQ and epigastric pain
    - Nausea, vomiting, and malaise
  - Renal
    - Disseminated intravascular coagulopathy (DIC) → acute kidney injury (AKI)

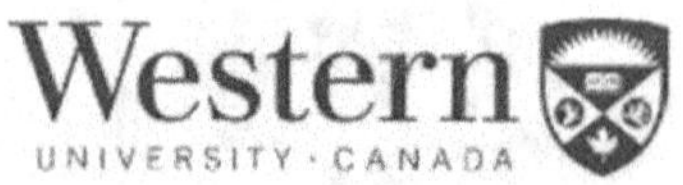

- CVS
  - Hypertension and proteinuria (in up to 85% of cases)
- Lung
  - Pulmonary edema (6%), ascites (8%), AKI in DIC (20%)
- Maternal mortality ~1%
- Perinatal mortality 7-22%
  - Premature detachment of the placenta
  - Intrauterine (IU) asphyxia
  - Prematurity
- Cornerstone of tx: delivery (Lee NM and Brady CW.World J Gastroenterol 2009;15(8):897-906)

➢ Diagnosis

- Hemolysis
  - MAHA, with schistocytes
- Elevated liver tests
  - Total bilirubin
  - AST> 70
- Low platelets (<100,000)

➢ Treatment

- Cornerstone of treatment: delivery
  - Delivery > 34 weeks; steroids for 48 hrs, then delivery if 24-34 weeks
- Gestational weeks
  - 24 to 34 weeks delivery
  - > 34 weeks delivery

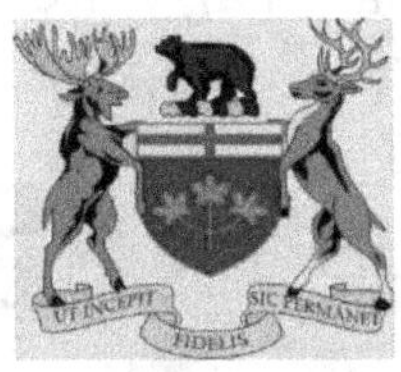

Acute Fatty Liver of Pregnancy (AFLP)

- Definition
  - Acute liver failure (hepatic encephalopathy, coagulopathy, jaundice) in second half of pregnanc (usually T3) due to an inherited deficiency of LCHAD (long-chain 3-hydroxyacetyl=CoA dehydrogenase), leading to a
    - Defect in mitochondrial beta-oxidation of fatty acid
    - ↓ breakdown of long chain fatty acids in the liver → microvesicular fatty infiltration of hepatocyte

- Demography
  - Occurs in T3
  - 1/10,000 to 1/15,000 pregnancies
  - Maternal and fetal mortality up to 20% (may be less with inclusion of all cases, including mild cases identified by ↑ suspicion and better diagnosis)
  - Risk factor
    - Nulliparious
    - Twins

- Pathophysiology
  - Association btw AFLP and an inherited defect in mitochondrial beta-oxidation of fatty acids[1]
    - Long-chain 3-hydroxyacyl-CoA dehydrogenase (LCHAD) deficiency
  - LCHAD (1 of 4 enzymes) responsible for the breakdown of LC fatty acids in the liver[1]
    - Accumulation of unbroken down metabolites (from fetus/placenta) → liver toxicity in mother

- Mutations: E474Q (genetic testing is available for affected mother, fathers, infants) (Ibdah JA, et al. N Engl J Med. 1999;340(22):1723-31)
  - Infants with E474Q mutation are at risk for the following:
    - Fatal nonketotic hypoglycemia
    - DCM
    - Progressive neuromyopathy

➢ Pathology

- In diagnostic uncertainty, liver biopsy is indicated
- Histology
  - Microvesicular fatty infiltration
  - Pericentral pallor with lobular disarray
  - Vacuolization of the central zone hepatocytes

➢ Clinical Presentation

- Non specific presentation, with progression to fulminant liver failure
- 1-2 weeks of non-specific symptoms
  - Nausea, vomiting
  - Abdominal pain
  - Fatigues
- 50% have sxs of pre-eclampsia
- Hepatic manifestations:
  - Encephalopathy
  - Coagulopathy
  - Jaundice
  - Hypoglycemia

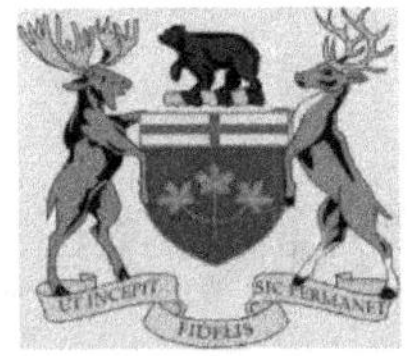

- Extra-hepatic manifestations:
  - Intraabdominal bleeding
  - Infection
  - DI
  - AKI

(Mackillop L and Williamson C. Postgrad Med J. 2010;86(1013):160-4)

- Laboratory
  - ↑ AST/ALT
  - ↑ conjugated bilirubin
  - ↑ WBC
  - ↑ INR
  - Platelets
    - If no DIC Normal
    - DIC ↓
  - ↑ serum NH_3
  - Hypoglycemia

- Differential

- Give the differentiation between AFLP and HELLP.

Symptoms	AFLP	HELLP
Parity	Nulliparous, twins	Multiparous, older
Encephalopathy	+	-
Jaundice	Common	Uncommon
Ammonia	High	Normal

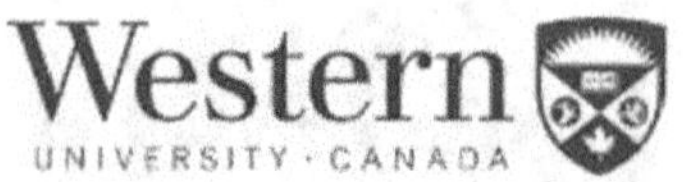

Symptoms	AFLP	HELLP
o Platelets	Low-normal	Low
o Prothrombin time	Prolonged	Normal
o APTT	Prolonged	Normal
o Fibrinogen	Low	Normal or increased
o Glucose	Low	Normal

Abbreviations: AFLD, acute fatty liver of pregnancy; HELLP, hemolysis elevate liver enzymes low platelets; PTT, partial thromboplastin time

- Treatment
  - Mild / moderate causes
    - Delivery after maternal stabilization (Kondrackiene J1 and Kupcinskas L. Medicina (Kaunas). 2008;44(5):337-45)
    - INR usually normalizes shortly thereafter
  - Severe cases
    - Supportive care post-partum in an ICU setting for complications of liver failure
      - Mechanical ventilation
      - Dialysis
      - Parenteral nutrition
      - Surgery for post C-section bleeding
  - Most patients recover with no sequelae of liver disease[2]
    - Mortality rates
      - Maternal – 12%
      - Fetal 20%

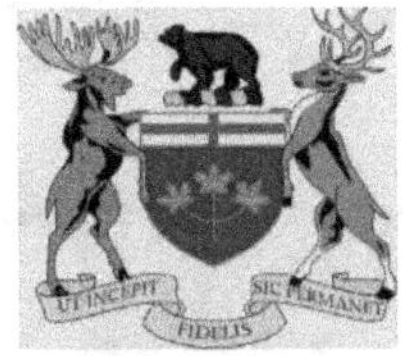

Liver Transplantation for Pregnancy - Unique Liver Disease

- Demography
  - Patient
    - Median age 30 yr
    - Median gestation 35 wk
  - Liver disease
    - ~2/3 HELLP
    - 1/3 AFLD

- Predictors of need for liver transplantation / death
  - Presence of hepatic encephalopathy (HE) (↑ RR~2x)
  - ↑ serum lactate (↑ RR~2x)
  - HE plus ↑ lactate (identified correctly 90% of patients needing LT or who died)
  - Unfavourable etiology
  - Interval of
    - HE
    - Jaundice
  - Age
    - INR
  - King`s College Criteria (KCC)
    - May **not** identify patients at risk of death without LT in this clinical setting.

(Westbrook RH, et al. Am J Transplant. 2010;10(11):2520-2526)

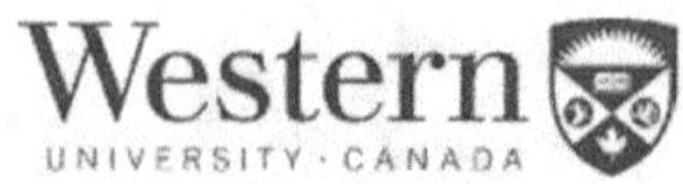

- Medical survivors vs LT/death (Westbrook RH et al. Am J Transplant. 2010;10(11):2520-6)
  - Presence of encephalopathy (43% vs 80-100%)
  - Lactate (2.5 survivors vs 7 OLTx/death)
  - Combination identified 90% of patients who died or needed OLTx
  - Of LT listed patients, none fulfilled non-acetaminophine KCC (INR, age, bili, unfavourable etiology or interval of jaundice to encephalopathy)

- Prognosis
  - Maternal survival, 87%
  - Maternal death
    - HELLP ~ 10%
    - AFLD ~ 25%
  - Predictors of poor LT outcome

"Health is the greatest gift,
contentment the greatest wealth,
faithfulness the best relationship."
Buddha

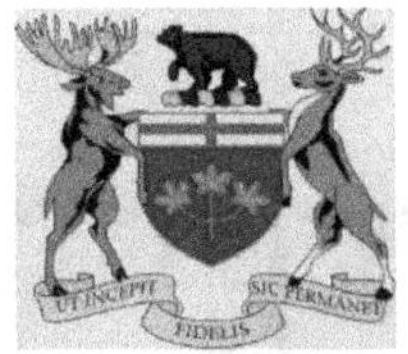

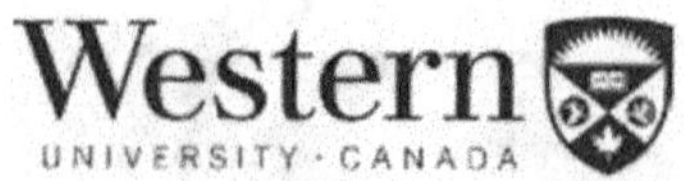
Western
UNIVERSITY · CANADA

MINI UPDATE

Autoimmune Hepatitis, and Variant (Overlap) Syndromes

Mark A Levstik

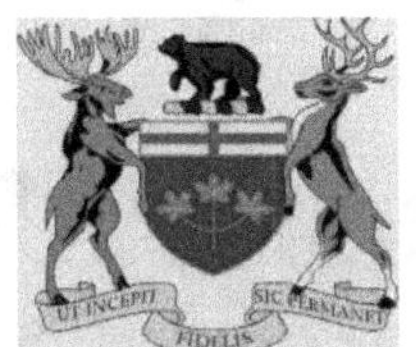

Autoimmune Hepatitis (AIH)

- Definition: "AIH is a disorder of unknown cause characterized by unresolving inflammation of the liver and by the presence of interface [limiting plate of the portal tract is disrupted by a lymphoplasmacytic infiltrate] on histologic examination, … hypergammaglobulinemia" (Feldman M., et al. Sleisenger and Fordtran's Gastrointestinal and Liver Disease. 9th Edition. Saunders/Elsevier, Philadelphia, 2010, page 1461), and autoantibodies".

- Demography
  - Occurs in all countries and races
  - Different HLA-associations (Europe B8, DR3 or DR4)
  - Prevalence > 1: 10,000
  - 75% women
  - All age groups

Age distribution at first manifestation

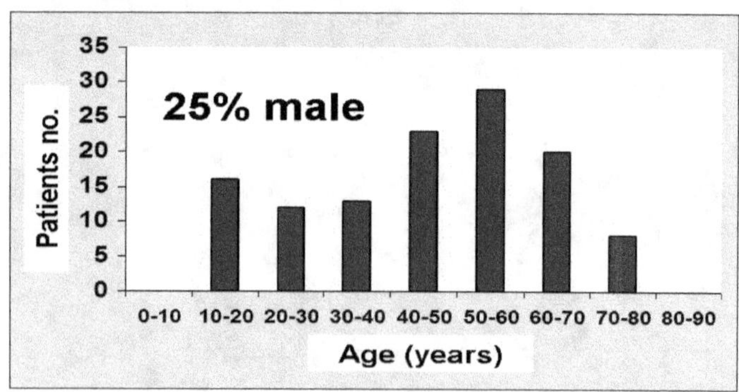

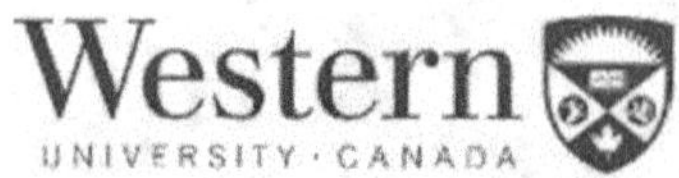

AUTOIMMUNE HEPATITIS, AND VARIANT (OVERLAP) SYNDROMES

➢ Types

- Give a classification of autoimmune hepatitis (AIH) based on autoantibody profiles of patients
  - Type 1 AIH
    - Sudden onset of symptoms in 40%, including fulminant hepatic failure
    - 38% have associate "autoimmune" disorders
    - F:M ratio of 3.6:1
    - Usual age of presentation, 50 years
    - Serum antibodies
      - ANA (anti-nuclear antibody)
      - SMA (smooth muscle antibodies
      - ANA plus SMA
      - Anti-actin
      - PANCA (perinuclear anti-neutrophil cytoplasmic antibodies; aka ANNA, anti-neutrophil nuclear antigens)
      - ↑ IgG

Adapted from: Czaja AJ. *Sleisenger and Fordtran's Gastrointestinal and Liver Disease* 2006. pg. 1872-1875; and 2010, pg. 1467.

- Give 4 forms or types of AIH.
  - I (f, 50) ANA+ ASM+ IgG↑
  - II (children) ALKMI+
  - III (M, 30) ASLA/LP+
  - Overlap syndrome AMA-neg. PBC, PSC, AMA-

In Germany, 20% of AIH type 2 occur in adults. Please see Feldman M., et al. Sleisenger and Fordtran's Gastrointestinal and Liver Disease. 9th Edition.

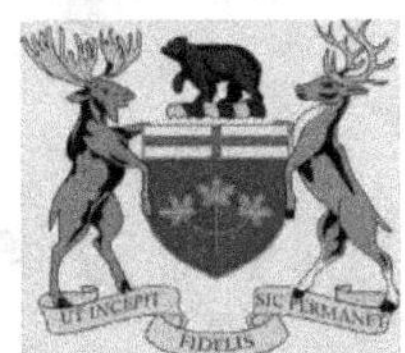

Saunders/Elsevier, Philadelphia, 2010, Table 88.3, page 1464, "Classification of Autoimmune Hepatitis Based on Autoantibodies".

Adapted from: Czaja AJ. *Sleisenger and Fordtran's Gastrointestinal and Liver Disease* 2006. pg. 1872-1875; and 2010, pg. 1467.

- Give the distinction between type I and 2 AIH.

Feature	Type 1 AIH	Type 2 AIH
Geographical variation	Worldwide	Worldwide
Age at presentation	All ages	Usually childhood and young adulthood
Sex (F:M)	3:1	10:1
Clinical phenotype	Variable	Generally severe
Characteristic autoantibodies	ANA ASMA Anti-actin antibody Anti-SLA/LP antibodies 25% of patients negative ANA	Anti-LKM-1 antibody Anti-LC-1 antibody
Histopathological features at presentation	Broad range: mild disease to cirrhosis	Generally advanced, ↑ inflammation/cirrhosis common
Treatment failure	Rare	Common
Relapse after drug withdrawal	Variable	Common
Need for long-term maintenance	Variable	Approximately 100%

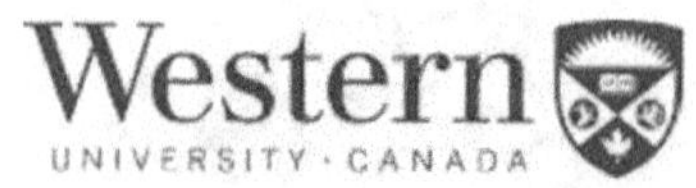

AUTOIMMUNE HEPATITIS, AND VARIANT (OVERLAP) SYNDROMES

Abbreviations: ANA, antinuclear antibody; ASMA, anti-smooth muscle antibody; anti-LC, anti-liver cytosol; anti-LKM, liver kidney microsomal antibody; anti-SLA/LP, soluble liver antigen/liver pancreas antigen.

Printed with permission: Gleeson D, Heneghan MA; British Society of Gastroenterology. British Society of Gastroenterology (BSG) guidelines for management of autoimmune hepatitis. Gut. 2011;60(12):1611-29, Table2.

Please see: Swan MG. Chapter 58. In: Therapeutic Choices. Grey J, Ed. 6th Edition, Canadian Pharmacists Association: Ottawa, ON, 2011, Table 5: Autoimmune Hepatitis, page 778

➢ Pathophysiology

- Give the pathophysiology of primary / idiopathic AIH.
    - Unknown and possible environment antigenic peptide (molecular mimicry) --→ inciting antigen fits in the antigen-binding groove of the class II DR molecule of the MHC antigen presenting cells (in USA / Canada, DRB1 gene, susceptibility alleles DRB1*0301 and DRB1*0401)
    - The DR molecule-antigen complex of the APC (antigen-presenting cell) interacts with the antigen receptor of CD4+ T-helper cells (1st signal).
    - The CD28 molecule on the surface of CD4+ t-helper cell binds to the B7 ligand on the surface of the APC" (2nd signal) (Feldman M., et al. Sleisenger and Fordtran's Gastrointestinal and Liver Disease. 9th Edition. Saunders/Elsevier, Philadelphia, 2010, page 1464).
    - CD4+ T-helper cells differentiate into Th1 or Th2 T-cells

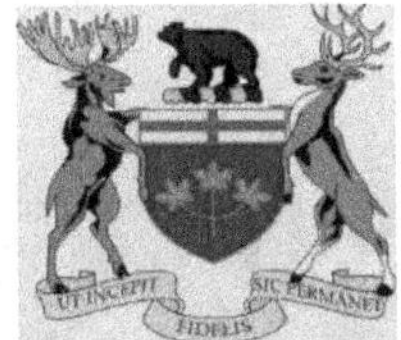

- The cytokine milieu of Th1 and Th2 cytokines is regulated
- This balance between Th1 and Th2 may be disturbed by
  - ↓ NKT (intrahepatic natural killer T cells)
  - ↓ regulation of CD8+ T cell proliferation by
  - T-reg (T-regulatory CD4+ CD25+) cells
- Hepatocyte damage is caused by
  - Cell-mediated cytotoxicity (regulated by type 1 cytokines), or
  - Antibody-dependent cell-mediated cytotoxicity (regulated by type 2 cytokines), or by
  - Both mechanisms
- Th1 (type 1 cytokine) pathway of activated CD4+ t-helper cells is stimulated by polymorphism of
  - TNF A*2 (TNF gene)
  - TNF receptor superfamily gene (FAS)
  - CTLA4 (the cytotoxic T lymphocyte antigen 4 gene)
  - TNFRSF6 (FAS gene phenotype at position –670)
- These polymorphisms and Th1 T-cells
  - Sensitize cytotoxic T cells
  - ↑ cell-mediated cytotoxicity
  - ↑ apoptosis of hepatocytes
- The cytokine pathways are increase by ↓ activity of T-reg (T-regulatory) cells
- Th

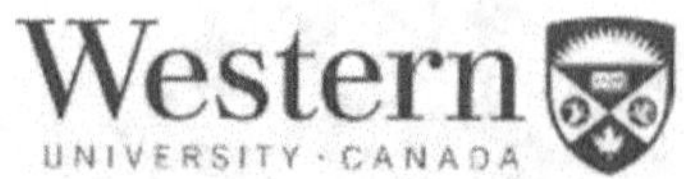

- 2 (type 2 cytokine) pathway of activated CD4+ T-helper cells causes differentiation of B cells into plasma cells
  - Plasma cells → ↑ production of immunoglobulin
  - Immunoglobulins → antibody-mediated cellular toxicity

SO YOU WANT TO BE A HEPATOLOGIST!

Persons with drug-associated AIH (autoimmune hepatitis) closely resembles non-drug associated AIH, including the presence of antinuclear anti-smooth muscle antibodies.

Apart from the historical aspects of time-associated clinical or laboratory changes, give the clues in an individual patient that the AIH is drug-associated.

- Drug-associated AIH is not associated with
  - History of other autoimmune diseases
  - HLA-B8 and HLA-DR alleles

➢ Causes / associations

- List 5 prescription medications, OTC preparations or herbs which may induce or unmask an AIH-like syndrome.
  - Antibiotics
    - Minocycline
    - Nitrofurantoin

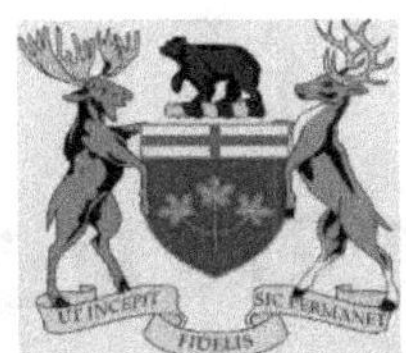

- Rifampin
- Interferon
- INH

- Metabolic
  - Orlistat
  - Statins
  - Propyl thiouracil
- Antihypertensives
  - Alpha methyldopa
- Herbs
  - St. John's Wort
  - Chapannal leaf
  - Black cohosh
- Immune
  - Anti-TNF therapy

Printed with permission: Heathcote EJ. *2007 AGA Institute Spring Postgraduate Course Syllabus*: 96.

➢ Clinical presentation
- Often asymptomatic (cryptogenic cirrhosis)
- 25% acute hepatitis (sometimes fulminant)
- Often fluctuating course
- Fatigue
- Arthalgias

AUTOIMMUNE HEPATITIS, AND VARIANT (OVERLAP) SYNDROMES

- Give 5 clinical presentations of AIH.
  - Acute hepatitis
  - Fulminant hepatitis
  - Asymptomatic chronic hepatitis +/- cirrhosis
  - Symptomatic chronic hepatitis +/- cirrhosis
  - "Burned out" decompensated cirrhosis +/-
  - *De novo* or recurrent AIH after liver transplantation (alloimmune)
  - AIH with overlapping PBC/PSC/AMA-neg PBC
  - Suspected from liver disease associated with other conditions
  - HCC

- Give 15 **immune diseases/disorders** which are associated with AIH.
  - Skin, eye
    - Iritis
    - Gingivitis
    - Dermatitis herpetiformis
    - Erythema nodosum
    - Lichen planus
    - Pyoderma gangrenosum
  - CNS/PNS
    - Peripheral neuropathy
    - Myasthenia gravis
  - Thyroid
    - Autoimmune thyroiditis
    - Graves' disease*

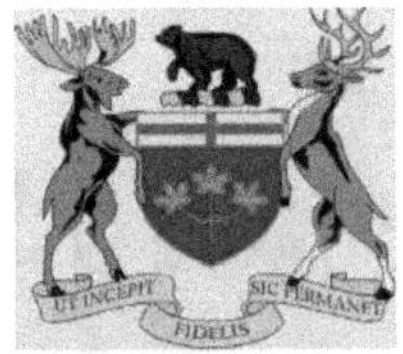

- Heart, lung
  - Pleuritis
  - Fibrosing alveolitis
  - Pericarditis
- Pancreas
  - Insulin-dependent diabetes
  - Autoimmune pancreatitis
- Gut, liver
  - Celiac disease
  - Ulcerative colitis
  - Autoimmune sclerosing cholangitis
  - Pernicious anemia
  - Autoimmune cholangitis (PSC)
- Kidney
  - Glomerulonephritis (immune complex)
- Blood
  - Coombs- positive hemolytic anemia
  - Cryoglobulinemia
  - Idiopathic thrombocytopenic purpura
  - Pernicious anemia ITP+ PA (Evan's syndrome)
  - Neutropenia
- MSK
  - Rheumatoid arthritis
  - Sjögren's syndrome
  - Synovitis
  - Systemic lupus erythematous
  - Focal myositis

Printed with permission: Czaja AJ. *Mayo Clinic Gastroenterology and Hepatology Board Review* 2008: pg. 398.

AUTOIMMUNE HEPATITIS, AND VARIANT (OVERLAP) SYNDROMES

Clinical Cautions

- The presence of symptoms of AIH does not refect the hepatic histology – "histological findings, including the frequency of cirrhosis, are similar in asymptomatic and symptomatic patients….."
- "the asymptomatic state does not preclude the need for glucocorticoid therapy if other objective manifestations of disease activity are present or emerge, and close surveillance of these patients for worsening inflammation is justified".
- Untreated asymptomatic mild AIH still progress, and there are no clinical indices that predict the course of the disease".

(Feldman M., et al. Sleisenger and Fordtran's Gastrointestinal and Liver Disease. 9th Edition. Saunders/Elsevier, Philadelphia, 2010, page 1471).

- Clinical Course
  - Asymptomatic ~ 40% (70% later become symptomatic)
  - Spontaneous resolution ~ 15%
  - Compensated cirrhosis ~ 40%
  - Esophageal varices (EV) ~ 55%
- Diagnostic dilemma
  - In principle, any elevation of liver enzymes could be due to AIH
  - There is no single test to exclude AIH

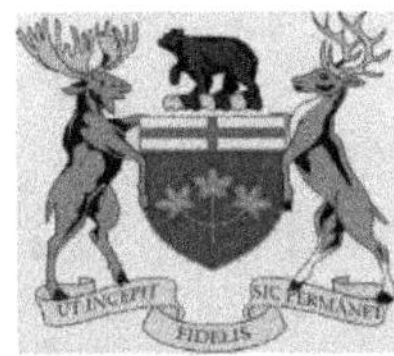

- The diagnosis of AIH is based on exclusion and probabilities expressed through the use of scoring systems.
- Other causes of chronic liver disease with similar features need to be excluded, including conditions, which overlap with AIH (PBC, PSC, AIH with cholestatic features, autoantibody-negative AIH).
- There are scoring systems which may be used to assist in making a definite or a probable diagnosis: please see Feldman M., et al. Sleisenger and Fordtran's Gastrointestinal and Liver Disease. 9th Edition. Saunders/Elsevier, Philadelphia, 2010, Table 88.1, page 1463, "Revised Original Scoring system for the Diagnosis of Autoimmune Hepatitis", and Table 88.2, "Simplified Scoring System for Diagnosis of Autoimmune Hepatitis"

- Give the **definite and probable criteria** for the diagnosis of AIH

Definite AIH	Probable AIH
➢ Exclude other causes of chronic liver disease	
o Normal AAT phenotype	– Partial AAT deficiency
o Normal ceruloplasmin level	– Abnormal copper or ceruloplasmin level but Wilson disease excluded
o Normal iron and ferritin levels	– Nonspecific iron or ferritin abnormalities

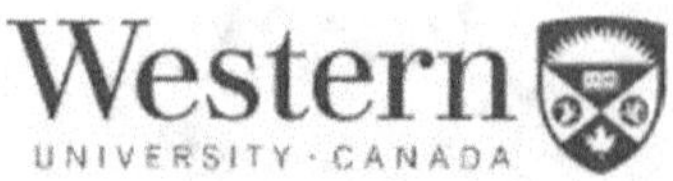

AUTOIMMUNE HEPATITIS, AND VARIANT (OVERLAP) SYNDROMES

Definite AIH	Probable AIH
No active hepatitis A, B, or C infection	No active hepatitis A, B, or C infection
Daily alcohol <25 g	Daily alcohol < 50 g
No recent hepatotoxic drugs	No recent hepatotoxic drugs
Predominant serum aminotransferase abnormality	Predominant serum aminotransferase abnormality
Suggestive lab tests	
Globulin, γ-globulin, or IgG level $\geq$1.5 times normal	Hypergammaglobulin emia of any degree
ANA, SMA, or anti-LKM1 $\geq$1:80 in adults and $\geq$1:20 in children; no AMA	ANA, SMA, or anti-LKM1$\geq$1:40 in adults; other autoantibodies
Liver biopsy	
Interface hepatitis–moderate to severe	Interface hepatitis–moderate to severe
No biliary lesions, granulomas, or prominent changes suggestive of another liver disease	No biliary lesions, granulomas, or prominent changes suggestive of another disease

Printed with permission: Czaja AJ. *Mayo Clinic Gastroenterology and Hepatology Board Review* 2008: pg. 392.

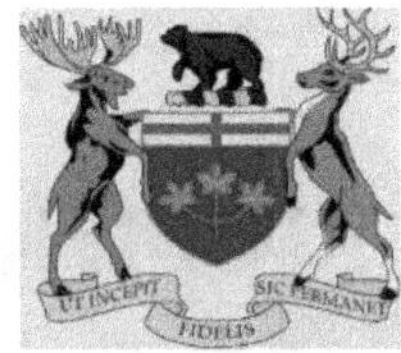

AUTOIMMUNE HEPATITIS, AND VARIANT (OVERLAP) SYNDROMES

Definite AIH	Probable AIH

- Autoantibodies in AIH

ANA: Anti-Nuclear Antibodies	50-60%
SMA: Smooth Muscle Antibodies	50-60%
LKM: Liver Kidney Microsomal antibodies	< 5%
SLA / LP: Soluble Liver Antigen / Liver-Pancreas	20-30%
Other (ANCA, LC1, SS-A, gp210, Sp100....)	

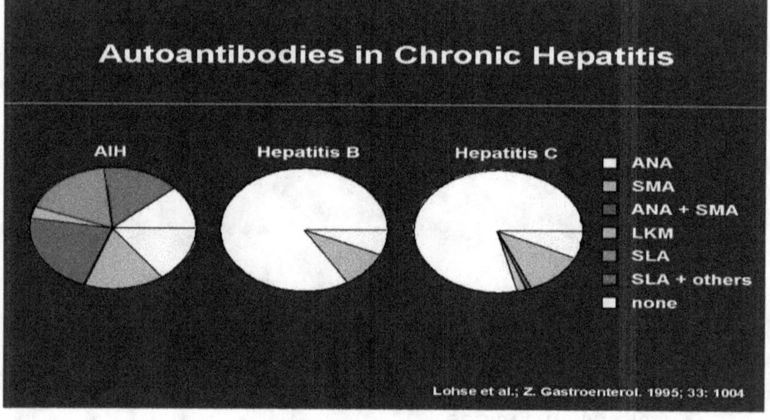

Source: Lohse Z, et al; Gastroenterol 1995: 33: 1004

Note: Although immunofluorescence is the traditional method for measuring the repertoire of conventional autoantibodies in AIH, many laboratories (especially those in the USA) are increasingly using ELISA-based methods, especially for anti-LKM antibodies.

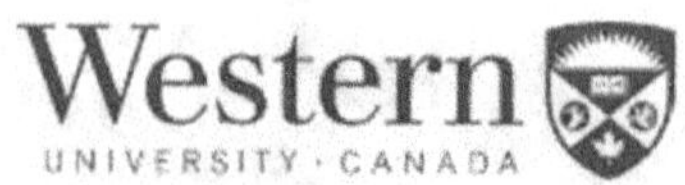

- In relation to anti-LKM-1 antibodies, these may be erroneously reported as detectable anti-mitochondral antibodies.

Clinical Words of Wisdom – the need for liver biopsies in AIH

"evaluation of liver tissue [doing a liver biopsy] before drug withdrawal is essential to establish remission because histologic activity may be present in 55% of patients who satisfy other requirements for remission".

"...histological improvement lags behind clinical and histologic resolution by three to eight months....."

"......complete resolution of the clinical and histological manifestations of the disease [AIH] does not preclude relapse after drug withdrawal" (Feldman M., et al. Sleisenger and Fordtran's Gastrointestinal and Liver Disease. 9th Edition. Saunders/Elsevier, Philadelphia, 2010, page 1473).

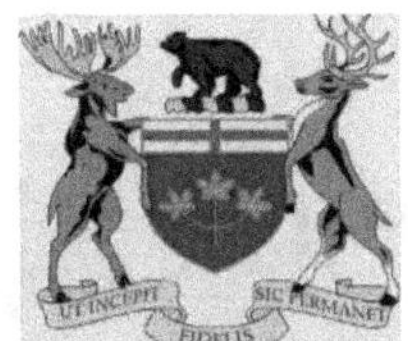

"Praise improves work ethic and motivation.

When were you last given this kind of praise on your annual assessments?"

"Praise may be more effective than rewards."

(Bribes, money)

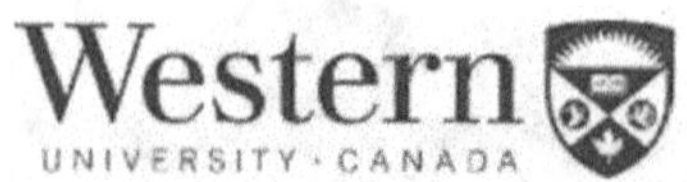

Simplified scoring system for diagnosis of autoimmune hepatitis

Category	Variable	Score
➢ Autoantibodies		
○ Antinuclear antibodies	1:40	+1
○ Smooth muscle antibodies	>1:80	+2
○ Antibodies to liver kidney microsome type 1	>1:40	+2
○ Antibodies to soluble liver antigen	Positive	+2
➢ Immunoglobulin level		
○ Immunoglobulin G	>Upper limit of normal	+1
	>1.1 times upper limit of normal	+2
➢ Histologic findings		
○ Morphologic features	Compatible with autoimmune hepatitis	+1
	Typical of autoimmune hepatitis	+2
➢ Viral disease		
○ Absence of viral hepatitis	No viral markers	+2
➢ Pre-treatment aggregate score		
○ Definite diagnosis		>7
○ Probable diagnosis		6

Adapted from: Hennes EM, Zeniya M, Czaja AJ, et al. Simplified diagnostic criteria for autoimmune hepatitis. *Hepatology* 2008;48:169-76.

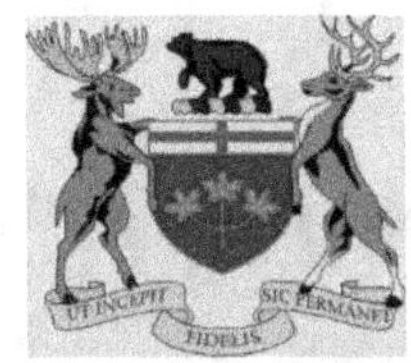

Useful background: Revised original scoring system for the diagnosis of autoimmune hepatitis

Category	Variable	Score
○ Gender	Female	+2
○ AP/AST	>3	-2
	<1.5	+2
○ Gamma globulin or IgG level above normal	>2.0	+3
	1.5-2.0	+2
	1.0-1.5	+1
	>1.0	0
○ ANA, SMA, or anti-LKM1 titer	>1:80	+3
	1:80	+2
	1:40	+1
	<1:40	0
○ AMA	Positive	-4
○ Viral markers	Positive	-3
	Negative	+3
○ Drug history	Yes	
	No	
○ Alcohol	<25 g/day	
	>60 g/day	

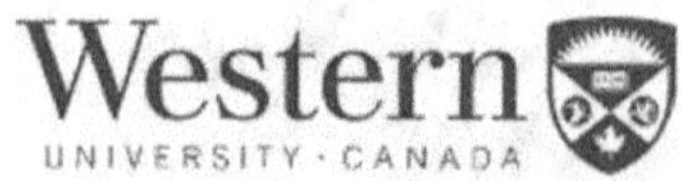

AUTOIMMUNE HEPATITIS, AND VARIANT (OVERLAP) SYNDROMES

Category	Variable	Score
HLA	DR3 or DR4	+1
Immune disease	Thyroiditis, ulcerative colitis, synovitis, others	+2
Other liver define autoantibodies	Anti SLA, anti actin, anti LC1, Panca	+2
Histologic features	Interface hepatitis	+3
	Plasmacytic	+1
	infiltrate	+1
	Rosettes	-5
	None of above	-3
	Biliary changes	-3
	Other features	
Treatment response	Complete	+2
	Relapse	+3
Pre-treatment score		
- Definite diagnosis	>15	
- Probable diagnosis	10-15	
Post treatment score		
- Definite diagnosis	>17	
- Probable diagnosis	12-17	

Adapted from: Alvarez F, Berg PA, Bianchi FB, et al. *J Hepatol* 1999; 31: 929-38.

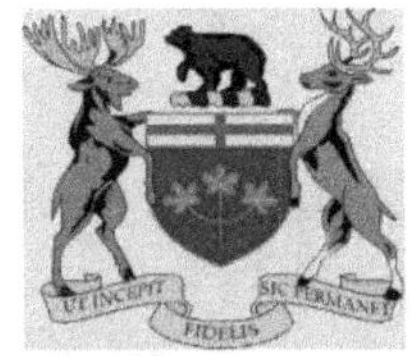

- Note on the revised diagnostic criteria of the International AIH group
  - Intended for use in scientific studies
  - Limited clinical validation data
  - Too complicated
  - Biased (.g. female)
  - False positive and false negative

➢ New Criteria for Autoimmune Hepatitis (International Autoimmune Hepatitis Group)

- Elevation of serum total IgG
  - IgG > 16 g/L — 1 point
  - IgG > 18.5 g/L — 2 points

- Autoantibodies
  - ANA, SMA or LKM > 1: 40 — 1 point
  - > 1: 80, or SLA/LP positive — 2 points

- Histology of chronic hepatitis
  - Compatible with AIH — 1 point
  - Typical of AIH — 2 points

- Absence of viral hepatitis

- Essential to make or confirm diagnosis
- Excludes other diagnoses (e.g. NASH)
- Findings must be compatible, can be typical
- Best measure of disease activity
- Macronodular nature makes staging unreliable
- (Mini-) laparoscopy superior in staging

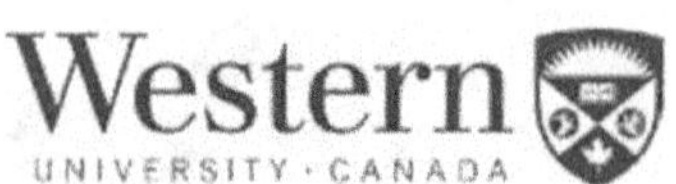

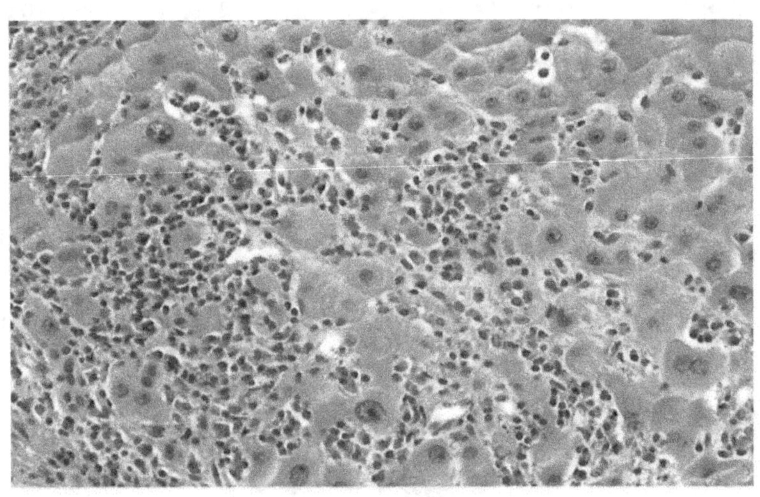

- Immunofluorescence: ANA

ANA Immunohistochemistry in AIH

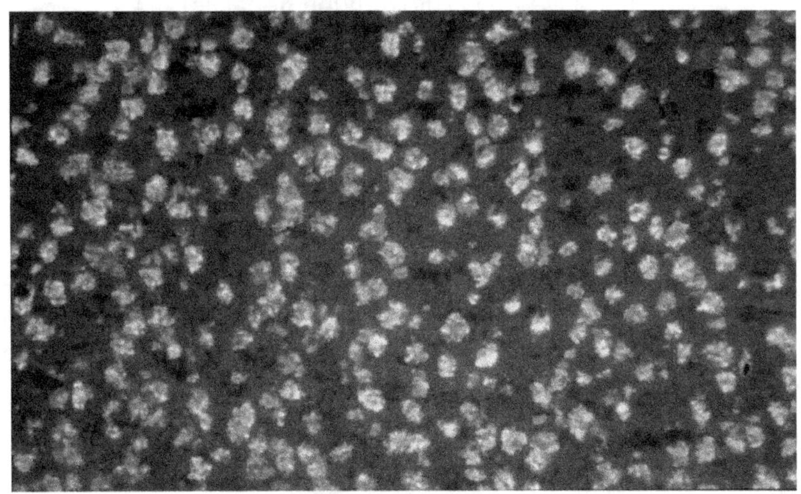

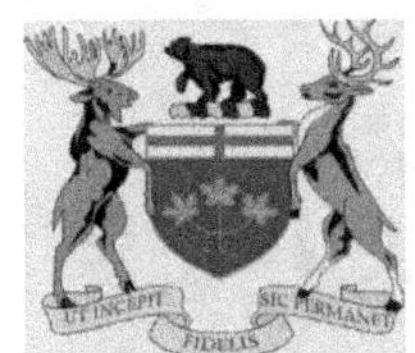

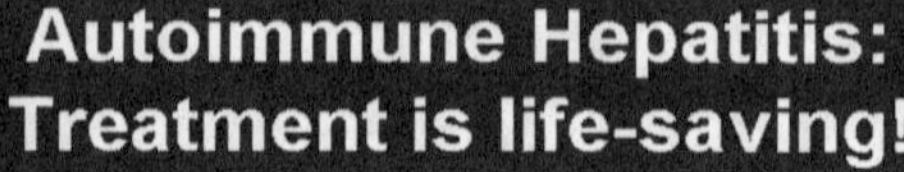

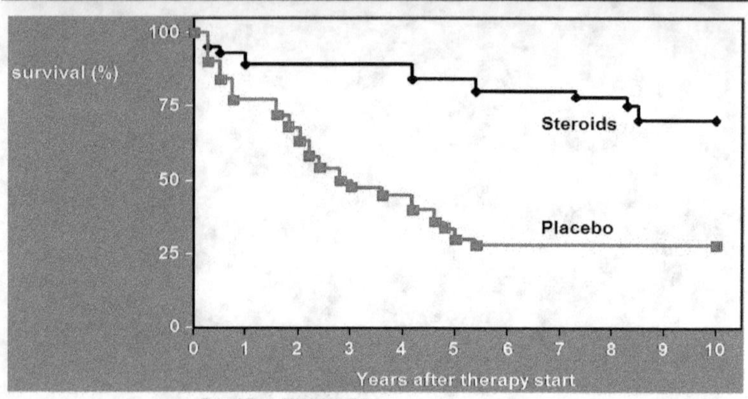

Royal Free Hospital Trial:
AP Kirk, S Jain, S Pocock, HC Thomas, and S Sherlock: Gut 1980; 21: 78-83

- Treatment of AIH

- Give the difference in the treatment of AMA-positive and –negative AIH (autoimmune hepatitis)
    - AIH ⇄ PBC in 10% to 15%, causing 2 overlap syndromes
    - AMA-positive AIH steroids, azathioprine (treat as per guideline for AIH, type I; may also be ANA-positive)
    - AMA- negative PBC steroids, UDCA (ursodeoxycholic acid) (aka autoimmune cholangiopathy)

Please see: Swan MG. Chapter 58. In: Therapeutic Choices. Grey J, Ed. 6th Edition, Canadian Pharmacists Association: Ottawa, ON, 2011, Table 3 and 5, page 775-778.

- Induction

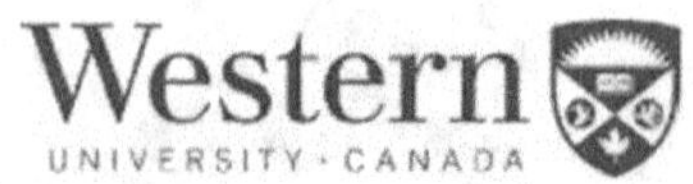

- 1 mg / kg prednisolone / day
  - Reduction by 10 mg/day per week to 20 mg/day
  - Slower reduction to 10 mg/day (response-dependent)
  - Reduction below 10 mg/day only in remission
- Budesonide 3 mg p.o. tid
- Tacrolimus 2 mg p.o. bid, aim level 5-8
- Cyclosporine 50 mg p.o. bid, aim level 100
- Imuran alternative:
  - Cellcept 250 – 1000 mg p.o. bid

- Give 10 preventative measures about which to advise patients with AIH treated with prednisone +/- azathioprine.

➢ General
- Monitor for weight gain
- Supplement with calcium, vitamin D, +/- bisphosphonates
- Monitor blood sugar, lipids, fat soluble vitamins
- Monitor CBC, ALT (if on Azathioprine)
- Annual checks for BP, cataract, glaucoma, BMD, Pap' smear, esophageal varices
- Check stools for ova/parasites after foreign travel
- "Stop" order on Rx
- Screening mammography, colonoscopy
- Access for depression
- Stress high doses of steroids, if necessary
- Wear medical alert bracelet

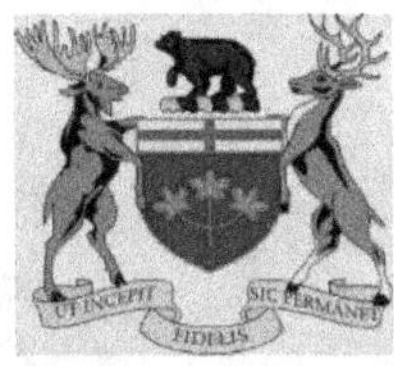

- Avoid stopping steroids suddenly (Addisonian crisis, recurrence of AIH)
- Avoid unplanned pregnancy; consider avoiding pregnancy if portal hypertension is marked; contraception
- Drug interactions
- Immunizations (see below)

➢ Specific

- If cirrhotic: avoid sedation, NSAIDs, anesthesia, interferon
- If cirrhotic, screen for HCC
- Avoid vaccination with varicella, MMR, yellow fever
- Vaccination for H. influenza, HAV, HBV, pneumococcus (hyposplenism)
- Assess for esophageal varices for primary prevention with banding or beta blockers (avoid use in pregnancy – fetal hypoglycemia)
- Assess for Ascites (SBP)

Adapted from: Heathcote J. *Am J Gastroenterol* 2006;101:S630–S632.

➢ Follow-up biopsies

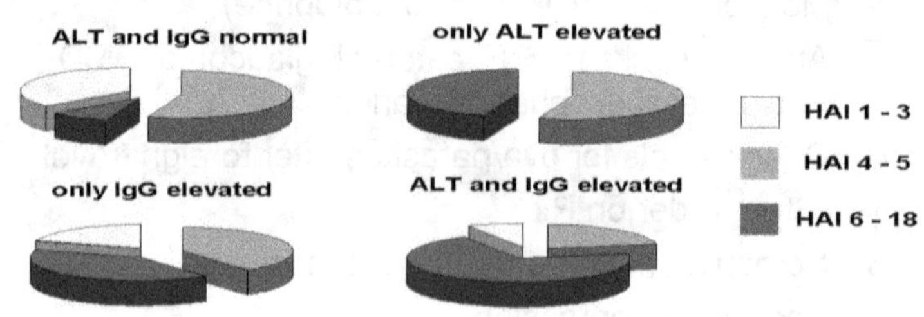

Source: Luth S, et al. J Clin Gastroenterol;43(1):75-80.

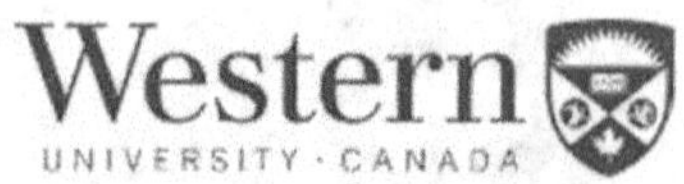

- Six month remission rates
  - Complete, 91%
  - Incomplete, 7%
  - None, 2%
- Maintenance
  - Azathioprine 1-1.5 mg/kg/d
    - +/- 5 mg (-10 mg) / day prednisolone
    - Aim: normal transaminases, normal IgG (normal histology or minimal hepatitis)
    - Duration: minimum 3-4 years
  - Outcome during maintenance therapy (mean follow-up, 95 months)
    - Remission 2/3
    - Relapse 1/3
- Treatment failure
  - Check diagnosis!
  - Check compliance
  - Refer to expert centre
  - Prednisolone IV 100 mg/day
  - Consider cyclophosphamide 100 mg / day IV
- Withdrawal of steroids
  - Only after minimum of one year
  - Risk of reactivation Ca 50%
  - Risk of reacitivation can be reduced by increasing azathioprine to 2 mg/kg
  - Choice dependent on risk profile
  - Outcome after treatment withdrawal
    - Sustained remission ¼
    - Relapse ¾
- Complete withdrawal of immunosuppression
  - Relapse common
  - Relapse mostly during first 12-18 months
  - Histological activity best predictor

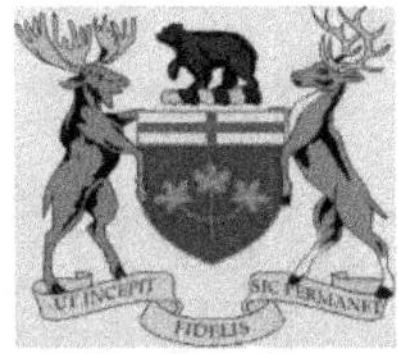

- > 3 years stable remission prior to treatment cessation
- HAI < 3

- Therapeutic Plan-Individualize
  - Prednisone 0.5 mg/kg or
  - Budesonide 3 mg tid
  - Imuran 1-2 mgkg or
  - Cellcept 500 mg bid
  - Once ALT and IgG normal
    - Taper steroid, then immunomodulator
    - Timeline 6 months each
  - Normal expectancy with individualized therapy

➢ Liver transplantation

Clinical Tip – Early Failure of Treatment and Need for Liver Transplantation.

- Profile of patient with needs to be considered early for liver transplantation include:
  - Decompensated patients with biopsy evidence of multilobular necrosis, in whom
  - Hyperbilirubinemia does not improve, and
  - At least one other lab test does not return to normal

➢ Therapy: continue steroids until

- Remission
  - "……absence of symptoms, resolution of all laboratory indices of active inflammation and histologic improvement of normal liver tissue or inactive cirrhosis" ((Feldman M., et al. Sleisenger and Fordtran's Gastrointestinal and Liver Disease. 9th Edition. Saunders/Elsevier, Philadelphia, 2010, page 1473).

- Treatment failure

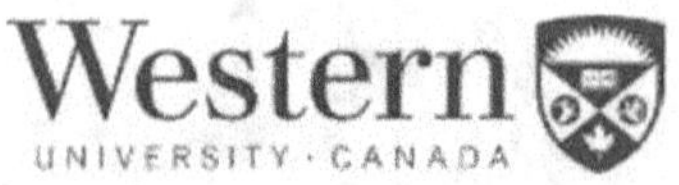

  - "worsening of the serum AST or bilirubin levels by at least 67% of previous values, progressive histological activity, or onset of ascites or encephalopathy"

- Incomplete response: "….improvement that is insufficient to satisfy remission criteria" (Feldman M., et al. Sleisenger and Fordtran's Gastrointestinal and Liver Disease. 9th Edition. Saunders/Elsevier, Philadelphia, 2010, page 1474).

- Drug toxicity

- Relapse
  - Occurs in 50% in 6 months
  - ~ 75% in 3 years
  - Defined as "… the reappearance of histologic disease after discontinuation of drug therapy" after previous achieved remission
  - Rational for maintenance therapy: repeated relapse and re-treatment leads to
    - ↑ cirrhosis
    - ↑ hepatic failure
    - ↑ need for liver transplantation
    - ↑ drug adverse effects
    - ↑ mortality

Obtain guidance from (Feldman M., et al. Sleisenger and Fordtran's Gastrointestinal and Liver Disease. 9th Edition. Saunders/Elsevier, Philadelphia, 2010, Table 88.5, page 1469).

> Tricks or Treats
>
> In patient with AIH (autoimmune hepatitis), if they are HLA-Dr3 positive, their therapeutic response may be lower.

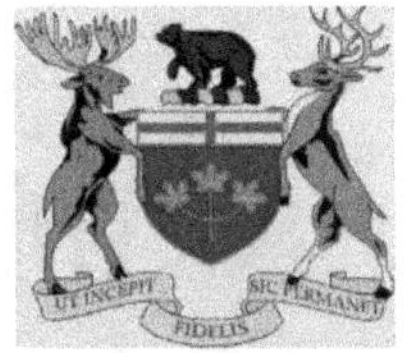

- Give the complications of liver transplantation (LT) which are more common for AIH than compared with non-autoimmune liver disease.
  - Acute rejection
  - Steroid-resistant rejection
  - Chronic rejection
  - Difficult in stopping steroids

➢ Clinical event	Conventional treatments		Possible empiric treatments	
	1st choice	2nd choice	3rd choice	4th choice
Treatment Failure	Prednisone (30 mg daily) and Azathioprine (150 mg daily), or prednisone alone (60 mg daily)	Prednisone (30 mg daily) Plus Mercaptopurin (1.5 mg/kg body weight daily)	Ciclosporin (5-6 mg/kg body weight daily) or prednisone (30 mg daily) plus Mycophenolate mofetil (2 g daily)	Tacrolimus (4 mg twice daily)
Drug toxicity	Azathioprine (2 mg/kg body weight daily) if prednisone intolerant	Prednisone (20 mg daily) if Azathioprine Intolerant	Budesonide (3 mg twice daily)	UDCA (13-15 mg/kg body weight daily)
Incomplete Response	Prednisone maintenance (≤ 10 mg daily) if serum AST level < three times normal value	Azathioprine maintenance (2 mg/kg body weight daily) if serum AST level <3 times normal value)	Budesonide Maintenance (3 mg twice daily)	UDCA Maintenance (13-15 mg/kg body weight daily)

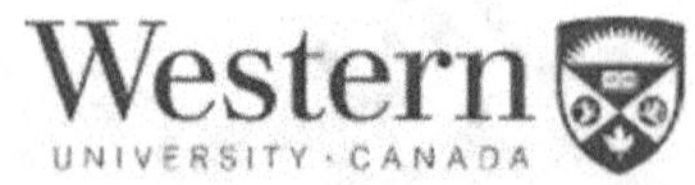

	1st choice	2nd choice	3rd choice	4th choice
Relapse	Azathioprine maintenance (2 mg/kg body weight daily) if serum AST level <three times normal value	Prednisone Maintenance reduced to (≤ 10 mg daily) if serum AST level <three times normal value	Mycophenolate mofetil maintenance (2 g daily)	Ciclosporin Maintenance (5-6 mg/kg body weight daily)

Abbreviations: AST, aspartate aminotransferase; UDCA, ursodeoxycholic ai

Printed with permission: Loza A, et al. *Nat Clin Pract Gastroenterol Hepatol* 2007; 4(4): pg. 206.

- Prognosis
  - Death from bleeding EV (esophageal varices) ~ 20%
  - Relapse may occur after drug withdrawal
  - The clinical course is influences by the level of ALT and gamma globulins, serology (anti-soluble liver antigen (SLA), anti-asialoglycoprotein receptor (ASGPR), anti-chromatin), liver biopsy (bridging or multilobular necrosis, or cirrhosis), HLA status, and response to treatment. Each of the above is associated on adverse outcome
  - The MELD (model for end-stage liver disease) score predicts survival
    Based on degree of impaired liver function, not affected by cause or presence of cirrhosis
    MELD ≥ 12 9 at presentation), 97% of these persons will fail steroid therapy

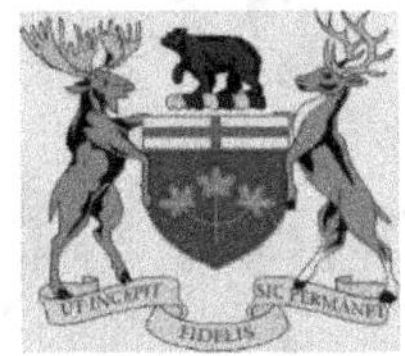

- New predictors of response to treat in autoimmune hepatitis type 1
  - Low levels of anti-α-actinin at baseline are independent predictors of response.
  - Autoantibodies against filamentous-actin and α-actinin.
  - Can be used as predictors of response to treatment in patients with AIH 1

For the details of these prognostic factors and outcome, please see Feldman M., et al. Sleisenger and Fordtran's Gastrointestinal and Liver Disease. 9th Edition. Saunders/Elsevier, Philadelphia, 2010, Table 88.5, page 1469, "Prognostic Factors and Associated Reported Outcomes in Autoimmune Hepatitis".

Please see Feldman M., et al. Sleisenger and Fordtran's Gastrointestinal and Liver Disease. 9th Edition. Saunders/Elsevier, Philadelphia, 2010, Table 88.4, page 1467, for a summary of the 4 "Variant Forms of Autoimmune Hepatitis".

Factors associated with clinically significant **endpoints** in autoimmune hepatitis (AIH)

Endpoint	Relapse (off treatment)	Progressive fibrosis or development of cirrhosis	Liver-related death or transplantation
o Frequency	- 50–90%	▪ 10–50%	10–20%
o Factors			

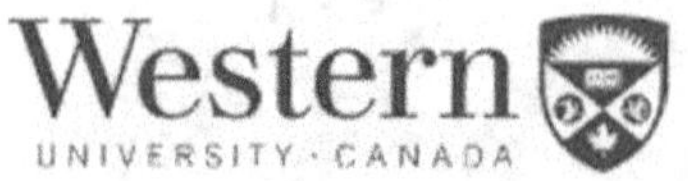

Endpoint	Relapse (off treatment)	Progressive fibrosis or development of cirrhosis	Liver-related death or transplantation
At presentation	- Long symptom duration - High serum globulin - LKM antibody positive - SLA/LP positive or no immune markers	▪ Low serum albumin and coagulopathy ▪ Confluent necrosis on biopsy	Females African-American men Type 2 AIH and SLA positive AIH Cirrhosis Confluent necrosis
On treatment	- Short treatment duration - Long time to remission	▪ Persistent AST elevation (failure of AST to halve in 6 months) ▪ Failure to achieve remission over 2 years ▪ Persistent inflammation on liver biopsy	Poor response, long time to achieve remission, persistent serum AST elevation
Pretreatment withdrawal	- Raised serum ALT or AST - Raised serum globulin IgG - Liver biopsy with any inflammation, or with portal tract plasma cells		
Subsequently		▪ Multiple relapses	Multiple relapses Development of cirrhosis

Abbreviations: ALT, alanine aminotransferase; AST, aspartate aminotransferase; LKM-1, liver kidney microsomal-1 antibody; SLA/LP, soluble liver antigen/liver pancreas antigen.

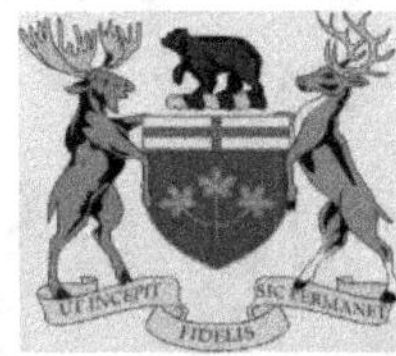

Printed with permission: Gleeson D, et al. Gut. 2011;60(12): 1611-29, Table 6.

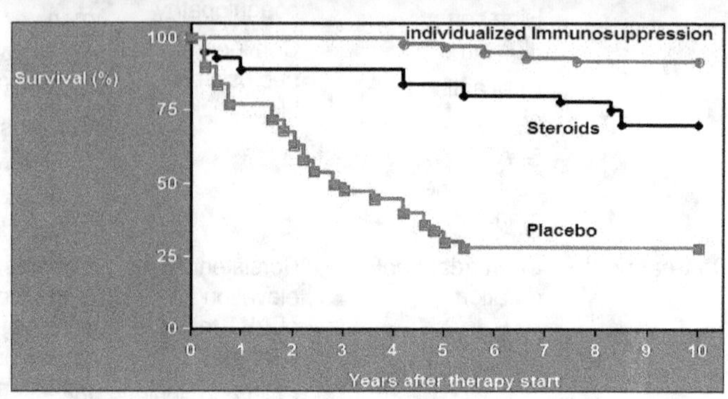

Kanzler et al.; Z. Gastroenterol. 2001, 39: 339-348

SO YOU WANT TO BE A HEPATOLOGIST!

- Give the comparison of non-hereditary versus hereditary AIH (aka APECED*)

Feature	Non-hereditary	Hereditary
Gender effect	F > M	F = M
Gene mutation	No	Single-gene mutation of AIRE (autoimmune regulator), autosomal recessive, complete gene penetrance
HLA predisposition	HLA-DR3 (DRB1*0304)	No
Response to therapy	65% achieve remission within 3 years; therapy improves 10-year survival rate to 93%	Poor

Abbreviation: APECED, autoimmune polyendocrinopathycandidiasis – ectodermal dystrophy

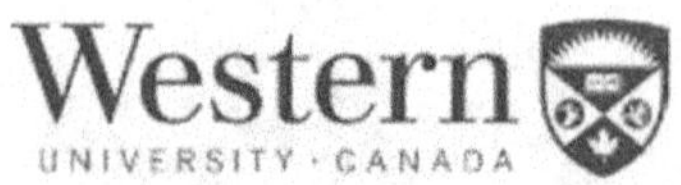

AIH plus HCV

- About 10% of persons with AIH also have HCV infection, and about half of HCV patients have features suggestive or AIH, such as
  - Autoantibodies
  - Other immune diseases, or
  - Both of above
- The treatment of AIH will affect the HCV, and vice versa. Treatment is usually focused on the predominant component, AIH or HCV.
- It is often best to first treat the AIH, because the interferon used in the treatment of HCV would worsen the AIH.

- Give the 3 infectious agents, which have homology with epitopes of CYP2D6, and are recognized by anti-LKM1.

Organisms showing molecular mimicry / molecular footprint / share motif with anti-LKM1 include

- HCV
- CMV
- HSV

This is outrageous; why would any sober person in their right mind need to know these molecular mimicries?

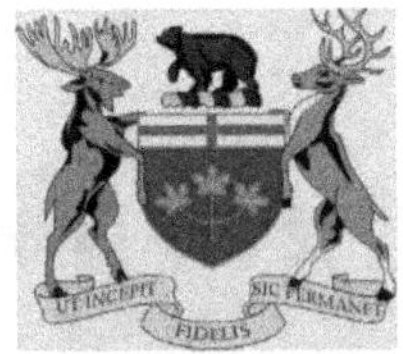

AUTOIMMUNE HEPATITIS, AND VARIANT (OVERLAP) SYNDROMES

- Give the features which help to distinguish between autoimmune predominant, or AIH plus HCV.

Feature	AIH predominant	HCV predominant
○ Associated diseases	– "autoimmune" disorders in 38%	▪ "immune complex"
○ Autoantibodies	– Multiple	▪ One
○ Symptomatic cryoglobulinemia	– Rare	▪ Yes
○ AST, IgG	↑↑	↑
○ Histology**	– Panacinar hepatitis – Interface hepatitis – Portal plasma cells	▪ Steatosis ▪ Portal lymphoid aggregates
○ Immune complex disorders	– Vasculitis – Glomerulo-nephritis – Symptomatic cryoglobulineia	

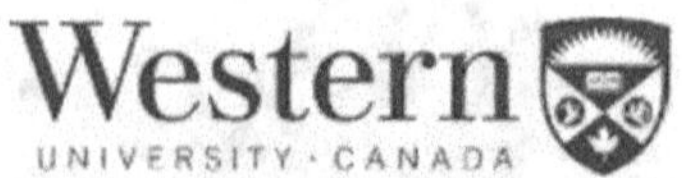

Variant (Overlap) Syndromes

- Laboratory
  - AIH plus PBC
    - Low titres of PBC-specific M2 mitochondrial antigens
    - AMA may come and go in 18% of persons with AIH
  - AIH plus PSC / PSC in adults, 41% of AIH who have
    - Cholestatic 'la' findings
    - Associated IBD (especially UC)
    - Failure to respond to steroids
    - Have cholangiographic changes of PSC
    - 54% of persons with PSC have features supporting a diagnosis of AIH (definite, or probable)
    - The duct changes in AIH plus PSC may be only in the small ducts ("small duct PSC")
    - In children with AIH
    - Large duct small duct PSC
    - AMI-positive PBC
    - AMA-negative PBC
    - Autoimmune cholangitis
  - Autoantibody negative AIH
    - No antibodies, but
    - Usually abnormal
    - HLA (HLA-D3 or DR4)
    - Interface hepatitis

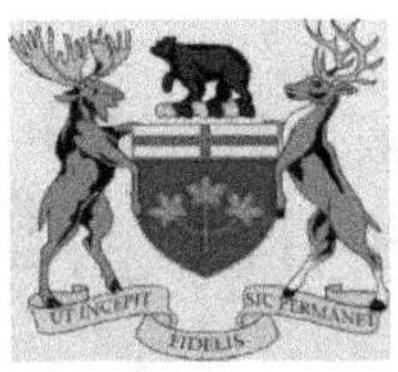

- Pathophysiology

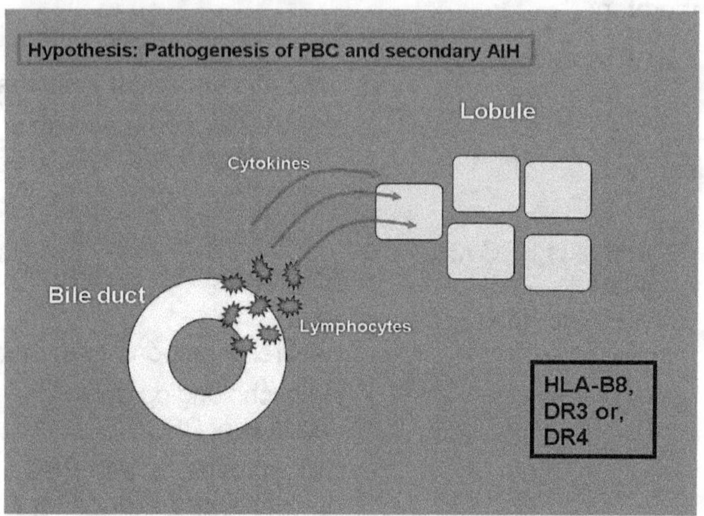

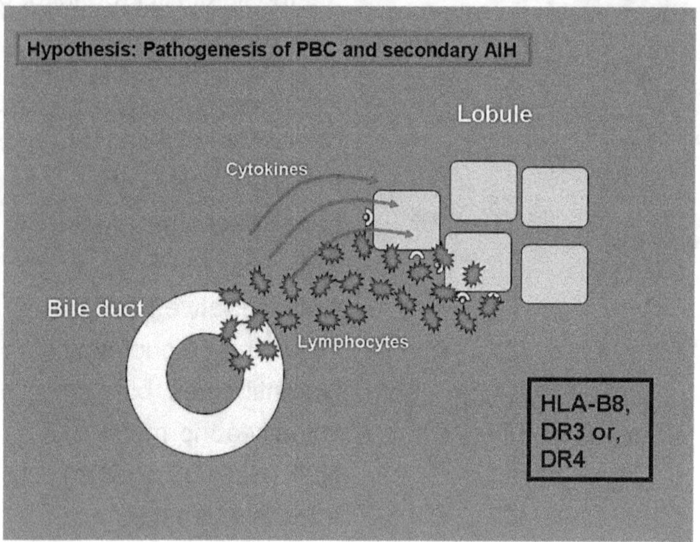

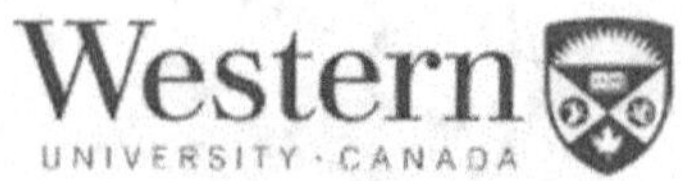

Overlap PBC / AIH ("Variant Syndrome")

- Occurs in 10-20% of PBC patients
- May develop sequentially, with either disease manifesting first
- Should always be considered in PBC not fully responding to UDCA
- Requires immunosuppression like AIH
- Overlap PSC / AIH
- Only small case series published
- Only few cases with initial ERCP
- AIH progressing to PSC (autoimmune sclerosing cholangitis, ASC) relatively common in children

Overlap AIH / PSC

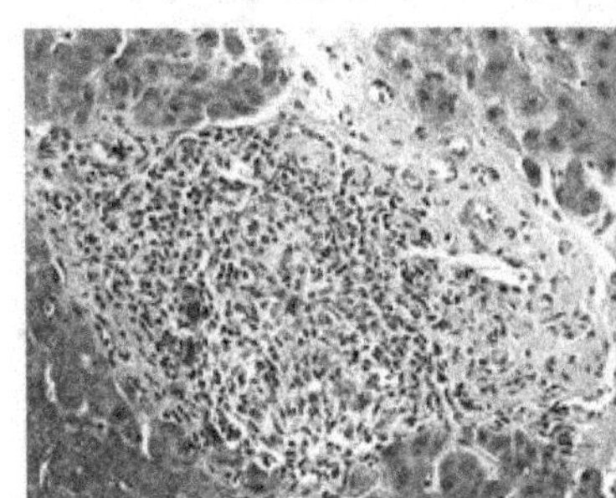

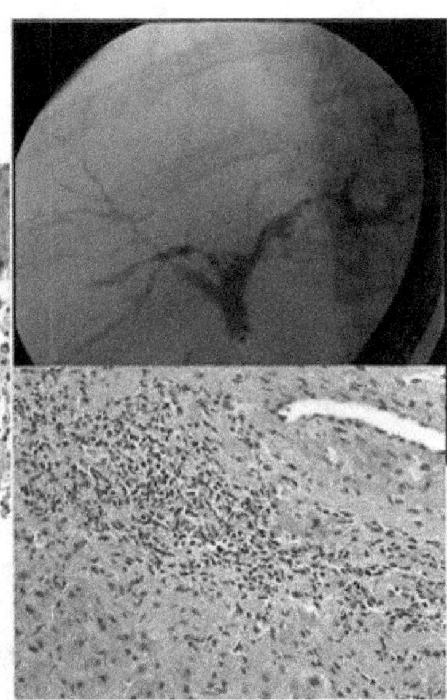

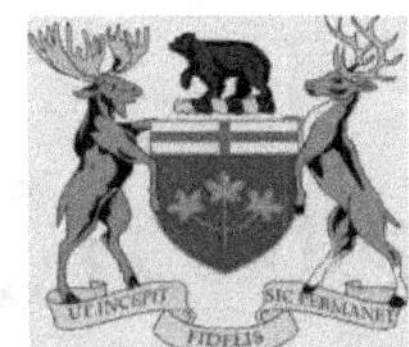

- Initial ALT and AP in 20 AIH patients, 20 PSC patients, and 16 patients who manifested features of both disease

- Give the treatments of the variant syndromes of AIH.

Variant syndrome	Salient features	Empiric treatment strategies
AIH and primary biliary cirrhosis (PBC)	- AMA positivity - Cholestatic and hepatitic tests - Increased serum IgM and IgG levels	▪ Corticosteroids if serum ALP is ≤ twice ULN ▪ Add ursodeoxycholic acid (UDCA) if serum ALP is > twice ULN and/or florid duct lesions in liver tissue ▪ Corticosteroids and UDCA
AIH and primary sclerosing cholangitis	- Ulcerative colitis - Pruritus - Cholestatic and hepatic tests - ALP:AST>1.5	▪ Prednisone, ursodeoxycholic acid, or both, depending on hepatic and cholestatic components
AIH and cholangitis (possibly AMA-negative primary biliary sclerosis)	- Abnormal cholangiogram - Fatigue - Pruritus - Cholestatic and hepatic tests - AMA negative - ANA and/or SMA positive	

- Normal cholangiogram

Abbreviations: ALP, Alkaline phosphatase; AMA, antimitochondrial antibodies; ANA, antinuclear antibodies; AST, aspartate aminotransferase; SMA, smooth muscle antibodies; ULN, upper limit of normal.

Adapted from: Czaja AJ. *Sleisenger & Fordtran's Gastrointestinal and Liver Disease: Pathophysiology/Diagnosis/Management* 2006 pg. 1874.

Useful background: The Mayo Clinic treatment schedules for adults with severe autoimmune hepatitis

Treatment duration (weeks)	Combination therapy Prednisone (mg daily)	Combination therapy Azathioprine (mg daily)	Prednisone monotherapy (mg daily)
1	30	50	60
1	20	50	40
2	15	50	30
Maintenance until end point	10	50	20

Printed with permission: Loza AJM, and Czaja AJ. *Nature Clinical Practice Gastroenterology & Hepatology* 2007; 4(4): pg. 204.

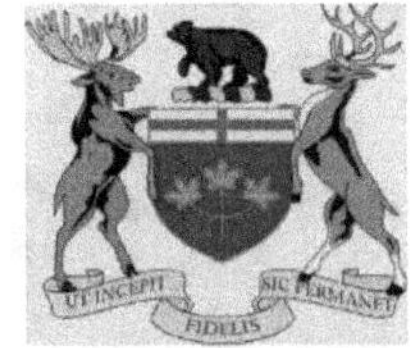

"Either I will find a way, or I will make one."

Philip Sidney

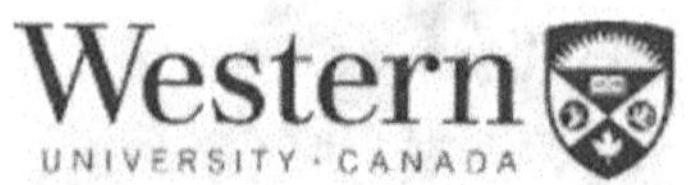

MINI UPDATE

Causality Assessment in Drug Induced Liver Injury

Mark A. Levstik

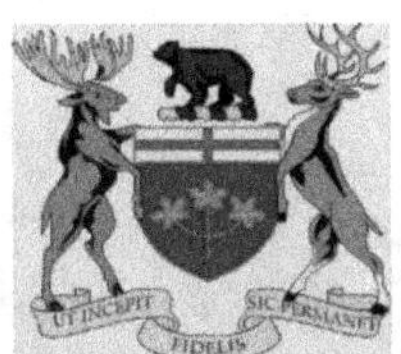

CAUSALITY ASSESSMENT IN DRUG INDUCED LIVER INJURY

- Demography

- Population-based study (81,300 French '97-'00)
  - 95 suspected cases
    - 34 probable DILI
      - 25% antibiotics 23% psychotropic 13% antilipid
    - 80% outpatients
    - 2 (7%) deaths
  - Incidence: 14 to 24 per 100,000
    - 8,000 annual cases, 500 deaths
    - 16 X > than ADR surveillance

- Pathophysiology

Drugs are metabolized by:

- Phase I reactions
  - Microsomal drug oxidases and the CYP gene superfamily
    - Involves the hemoprotein f the CYP gene
    - Drugs are converted to a toxic metabolite (e.g. acetaminophen → NAPQI)

- Phase II
  - Conjugation
    - Through glucuronic acid or inorganic sulfate by formation of ester links with the drug

- Phase III
  - Secretion of drugs or their metabolites by transporters
    - ATP-binding cassette (ABC) protein
    - MDR1 (multidrug resistance protein C1)
    - MRP1 (multidrug resistance-associated proteins)

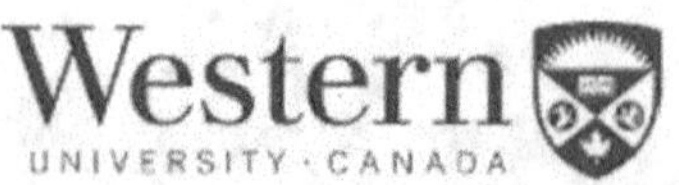

- MRP-3 sinusoidal membrane of hepatocytes
- MRP2 canalicular membrane (CM) of hepatocytes

- Give the reason why DILI resulting from drugs metabolized by phase I reactions (e.g. acetaminophen) is localized in zone 3 (around the terminal hepatic venules [THV]).
  - Phase 1 reactions are catalyzed by microsomal drug oxidase, the key component of when is a hemoprotein of the CYP gene superfamily.
  - CYP2E1 is located in hepatocytes which form a 1 to 2 hepatocyte thick rim around the THV.

- Give 5 drugs that have been reported to have an increased risk of hepatotoxicity in patients with chronic liver disease.

Drug	Underlying liver disease as a risk factor
Antiandrogens	Chronic viral hepatitis B, C
Antiretrovirals (e.g. zalcitabine, saquinavir)	Hepatitis B, C
Ibuprofen (NSAIDs)	Hepatitis C
Methimazole	Chronic hepatitis B
Methotrexate	Alcoholic liver disease, NAFLD

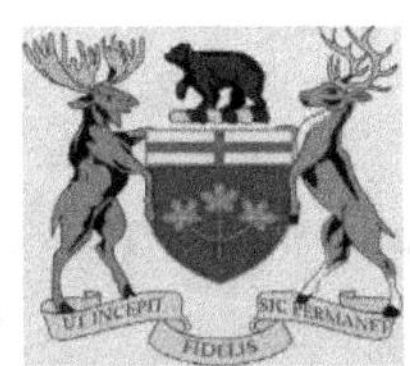

Drug	Underlying liver disease as a risk factor
o Oral contraceptives	- Women with liver tumours, or history of jaundice of pregnancy
o Rifampin	- Primary biliary cirrhosis
o Vitamin A (high doses)	- Alcoholic liver disease

Adapted from: Gupta NK, and Lewis JH. *Aliment Pharmacol Ther* 2008; 28(9): 1021-41.

- Give 5 major toxic mechanisms of drug-induced liver injury, leading to hepatocyte apoptosis and necrosis.
  - Direct hepatotoxicity
    - Injury to
      - Mitochondria
      - Plasma membrane
  - ROS (reactive oxygen species)
    - "the liver is exposed to oxidative stress by the propensity of hepatocytes to reduce oxygen…."
    - Some drugs (e.g. acetaminophen) may be converted by CYP into pre-oxidant reactive metabolites
    - CYP-mediated metabolism → formation of reactive metabolites → ↓ glutathione → injury to mitochondria → 1) release of cytochrome C and 2) operation of MPT (mitochondrial permeability transition) → activation of caspase → apoptosis

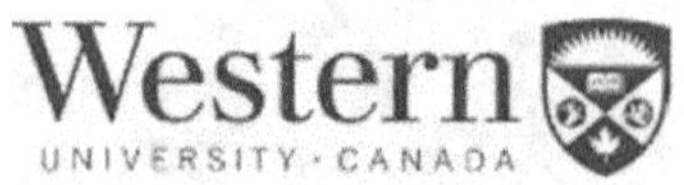

- Formed from injured hepatocytes and kupffer cells
- Reactive metabolites undergo covalent binding to proteins
- Protein-drug adducts
  - Inactive important enzymes
  - May be acted upon by immunodestructive processes

➤ Glutathione system

- Pro-oxidants signal Nrf (the redox-sensitive transcription factor)
- Nrf → ↑ CYP 2E1 expression → ↑ hepatic glutathione synthesis (from cysteine) → ↑ antioxidant effects
- Cystolic glutathione
  - In the reduced state, resulting from the effect of NADPH and glutathione reductase
  - Glutathione deficiency injures mitochondria, releases cytochrome C and MPT (mitochondrial membrane permeability transition), leading to activation of caspases and apoptosis

➤ Biochemical pathways of cellular damage

- Covalent binding of drug to cellular proteins
- Oxidation of proteins
- Post-translational modification of proteins
- Lipid peroxidation
- Cleavage of DNA
- ↑ Ca_I^{2+} (intracellular concentration of Ca^{2+})

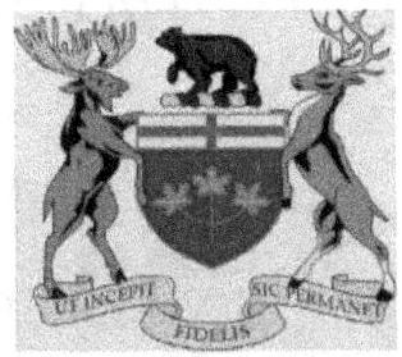

- Hepatic non-hepatocyte cells
  - Kupffer cells
    - Act as macrophages and antigen-presenting cells
    - Activated Kupffer cell may release TNF, ROS and as-L, which may lead to hepatocyte apoptosis / necrosis
  - Endothelial cells
    - Their low glutathione context make then susceptibility to vascular injury
  - Stellate cells
    - When activated, will deposit matrix and lead to fibrosis

- Immunologic mechanisms
  - Formation of ligands with death receptors
  - Porin-mediated introduction of granzyme
  - "altered antigen" drug metabolite interacts with cellular proteins to form drug-protein adducts (haptens)
  - Drug-induced autoimmunity

- Spectrum of DILI

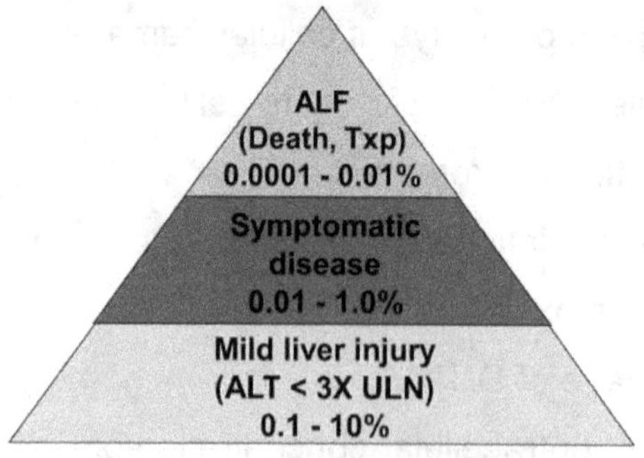

Abbreviations: ALF, acute liver failure; Txp, liver transplantation; ULN, upper limit of normal

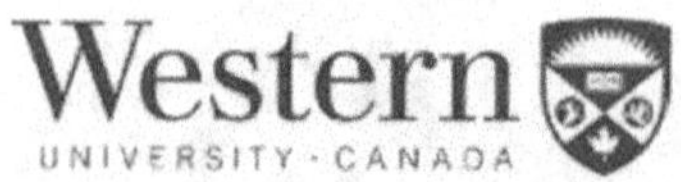

CAUSALITY ASSESSMENT IN DRUG INDUCED LIVER INJURY

Acute DILI

- Laboratory
  - Hepatocellular
    - $R > 5$
    - ALT > 2x ULN or baseline
  - Cholestatic
    - $R < 2$ and Alk > ULN
  - Mixed
    - $2 < R < 5$

R = (ALT / ULN) / (Alk / ULN)

Source: Bénichou C. J Hepatol 1990; 11: 272-6.

- Risk

- Give 15 factors which increase the risk of the development of DILI (drug-induced liver injury)

  - Older age
  - Female gender
  - Polypharmacy
  - Past history of adverse drug reaction
  - Alcohol
    - $\downarrow$ dose threshold and $\uparrow$ severity of hepatotoxicity of some drugs, e.g. acetaminophen, isoniazid, niacin, methrotrexate

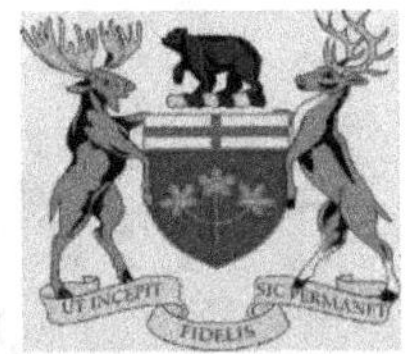

- Nutritional status
  - Obesity
  - Halothane
  - Malnutrition
  - Methotrexate
  - Tamoxifen
- Pre-existing liver disease
  - Methotrexate
  - HBV, HCV, HIV / AIDs
    - Anti-TB drugs
    - HAART therapy
    - Anti-cancer drugs
    - Ibuprofen
    - Myeloablation
    - Anti-androgens
    - Sulfonamides
  - HCV sinusoidal obstruction syndrome
- Other diseases
  - Rheumatoid arthritis
    - Salicylates
    - Sulfasalazine
  - Diabetes, obesity
    - Methotrexate
  - Chronic renal disease
    - Methotrexate → fibrosis
    - Renal transplantation → azathioprine-associated hepatic vascular damage

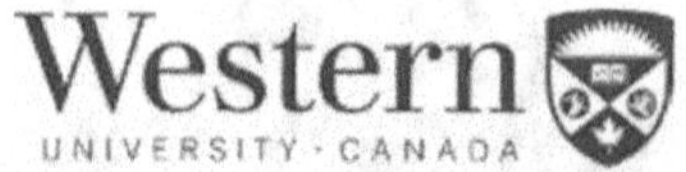

CAUSALITY ASSESSMENT IN DRUG INDUCED LIVER INJURY

- Pathology

- Give 7 types of histopathological changes seen in DILI
  - Acute hepatitis
  - Fulminant hepatic failure
  - Chronic granulomatous hepatitis
  - Chronic hepatitis
  - Autoimmune hepatitis
  - Cholestasis with/without hepatitis
  - Steatohepatitis with / without fibrosis
  - Vascular toxicity
    - SOS (sinusoidal obstruction syndrome; aka veno-occlusive disease)
    - Sinusoidal dilation
    - Cavernous hemangioma
    - NRH (nodular regenerative hypertension
    - Peliosis hepatitis
  - Tumor
    - FNH
    - Hepatic adenoma
    - HCC
    - Cavernous hemangioma

- Hepatic manifestations
  - Hepatitis
    - Acute hepatitis
    - Chronic hepatitis
    - Granulomatous disease

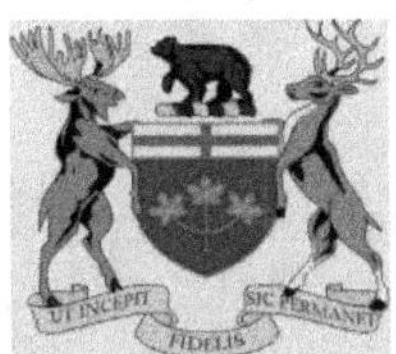

- Cholestasis
  - Acute cholestasis
- Fat
  - Fatty liver/ NASH
- Fibrosis/ cirrhosis
- Vessels
  - Vanishing bile duct
  - VOD, peliosis
- Tumors
  - Benign & malignant neoplasia

➢ Diagnosis

- Temporal relationship
  - Not dose related
  - ? Clinical risk factors
- Biochemical injury pattern
  - "Signature" vs protean
  - Prior reports/ cases
  - Exclude other likely causes
- Improvement with discontinuation
- DILI is a diagnosis of exclusion based on circumstantial evidence due to lack of objective confirmatory lab test, rechallenge, or "GOLD" standard
  - Requires a high index of suspicion
- DILI diagnosis is usually retrospective
  - Exclude other causes
  - Dechallenge requires follow-up

➢ Causality assessment

- Generic instruments
  - WHO (World Heath Organization)
  - Bayesian

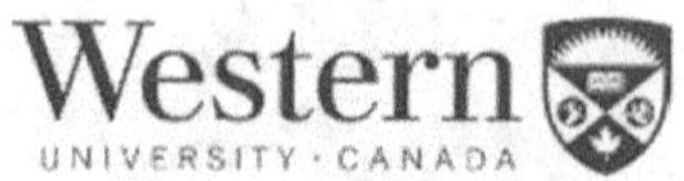

CAUSALITY ASSESSMENT IN DRUG INDUCED LIVER INJURY

- Liver specific
  - Expert opinion
  - Roussel Uclaf Causality Assessment Method (RUCAM) '89
  - Clinical Diagnostic Scale (CDS) '97
  - DILIN approach

- DILI Causality Instrument
  - Sensitive
  - Specific- Low probability in non-drug cases
  - Reproducible
  - Content validity- weighting is evidence based
  - Criterion validity- "Gold Standard" expert panel
  - Discrimination- a semi-quantitative estimate
  - Validated in independent groups
  - Generalizability- Young vs old, mild vs severe, hepatocellular vs cholestatic, normal vs abnormal baseline LFT's
  - Ease of use

- RUCAM (Roussel Uclaf Causalty Assessment Method)
  - Temporal relationship (0 to 2)
  - Course (-2 to 3)
  - Risk factors (0 to 2)
  - Concomitant drug (0 to -3)
  - Non-drug causes (-3 to 2)
  - Prior reports/ information (0 to 2)
  - Re-challenge (-2 to 3)

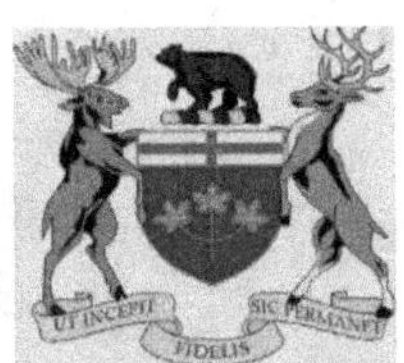

Score (-8 to 14)
  - Highly probable >8
  - Possible 3-5 Excluded ≤0
  - Probable 6-8
  - Unlikely 1-2

- RUCAM limitations
  - Ambiguous instructions
  - Criteria for competing cause/drug not clear
  - Onset > 30 days after d/c (e.g. Augmentin)
  - Derived from expert opinion rather than prospectively collected data set
    - Limited risk factors
    - Overweighting of rechallenge

- Clinical Diagnostic Scale
  - Temporal association
    - From initiation (1 to 3)
    - From cessation (-3 to 3)
    - Normalization (0 to 3)
  - Non-drug causes (-3 to 3)
  - Extrahepatic manifestations (0 to 3)
  - Rechallenge (0 to 3)
  - Prior reports (-3 to 2)

- Comparison CDS vs RUCAM
  - RUCAM performed better overall
  - CDS performed poorly if
    - Delayed onset (> 15 days)
    - Prolonged recovery (Cholestasis)
    - ALF/ Death (6%)
      - CDS: 6 possible 7 unlikely/ excluded
      - RUCAM: 6 definite 6 probable 1 possible
    - Idiosyncratic (75%)

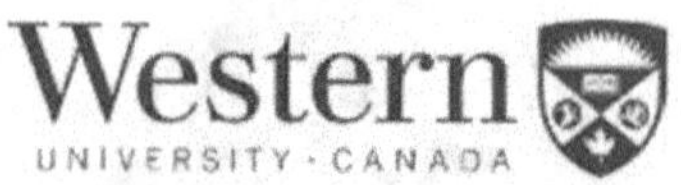

Abbreviations: CDS, clinical diagnostic scale; RUCAM, Roussel Uclaf Causality Assessment Method

Source: Hepatology 2011; 33: 123; Weiler-Normann, **J** *Hepatol***.** *2011*;55(4):747-9.

Gold standard: Expert panel (l228 Spanish cases '94-'00)

		CDS			
RUCAM	Exclude	Unlike	Poss	Prob	Def
Exclude	21	2			
Unlike		4	3		
Possible			8	1	
Probable		1	30	43	16
Definite		5	40	53	1

Source: Lucena MI, et al. Hepatology. 2001;33(1):123-30.

SO YOU WANT TO BE A HEPATOLOGIST!

- In the context of DILI, give the meaning of the Hy law.
    - In DILI, the finding of clinical jaundice plus increased ALT or AST has a mortality ratio of ~ 10%.

Please see Feldman M., et al. Sleisenger and Fordtran's Gastrointestinal and Liver Disease. 9th Edition. Saunders/Elsevier, Philadelphia, 2010, Table 86.3, page 1427 for "Risk Factors for Acetaminophen Induced Hepatotoxicity"; also Table 86.4, page 1431, "Type of Drug-Induced cute Hepatitis: Immunoallergic Reaction Versus Metabolic Idiosyncrasy".

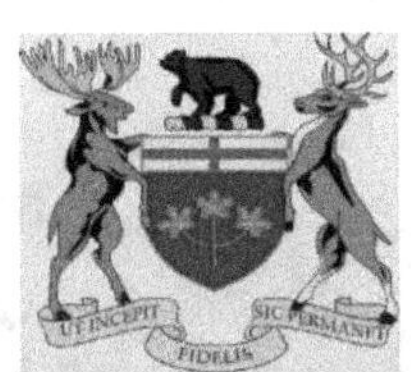

Clinical Tip

"……the presence of underlying liver disease does not predispose to acetaminophen hepatotoxicity" (Feldman M., et al. Sleisenger and Fordtran's Gastrointestinal and Liver Disease. 9th Edition. Saunders/Elsevier, Philadelphia, 2010, page 1427).

- Differential diagnosis

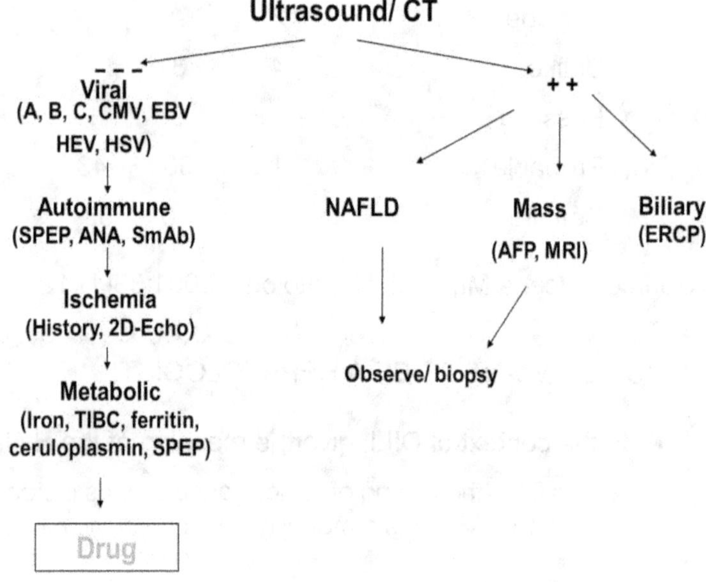

- Feldman M., et al. Sleisenger and Fordtran's Gastrointestinal and Liver Disease. 9th Edition. Saunders/Elsevier, Philadelphia, 2010, Table 86.7, page 1443, "Risk Factors for Methotrexate-Induced Hepatic Fibrosis".

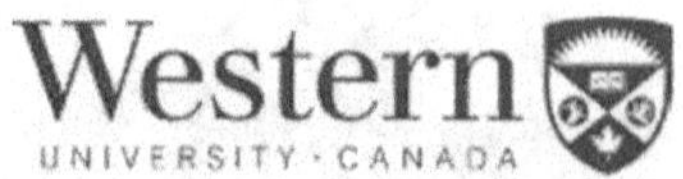

- Feldman M., et al. Sleisenger and Fordtran's Gastrointestinal and Liver Disease. 9th Edition. Saunders/Elsevier, Philadelphia, 2010, Table 86.8, page 1445, "Types of Drug-Induced Hepatic Vascular Disorders: Clinics Pathologic Features, Outcome, and Implicated Etiologic Agents".
- Feldman M., et al. Sleisenger and Fordtran's Gastrointestinal and Liver Disease. 9th Edition. Saunders/Elsevier, Philadelphia, 2010, Table 87.1, page 1448, "Clinical Pathological Features of Halothane Hepatitis".

Drug Induced Liver Injury Network (DILIN) Objectives

- To collect biological samples from bonafide cases and controls to study pathogenesis using biochemical, serological and genetic techniques
- To develop standardized instruments, definitions, and terminology for drug and CAM induced liver injury

- Prospective study
  - Inclusion criteria
    - Age > 2
    - Liver injury due to a drug within 6 months of presentation
    - On 2 consecutive blood draws
      - AST/ ALT > 5 X ULN or baseline
      - Alk phos > 2X ULN or baseline
      - T bilirubin > 2.5 mg/dl

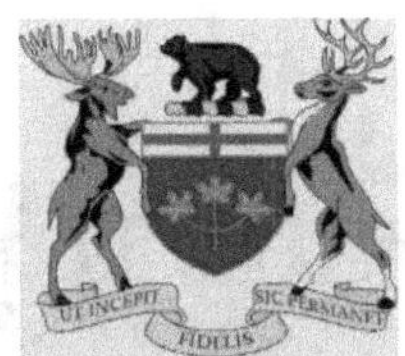

CAUSALITY ASSESSMENT IN DRUG INDUCED LIVER INJURY

- Exclusion criteria
  - Acetaminophen hepatotoxicity
  - Prior liver transplant
  - Pre-existing AIH, PSC, PBC which may confound ability to diagnose DILI
    - Chronic HBV, HCV allowed

- Baseline visit

- All patients
  - HAV (IgM)
  - HBsAg, HBcAb
  - HCV ab
  - ANA, SmAb
  - Monospot
  - HIV ab
  - Liver ultrasound
  - Ceruloplasmin (< 50)
  - AMA (Cholestatic)
- Chronic HBV
  - HBV DNA
  - HBeAg, HBeAb
  - HDV Ab
- Chronic HCV
  - HCV RNA

- Causality assessment
  - Causality committee
    - 5 site PI's, 1 DCC, 1 NIH

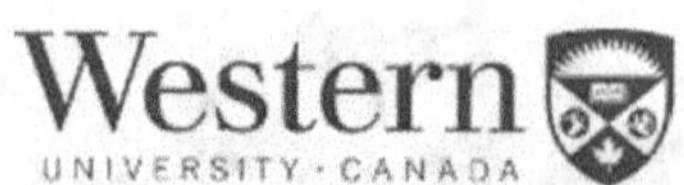

CAUSALITY ASSESSMENT IN DRUG INDUCED LIVER INJURY

- 3 independent reviewers per case
  - Site PI and 2 others
  - Review clinical narrative, subset CRF, labs
  - Assess causality, RUCAM, Data completeness checklist
- Conference call if not unanimous

- Clinical narrative
  - Presentation
  - Detailed medication hx/ compliance
  - Concomitant meds/ CAM
  - PMH (past medical history)
  - Social and family history
  - Physical exam
  - Liver tests, enzymes & other lab measurements
  - Diagnostic tests
    - Central path review
  - Outcome

- Causality assessment

Likelihood	Category
> 95%	Definite
75 -95%	Likely
50 -75%	Probable
25 -50%	Possible
< 25%	Unlikely

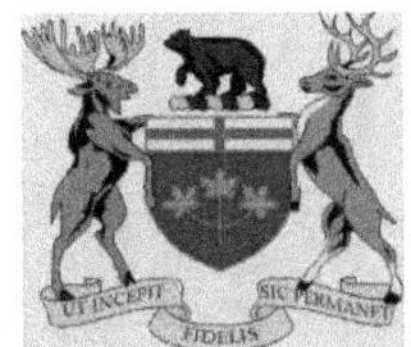

- What is needed?
    - Need Bonafide cases of DILI
        - ? Features ? Risk factors ? Mechanism ? Outcome
        - Surveillance system
    - Improved causality assessment instruments
        - Key data, sensitive/ specific, validated
        - User friendly, widely available
    - Objective lab test to confirm diagnosis
        - ? Lymphocyte proliferation assays/ biomarker
        - ? Genetic susceptibility test
    - Reference database for DILI

287 Japanese DILI cases '78-'02

- 55% hepatocellular 24% mixed 22% cholestatic

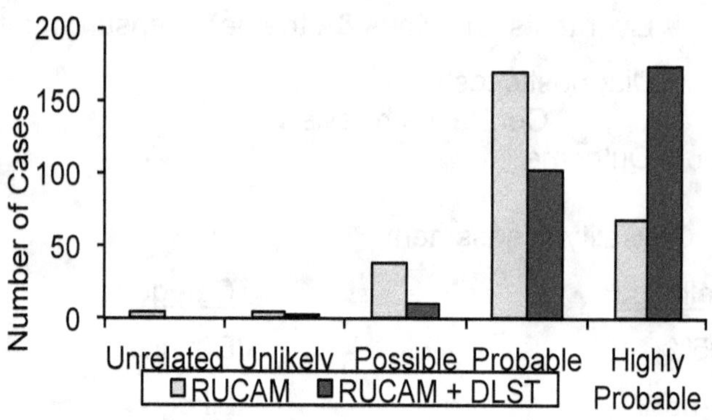

- Latency > 15 or 30 d changed, other drugs omitted,
- + DLST = +2 Eosinophils > 6% = + 1

Source: Hep Research 2003: 27: 191
Takikawa H., et al, Hepatology Research. Volume 27, issue 3, 11/2003. P.192-195

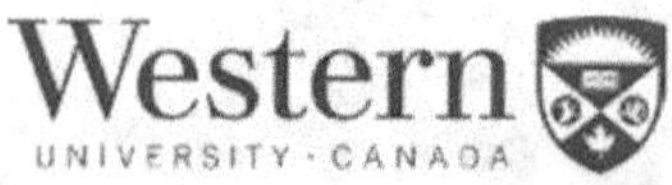

Fulminant DILI (USA)

- 138 DILI ALF LT recipients (15%) '90-'02
  - Mean age 35 75% female 70% Cau 26% AA
    - 17% INH 9 % PTU 7% dilantin 7% valproate
- 40 DILI (13%) ALFSG '98-'03
  - Med age 41 72% female 58% Cau
    - 27% antibiotics 10% troglitazone 10% bromfenac
    - 25% spont survival 53% transplant

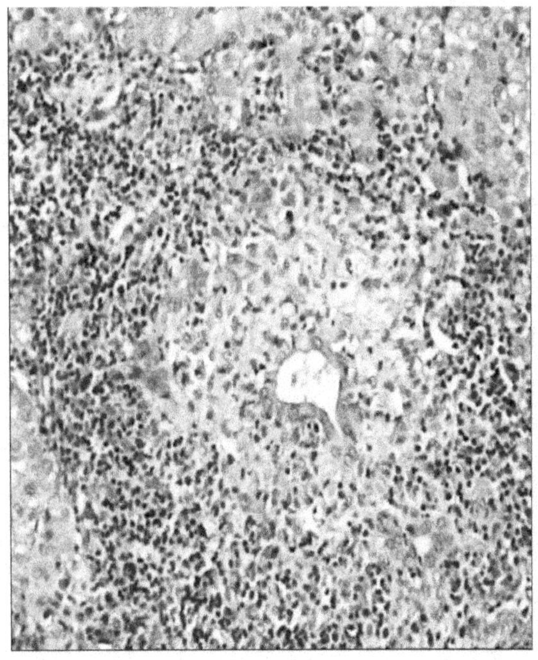

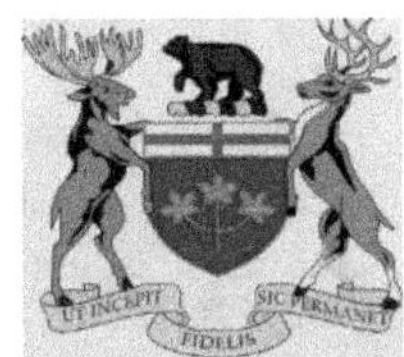

Idiopathic Hepatitis

- $2/10^5$ hospitalizations per medicaid- patient years for idiopathic acute hepatitis
  - HCV not excluded ('80-'87)
- Acute "non-A, non-B" hepatitis
  - 5- 8% of post-Tx hepatitis
- 17% of ALF is indeterminate

Source: Carson JL, et al. Arch Intern Med. 1993;153(11):1331-6.

ADR: Causality Assessment

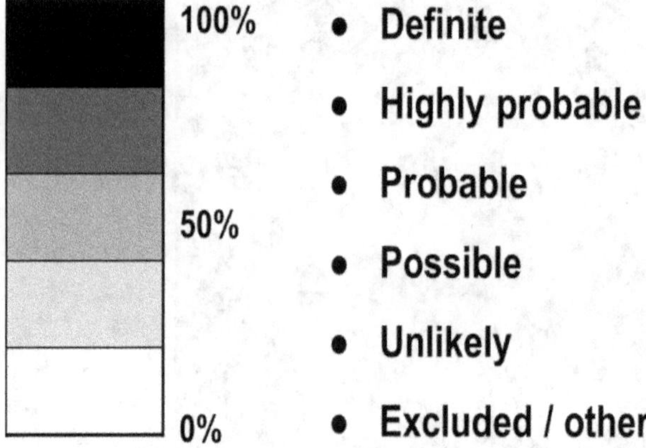

DILI Examples

- Give 6 risk factors for **methotrexate** induced hepatic fibrosis, their clinical importance, and their implications for prevention.

Risk factors	Importance	Implications for Prevention
○ Age	– Increased risk >60 yr, possibly related to renal clearance and/or biological effect on fibrogenesis	▪ Care in use of methotrexate in older persons
○ Dose	– Incremental dose	▪ 5-15 mg/wk is safe
	– Dose frequency	▪ Weekly bolus (pulse) safer than daily schedules
	– Duration of therapy	▪ Consider liver biopsy every 2 years
	– Cumulative (total) dose	▪ Consider liver biopsy after each 2 g methotrexate
○ Alcohol consumption	– Increased risk with daily levels > 15 g (1-2 drinks)	▪ Avoid methotrexate use if alcohol intake not curbed. ▪ Consider pre-treatment liver biopsy with relevant history of alcohol use.

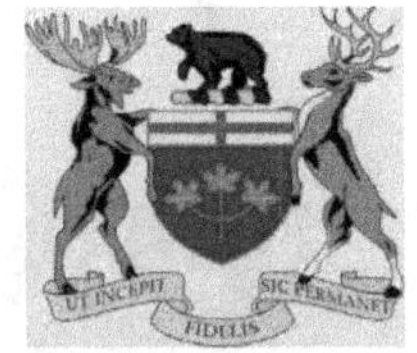

Risk factors	Importance	Implications for Prevention
○ Obesity	– Increased risk	▪ Consider pre-treatment and interval liver biopsies
○ Diabetes mellitus	– Increased risk in obese persons (type 2 diabetes mellitus)	▪ Consider pre-treatment and interval liver biopsies
○ Pre-existing liver disease	– Greatly increased risk, particularly related to alcohol, obesity, and diabetes (NASH)	▪ Pretreatment liver biopsy mandatory ▪ Avoid methotrexate, or used scheduled interval biopsies according to severity of hepatic fibrosis, total dose, and duration of methotrexate therapy
○ Systemic disease	– Possibly risk greater with psoriasis than rheumatoid arthritis (may depend on preexisting liver disease, alcohol intake)	▪ None
○ Impaired renal function	– Increased risk because of reduced clearance of methotrexate	▪ Reduced dose ▪ Greater caution with use
○ Other drugs	– NSAIDS, vitamin A and arsenic may increase risk	▪ Greater caution with use ▪ Monitor liver biochemical tests

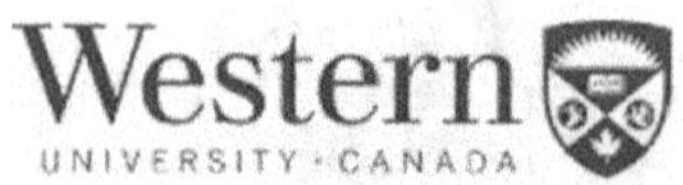

Abbreviations: Nash, non-alcoholic steatohepatitis; NSAIDS, nonsteroidal anti-inflammatory drugs

Printed with permission: *Sleisenger and Fordtran's Gastrointestinal and Liver Disease: Pathophysiology/ Diagnosis/ Management.* Ninth edition, 2010, Table 86.7, pg 1443.

- Give 7 hepatobiliary complications of the use of **oral contraceptive agents (OCAs).**
  - Gallstones
  - Cholestasis
  - Unmasking PBC, and other cholestatic diseases
  - Unmasking porphyria
  - Tumours
    - Adenomas
    - ↑ size of FNH (focal nodular hyperplasia)
    - Hepatocellular carcinoma (rare)
  - Increased risk of NASH
  - Vascular
    - Budd-Chiari syndrome
    - Peliosis hepatic (sinusoidal dilation)

- Give the antidote for the acute hepatotoxicity caused by the mushroom, **Amanita phalloides**.
  - Flavonoids (silybin [silymarin], or analogs of tocopherol; penicillin
  - That was a Canary!

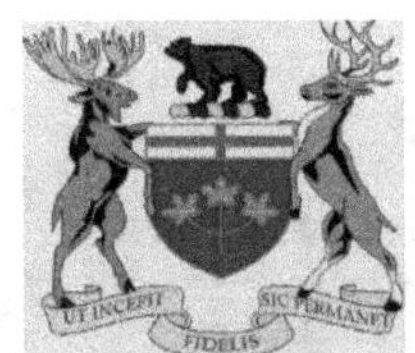

- Give the mechanism of hepatotoxicity of Amanita phalloides.

o Alpha-amatoxin	– ↓ mRNA – ↓ protein synthesis
o Phalloidin	– Interferes with polymerization of actin – Disrupts cell membranes

Comment from author: If you knew the answer to this question, you are studying too much, and you definitely need to get out more!

CLINICAL CHALLENGE

Jaw clenching and teeth grinding (bruxism) are not common extrahepatic manifestations of liver disease. In the patient with these signs plus tender hepatomegaly, sweating, fever and transaminases > 1000, give the likely diagnosis.

- o Acute hepatitis with sweating, fever, jaw clenching and teeth grinding would be suggestive of drug induced liver injury, for example from "ecstasy".

- For an extra mark, give the chemical name for ecstasy (clue: MDMA).
  - o Ecstasy is methylenedioxymethamphetamine.

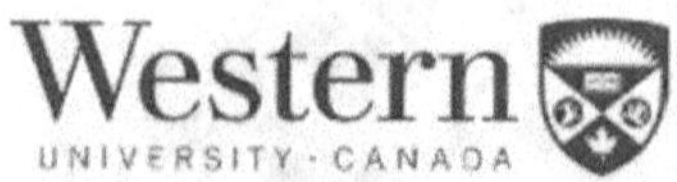

> CLINICAL PEARL: DILI
>
> The dose of acetaminophen which places the ordinary patient at risk for ALT is 8 gm, but the dose level may be lower, especially for the smaller person. It is better to remember the threshold as < 150 mg/kg, rather than 6-8 gm.

Liver Disease

- List 10 drugs, which are relatively contraindicated and must be used cautiously in persons with liver disease.
  - Clonazepam
  - Conjugated estrogen/medroxy-progesterone
  - Dantrolene
  - Felbarnate
  - Gemfibrozil
  - Lovastatin and other HMG-CoA reductase inhibitors (statins)
  - Metformin
  - Methotrexate
  - Naltrexone
  - Niacin
  - Pemoline
  - Phenelzine
  - Tacrine (in persons with prior jaundice)
  - Ticlopidine
  - Tolcapone
  - Valproic acid
  - Zalcitabine

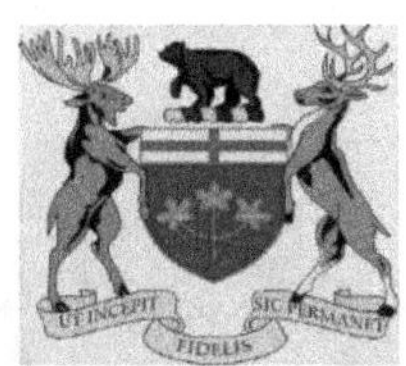

Suggestion from the author: you have better things to do than to memorize this list: In the patient with liver disease, look up this list, or look up the dugs to be used

Adapted from: Gupta NK, and Lewis JH. *Aliment Pharmacol Ther* 2008; 28(9): 1021-41.

- Give 10 drugs for which lower doses are recommended in patients with cirrhosis ("**hepatic dosing**").
    - Acetaminophen
    - Benzodiazepines
    - Beta blockers
    - Cetirazine
    - Fluoxetine
    - Indinavir
    - Lamotrigine
    - Losartan
    - Moricizine
    - Narcotics
    - PPIs
    - Repaglinide
    - Risperidone
    - Sertraline
    - Topiramate
    - Tramadol
    - Valproic acid
    - Venlafazine
    - Verapamil

Adapted from: Gupta NK, and Lewis JH. *Aliment Pharmacol Ther* 2008; 28(9): 1021-41.

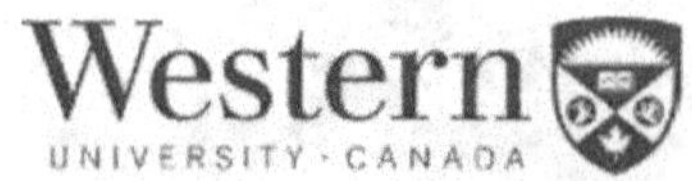

MINI UPDATE

Biliary Tract Motor Function and Dysfunction

Aze Wilson

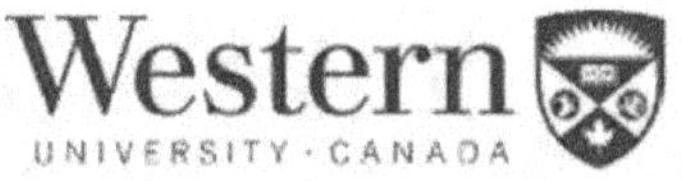

BILIARY TRACT MOTOR FUNCTION AND DYSFUNCTION

The Biliary Tree

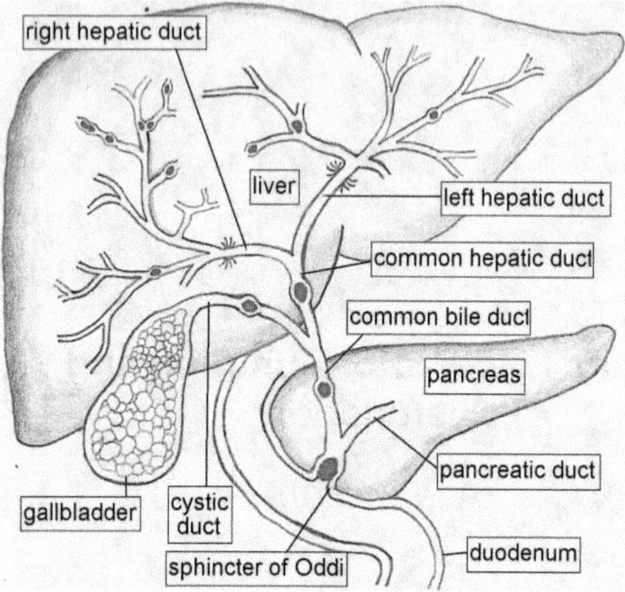

Muscle Layers

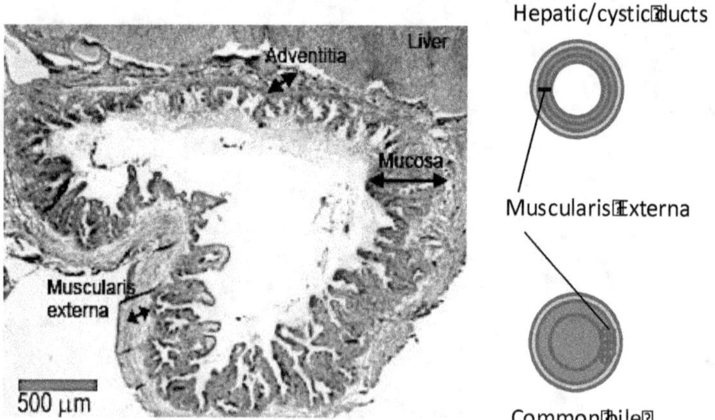

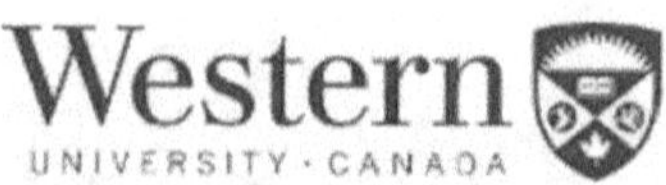

BILIARY TRACT MOTOR FUNCTION AND DYSFUNCTION

Sphincter of Oddi (SOD)

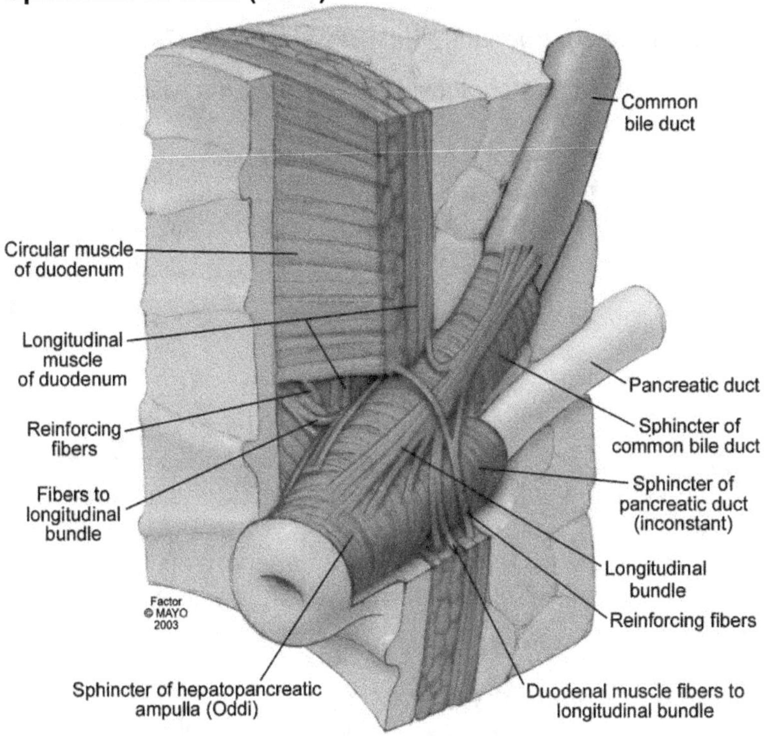

Common bile duct
Circular muscle of duodenum
Longitudinal muscle of duodenum
Reinforcing fibers
Fibers to longitudinal bundle
Pancreatic duct
Sphincter of common bile duct
Sphincter of pancreatic duct (inconstant)
Longitudinal bundle
Reinforcing fibers
Factor © MAYO 2003
Sphincter of hepatopancreatic ampulla (Oddi)
Duodenal muscle fibers to longitudinal bundle

➢ Definition

- Non-calculous obstructive disorder occurring at the level of the sphincter of Oddi
    - Fibrosis +/- inflammation (passive obstruction)
    - Muscle spasm (active obstruction)
- Also known as
    - Papillary stenosis
    - Biliary dyskinesia
    - Postcholecystectomy syndrome

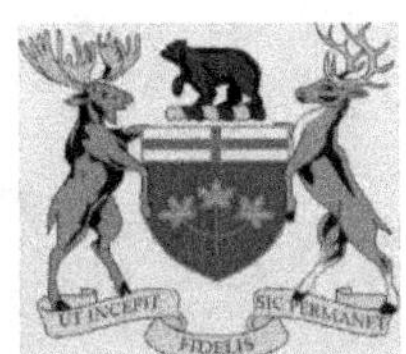

BILIARY TRACT MOTOR FUNCTION AND DYSFUNCTION

- Demography
  - Most common in middle-aged women (74-90%)
  - SOD in postcholecystectomy patients with persistent pain
    - 10-20% postcholecystectomy pain
    - SOD by SO manometry: 30% to 60%
    - Milwaukee Classification of SOD dysfunction

Type I	86%
Type II	55%
Type III	28%

Type I	- Typical biliary pain - Liver enzymes (AST, ALT or ALP) > 2 times x ULN, normal limit documented on at least 2 occasions during episodes of pain - Dilated CBD > 12 mm in diameter - Prolonged biliary drainage time (> 45 min)
Type II	- Biliary type pain, and - One or two of the above criteria
Type III	- Biliary type pain only

Abbreviation: ULN, upper limit of normal

- SO basal pressure
  - ↑SO basal pressures have been detected in
    - 40% of patients with gallstones (with or without pain)
    - 40% of patients with abnormal liver enzymes (no stones)
    - 50% of patients with pain and no gallstones

(Cicala et al Gut 2001; Ruffolo et al Dig Dis Sci 1994)

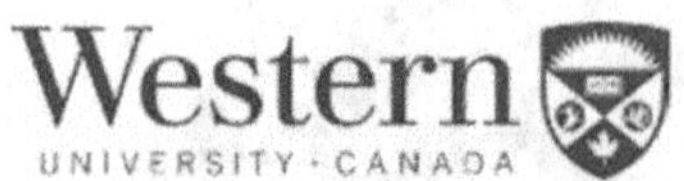

BILIARY TRACT MOTOR FUNCTION AND DYSFUNCTION

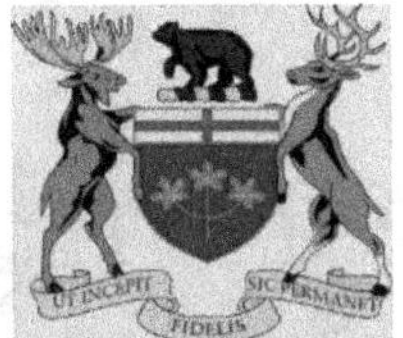

BILIARY TRACT MOTOR FUNCTION AND DYSFUNCTION

- Clinical
  - Types of biliary pain
    - Persistent or recurrent biliary pain in the absence of structural abnormalities following cholecystectomy (postcholecystectomy syndrome)
    - Idiopathic recurrent pancreatitis
    - Biliary pain with an intact GB but no stones (most controversial)
  - Typical biliary pain
    - Severe, epigastric or RUQ, radiating to back or shoulder
    - Lasts > 30 min
    - Occurs at least 1 time/year
- Laboratory
  - < 50% have abnormal liver enzymes
  - See above for liver enzymes and type of SOD (IIa)
- Sphincter of Oddi Manometry (SOM)
  - Performed during ERCP
    - Cannulate ampulla with manometry catheter
  - Stop all drugs that relax or stimulate the SO must be stopped
    - Nitrates, CCBs, anti-cholinergics
    - Narcotics, cholinergics
  - Measures basal SO pressures on TWO pull-throughs for confirmation

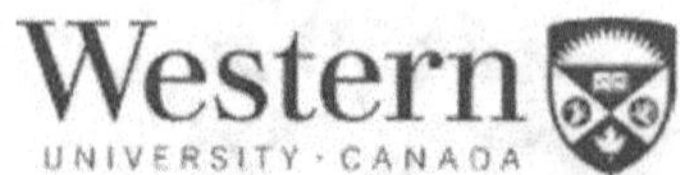

- Pancreatic sphincter manometry also mandatory when the indication for SOM is idiopathic recurrent pancreatitis

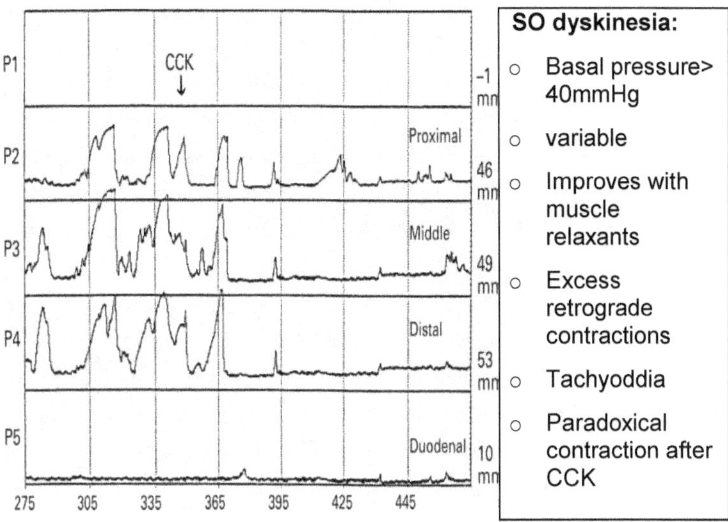

SO dyskinesia:

- Basal pressure> 40mmHg
- variable
- Improves with muscle relaxants
- Excess retrograde contractions
- Tachyoddia
- Paradoxical contraction after CCK

SO stenosis:

- Basal pressure> 40mmHg
- Reproducible
- No response to muscle relaxants

Normal Values of Sphincter of Oddi Manometry (SOM)

- Basal sphincter pressure < 35
- Intraductal pressure < 13
- Phasic waves
  - Amplitude < 22
  - Duration < 8
  - Frequency < 10

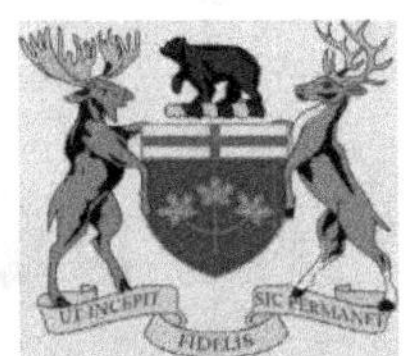

BILIARY TRACT MOTOR FUNCTION AND DYSFUNCTION

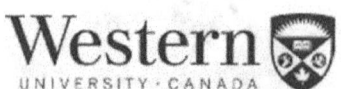

BILIARY TRACT MOTOR FUNCTION AND DYSFUNCTION

- Diagnosis:
  - Non-invasive evaluation:
    - Physical exam often normal
    - Serum transaminases
    - ↑ 3-4x ULN)
      - Lipase
      - Amylase
    - Abdominal imaging (CT or ultrasound)
    - Rule out other common causes of abdominal pain
    - Morphine-neostigmine provocative test (Nardi test): poor sensitivity and specificity
    - Fatty meal ultrasonography
    - Biliary scintigraphy
  - Invasive evaluation:
    - ERCP
      - Sessential to exclude organic disease eg.
        - stones
        - strictures
        - neoplasms
    - Note SOD patients have a high complication rate post-ERCP
    - Sphincter of Oddi Manometry (SOM)
      - Gold standard for SOD diagnosis
  - Manometry is specific but NOT sensitive
    - 42% symptom response SOD in type 2 SOD patients with normal SOM
    - Normal SOM in many type 1 patients with >90% response to sphincterotomy (may be different cause)

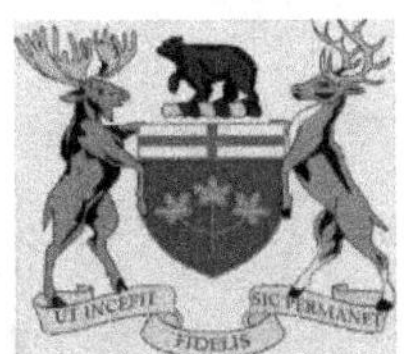

- SOD less common in type 3 patients (response 40-60%)
  - Pain alone is a poor predictor of SO dysfunction
- Pain with contrast injection at ERCP
  - Not predictive of SOD

- Treatment
  - Pharmaceutical
    - Low fat diet
      - ↓ pancreticobiliary stimulation
    - Smooth muscle relaxants (CCB, nitrates, octreotide) to ↓ SO pressure
    - Use for all type 3 and for mild-moderate type II SOD patients
  - Botulinum toxin injection
    - ↓ SO pressure by 50%
    - Predicts response to sphincterotomy
    - Requires 2nd ERCP

- Endoscopic Sphincterotomy
  - Biliary pain post cholecystectomy
  - Relief of biliary pain with sphincterotomy

	SOM	
Type	Normal	Abnormal
I	90-95%	90-95%
II	35-42%	85%
III	< 10%	55-60%

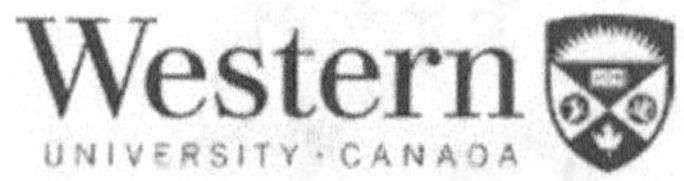

BILIARY TRACT MOTOR FUNCTION AND DYSFUNCTION

The Efficacy of Endoscopic Sphincterotomy after Cholecystectomy in Patients with Sphincter of Oddi Dysfunction

- Abnormal SOM > 85% vs. 25% response with placebo (sham ES)
- Normal SOM ~25% for both ES and SHAM

- Biliary pain intact gallbladder and no stones
- Possible causes for failure to achieve pain relief after sphincterotomy for presumed SOD:
  - Non biliary pain – functional gut disorder
  - Inadequate initial sphincterotomy
  - Residual pancreatic sphincter hypertension

- Placement of biliary or pancreatic stent
  - Advantage
    - Predict LT response to sphincterotomy (unlike SOM)
  - Disadvantage
    - High rate of induced pancreatitis

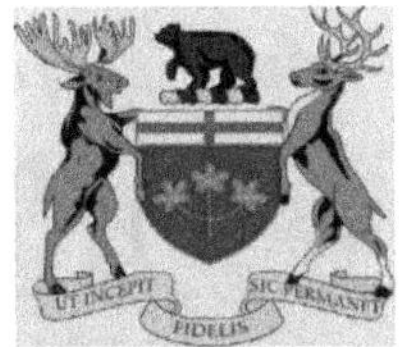

MINI UPDATE

Post-Transplant Lymphoproliferative Disorders

Aze Wilson

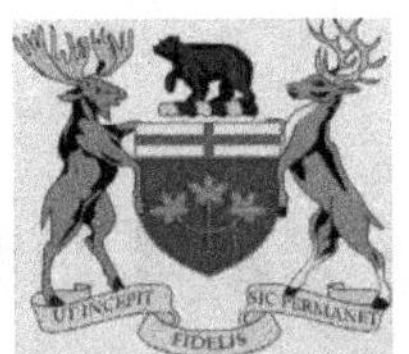

Post-transplant Lymphoproliferative Disorders (PTLD)

- Lymphoid and/or plasmacytic proliferations that occur in the setting of solid organ or allogeneic hematopoietic cell transplantation as a result of immunosuppression

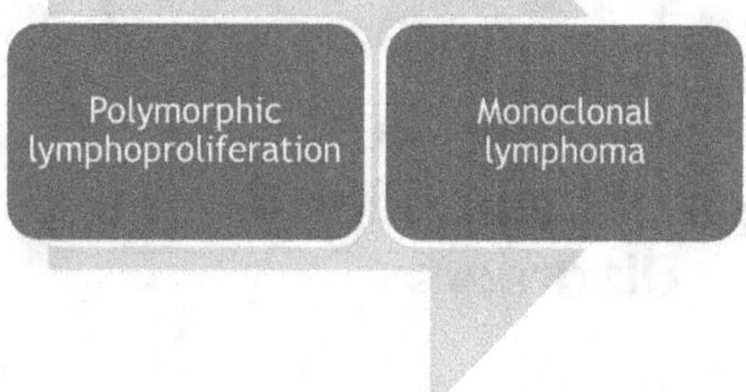

➢ Demography

- Major complication after liver transplantation (OLTx)
- Prevalence of PTLD post-OLTx (Taylor, Marcus & Bradley, Crit Rev Oncol Hematol, 2005)
  - 2.8% of adults
  - 15% of children
- Mortality = 50%
- 85% are of B-cell origin (Allen et al, Can J Infect Dis, 2002)
  - > 80% are EBV-associated
- 15% are T-cell origin[2]
  - 30% are EBV associated

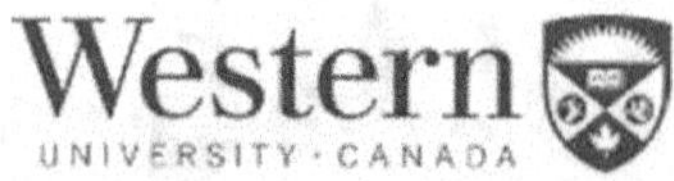

POST-TRANSPLANT LYMPHOPROLIFERATIVE DISORDERS

- Types of PTLD (WHO 2008)
  - These conditions lie along a continuum of disease and are categorized by the 2008 WHO classification system as PTLD
  - Spectrum of disease:
    - Plasmacytic hyperplasia
    - Polymorphic
    - Monomorphic
    - Hodgkin disease
  - Please note
    - Small B cell lymphoid neoplasms (eg, follicular lymphomas, small lymphocytic lymphoma)
    - Marginal zone (MALT) lymphomas arising in the post-transplant setting are **not** considered PTLD.

- **Early lesions**
  - Seen in 1st year, post orthoptic transplantation (post-OLTx, all other PTLDs have variable onset post-OLTx)
  - Monomorphic B cell lymphoma (DLBCL) [diffuse large B cell lymphoma] most common
  - Plasmacytic hyperplasia and infectious mononucleosis-like PTLD)
  - Presents as an infectious mononucleosis-type acute illness characterized by polyclonal B cell proliferation with no evidence to suggest malignant transformation.
  - Always EBV positive

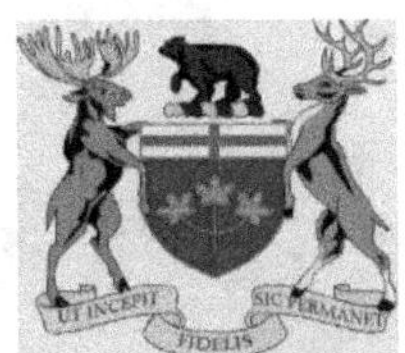

- **Polymorphic PTLD**
    - Polymorphic PTLD are polyclonal or monoclonal lymphoid infiltrates that demonstrate evidence of malignant transformation but do not meet all of the criteria for one of the B cell or T/NK cell lymphomas recognized in immunocompetent patients.

- **Monomorphic PTLD**
    - Most common (DLBCL)
    - Monoclonal lymphoid proliferations that meet the criteria for one of the B cell or T/NK cell lymphomas recognized in immunocompetent patients.
    - Diffuse large B cell lymphoma (DLBCL) and less commonly Burkitt lymphoma (BL) or a plasma cell neoplasm (eg, myeloma or extramedullary plasmacytoma).
    - Lymphomas of T cell or NK cell origin are uncommon, but, when seen, are usually classified as peripheral T cell lymphoma, not otherwise specified (PTCL, NOS).
    - Very few cases of T cell PTLD had been reported in kidney transplant recipients. The diagnosis of each of these lymphoma subtypes is described briefly below and presented

- **Classic Hodgkin – least common**
    - Usually seen in first year post OLTx
    - Variable onset post transplant
    - Monomorphic b cell lymphoma (DLBCL) most common

POST-TRANSPLANT LYMPHOPROLIFERATIVE DISORDERS

➢ Pathophysiology

- EBV-positive patients (more common)
  - EBV – gamma-herpes virus
    - Stimulates B-cell proliferation and transformation
  - In the immunocompetent host:
    - EBV infection targets oropharynx
    - Triggers a humoral and cellular immune response (IR)
    - After primary clearance:
      - EBV persists in infected B-cells = LATENT INFECTION
  - 4 types of latency:
    - Differentiated by Ag expression pattern in infected B-cells
  - The higher the number the more immunogenic.
  - In the immunocompetent host:
    - EBV reactivation is INHIBITED by cytotoxic T-lympphocytes (CTLs)
  - In the immunosuppressed host:
    - There is down-regulation of the cytotoxic T-cell response (Thorley-Lawson NEJM 2004)
    - EBV-driven lymphoproliferation can occur
      - Degree of PTLD depends on degree of virus inhibition of apoptosis.
      - Other factors may also play a role
        - microsatellite instability (MSI)
        - molecular alterations, etc.

- EBV-negative patient (less common)
  - Mechanism unclear
  - Associated with

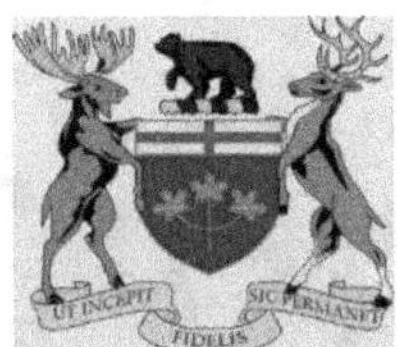

    - Later onset
    - Monomorphic histology
    - Aggressive clinical behaviour

  - Hypothesis:
    - EPV-negative PTLD is associated with an unidentified viral agent or the loss of EBV
    - With presumed EBV loss
    - Initial lymphoproliferation is stimulated by EBV
    - Mutations over time lead to EBV-independent replication

- Risk Factors

  - EBV- recipient with EBV-positive donor
    - Infected B cells are introduced in the donor
    - Recipient does not have abs to resis infection or control B-cell overgrowth in infected B cells
    - Young

  - Intensity of immunosuppression (especially with anti-T cell abs ATG or OKT3)

  - 1st year post transplant
    - Higher risk in organs with more B cells eg. small bowel

  - Pre-transplant steroids
    - May have an increased risk
    - mTOR inhibitors may have a decreased risk, but studies are inconclusive

- Clinical

  - Symptoms
    - Fever
    - Lymphadenopathy
    - Weight loss
    - Splenomegaly

POST-TRANSPLANT LYMPHOPROLIFERATIVE DISORDERS

  - Localized to one site, to the graft or can be diffuse with multi-organ dysfunction (MOD)
  - Can see bone marrow and central nervous system involvement

- PTLD
  - 20% had localized liver disease
  - 13% had multifocal disease
  - Lymphomas versus general lymphomas more likey to have
    - More extra-nodal involvement
    - High grade and aggressive behavior
    - Poor outcomes

- Predictors of poor outcomes[1]:
  - High grade
  - Poor performance status
  - EBV-
  - Graft involvement

(Parker et al Br J Haem, 2010;149(5):675-92)

- Diagnosis:
  - Early diagnosis is important
    - To prevent evolution to a more aggressive variant
  - Surveillance of EBV load by quantitative PCR
  - Frequency of surveillance unknown (highly sens, spec only 50%)
  - Progressively rising EBV DNA → further investigation
  - If high clinical suspicion → biopsy, and send tissue for EBV analysis and CD20 expression.
  - If PTLD discovered → staging with CT neck, chest, abdomen/pelvis
    - Evaluation of transplanted liver status
    - May need BM
      - CNS imaging or LP

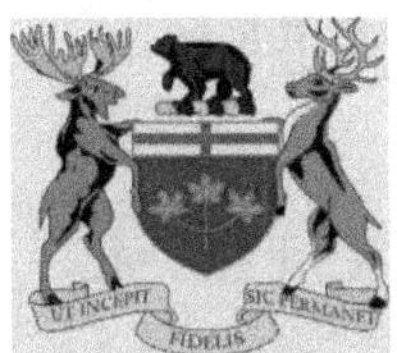

- Bone marrow aspiration

➢ Prophylaxis

- Intensity of immunosuppression (IS) is a modifiable RF
  - Risk factors for PLTD
  - ↓ IS may be considered if a ↑ EBV load seen post liver transplantation
    - Antiviral therapy may ↓ incidence of PTLD in EBV- paediatric recipients

➢ Treatment

- ↓ IS (~25-50%)
  - Restoration of T cell function
- Risk factors for failure
  - High LDH
  - Organ dysfunction
  - Multiorgan dysfunction
- If no risk factors, 90% response has been seen ↓ within 2-4 weeks with ↓ IS (immunosuppression)

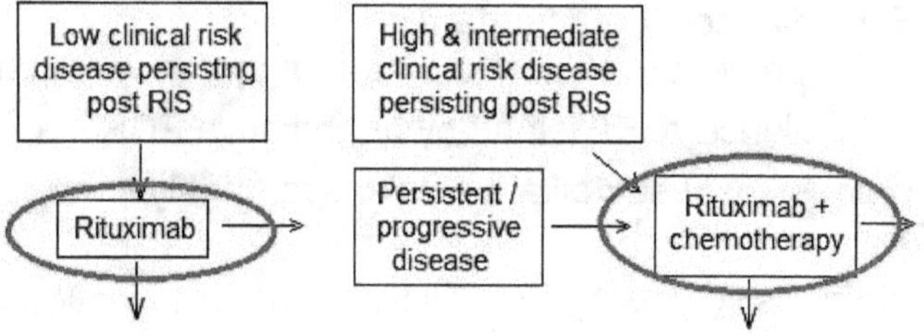

- **Rituximab**
  - Rituximab – remission rates of 44-65% in CD20-positive PTLD
  - Chemotherapy
    - ↑ liver transplant disease free survival
    - CHOR +/- Rituximab
    - ↑ remission rates = 65-100%
      - ↓ rates of graft loss

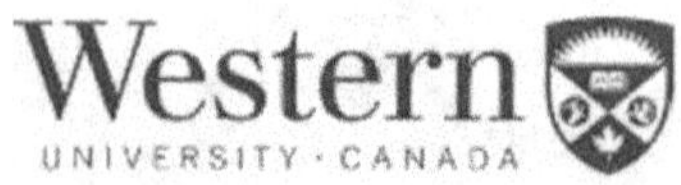

  - Should be initiated quickly in:
    - high grade ALD
    - inadequate response
    - progression despite other txs.

- Local control
  - Surgical resection vs radiotherapy
  - No demonstrated benefit as 1st line treatment
  - May be helpful in treatment of local complications
  - Radiation required for CNS or orbital disease

- Adaptive immunotherapy
  - Infusions of EBV specific CTLs from peripheral blood of recipient → ↓ EBV DNA, with no significant toxicity
  - LT EBV immunity is NOT maintained
  - Complex and expensive
  - Only available in clinical trials

Summary

- PTLD is a serious complication of OLTx
- Disease can occur along a spectrum, with possible evolution to more malignant variants
- Non-specific signs and symptoms
- Usually EBV-associated
- Literature recommends monitor EBV DNA levels q2weeks in high risk OLTx patients
  - Reduction in immune suppression if level is high
- If PTLD diagnosed – biopsy and pre-treatment imaging
  - Reduce immune suppression
  - If low risk B-cell disease = rituximab
  - Rituximab – non-responders, high risk disease
  - Multiorgan dysfunction = chemotherapy
  - Localized, stage 1 disease - surgical resection/radiotherapy

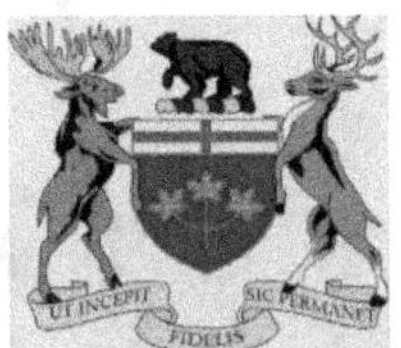

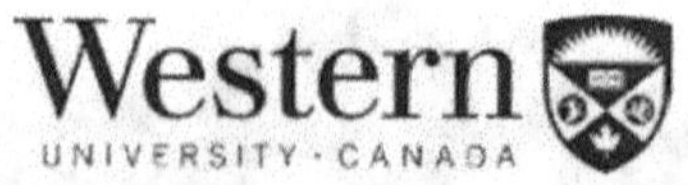
Western
UNIVERSITY · CANADA

PANCREAS

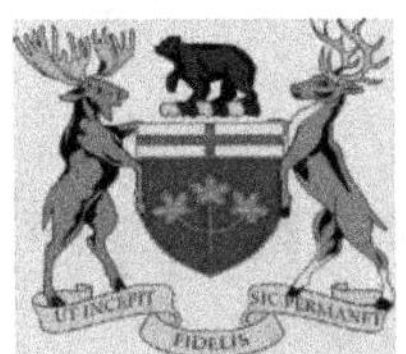

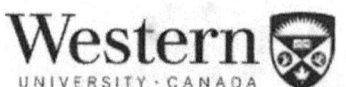

Acute Pancreatitis

Alan BR Thomson

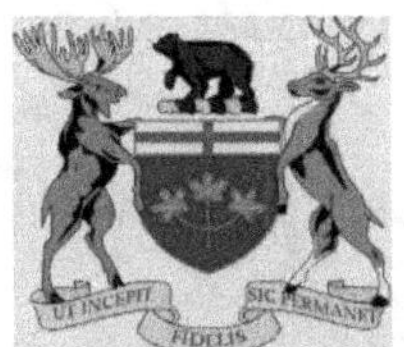

ACUTE PANCREATITIS

- Definitions
  - Acute pancreatitis is "……an event triggered by sudden pancreatic injury that is followed by sequential inflammatory responses" (Feldman M., et al. Sleisenger and Fordtran's Gastrointestinal and Liver Disease. 9th Edition. Saunders/Elsevier, Philadelphia, 2010, page 901).
    - Alternate definitions:….an acute inflammatory process of the pancreas with variable involvement of other regional tissue or remote organ systems" (Feldman M., et al. Sleisenger and Fordtran's Gastrointestinal and Liver Disease. 9th Edition. Saunders/Elsevier, Philadelphia, 2010, page 931).
    - "…best defined clinically by a patient with [or all of the following criteria: (1) symptoms such as epigastric pain, consistent with the disease; (2) a serum amylase or lipase greater than three times a year limit of normal; or (3) radiologic imaging consistent with the diagnosis, usually using computed tomography (CT) or magnetic resonance imaging (MRI) ((Feldman M., et al. Sleisenger and Fordtran's Gastrointestinal and Liver Disease. 9th Edition. Saunders/Elsevier, Philadelphia, 2010, page 960).
  - Acute pancreatitis is….. an event triggered by sudden pancreatic injury that is followed by sequential inflammatory responses (Feldman M., et al. Sleisenger and Fordtran's Gastrointestinal and Liver Disease. 9th Edition. Saunders/Elsevier, Philadelphia, 2010, page 901).
  - Chronic pancreatitis "…..is a process that usually begins with recurrent pancreatitis and ends with immune-related destruction of the pancreas and widespread glandular fibrosis" (Feldman M., et al. Sleisenger and Fordtran's Gastrointestinal and

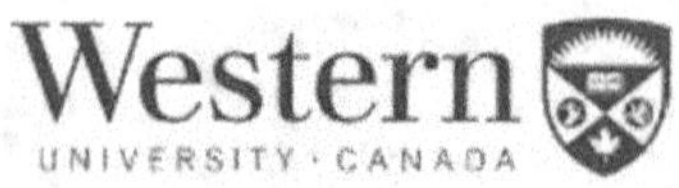

Liver Disease. 9th Edition. Saunders/Elsevier, Philadelphia, 2010, page 931).

- Hereditary pancreatitis is "……recurrent acute or chronic pancreatitis in an individual from a family in which the pancreatitis phenotype appears to be inherited through a disease-causing gene mutation expressed in an autosomal dominant pattern."
  - Caused by mutations in $PRSS_1$ (cationic trypsinogen) gene
  - Clinical phenotype: recurrent acute pancreatitis
  - Penetrance of genotype to phenotype 80%
- Familial pancreatitis is "….pancreatitis from any cause that occurs in a family with an incidence [of pancreatitis] that is greater than would be expected by chance alone, given the size of the family and incidence of pancreatitis within a defined population" (familial may or may not be caused by a genetic defect).
  - Usually caused by
    - SPINK1 mutations, or
    - CFTR – SPINK1 genotypes atypical (homozygous or atypical compound heterozygous.
- Tropical pancreatitis is "……a form of early age-onset, non-alcoholic chronic pancreatitis occurring in tropical regions what is often clustered among family members, and that has a complex genetic basis." SPINK1 N34S mutations are common

➢ Demography

- Wide variation in quoted incidence ~ $25/10^5$
- Incidence depends on causes

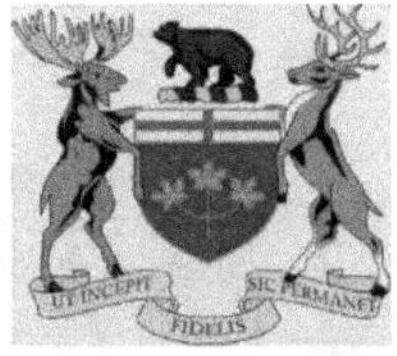

- Most common causes are alcohol excess and cholelithiasis

> Causes / associations

- Give 20 causes of acute pancreatitis.

o Idiopathic	– Pancreas divisum – Choledochocele
o Inherited	– CFTR, SPINK 1 & 2, CT gene and other mutations
o Infection	– Viral (mumps, Coxsackie, CMV, HSV, HIV) – Bacterial (Mycoplasma, Legionella, Leptospira, Salmonella) – Fungal (Aspergillus) – Parasitic (toxoplasma, cryptosporidium, Ascaris)
o Inflammation	– Penetrating gastroduodenal ulcer – Crohn disease
o Ischemic	– Ischemia – Vascular bypass surgery – Vasculitis
o Immune	– Idiopathic autoimmune pancreatitis

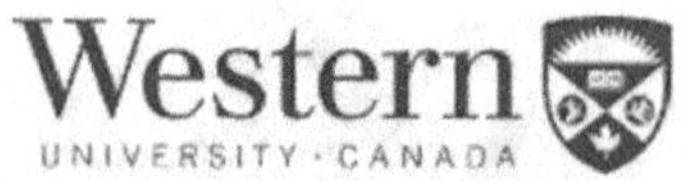

- Obstruction
  - Gallstones
  - Biliary sludge
  - ERCP
  - Juxta-ampullary diverticulum
  - Ampullary neoplasms
  - Pancreatic neoplasms
  - Ampullary stenosis
  - Sphincter of Oddi dysfunction (SOD)

- Trauma
  - Blunt trauma
  - Penetrating trauma
  - Post ERCP

- Metabolic
  - Hypertriglyceridemia
  - Hypercalcemia

- Medications/ toxin
  - Ethanol
  - Methanol
  - Scorpion venom
  - Drugs: immunosuppressant, pentamadine, DDI, furosemide, thiazides, sulfasalazine, 5-ASA, salicylates, L-asparaginase, azathioprine, valproate, estrogen, sulindac, and others (see next question please)

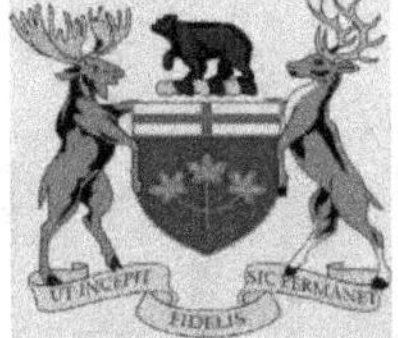

SO YOU WANT TO BE A GASTROENTEROLOGIST!

- Give systemic diseases associated with pancreatitis.
  - Endocrine
    - Diabetes (ketoacidosis)
    - Hypercalcemia
  - Hematology
    - HUS (hemolytic uremic syndrome)
  - MSK
    - SLE (systemic lupus erythematosus)
  - Transplantation
    - The surgery itself
    - Immunesuppressants

➢ Genetics

Acute pancreatitis may be caused by or associated with genetic defects, which disrupt mechanisms which normally protects the process from trypsin associated injury, and therapy increases the susceptibility of the pancreas.

- Give examples of four major **susceptibility genes,** which cause or predispose to pancreatic disease.
  - Cationic trypsinogen ($PRSS_1$) [protease serine 1]) gene mutations. There are 3 forms of trypsinogen
    - $mPRSS_1$
      - Cationic trypsinogen (65%)
      - Protease serine 1 gene
    - $PRSS_2$
      - Anionic trypsinogen (30%)

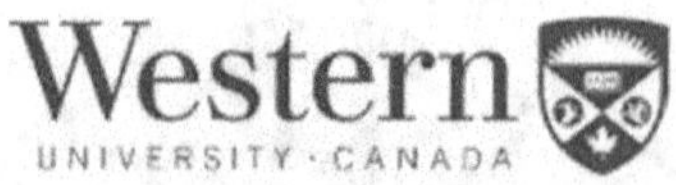

- $PRSS_3$
  - Mesotrypsin
- PST_1 (aka $SPINK_1$ [serine protease inhibitors Kazal type 1])
- Cystic fibrosis conductance regulator gene
- SBDS (Schwachman-Bodian-Diamond Syndrome) gene
- CASR (Calcium-sensing receptor) gene polymorphism
  - Trypsin
    - TAP (trypsinogen activation peptide) =

$$\text{Trypsinogen} \xrightarrow[\text{Trypsin (autoactivation)}]{\text{enterokinase}} \text{trypsin + TAP}$$

➢ Pathogenesis

- Inadvertent activation of trypsin in the pancreas is prevented by several protective mechanisms to prevent autodigestion

- Give 6 major factors involved in the pathogenesis of acute pancreatitis.
  - Failure of the normal mechanisms of protecting pancreas from autodigestion by trypsin and the pancreatic proenzymes activated by trypsin.
  - Activation of complement and Kinin systems
  - Associated genetic abnormalities
    - $SPINK_1$ (aka PSTI, pancreatic secretory trypsin inhibitor) mutations, resulting in loss of the

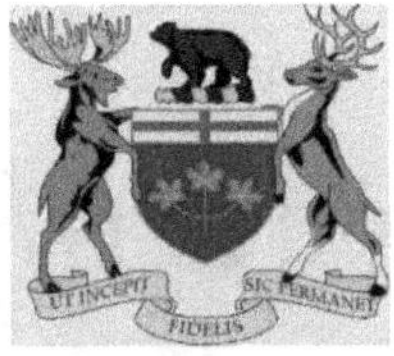

normal effect of inactivating 20% of trypsin activity.

- $PRSS_1$ (cationic trypsinogen gene)

- Associated metabolic abnormalities e.g.
  - ↑ serum triglyceride
  - ↑ serum Ca^{2+}
  - Acidosis
- Disassociation
  - Between continued synthesis but blocked secretion of pancreatic enzymes
  - Enzymes accumulate in acini, causing damage
  - Possible colocalization of pancreatic enzymes in the lysosomes
- Disruption of tight junctions
  - Pancreas: loss of paracellular barrier of acinar cells and intralobular pancreatic duct cells
  - GI tract: ↑ translocation of gut bacteria
- Microcirculatory changes
  - Vasoconstriction
  - Release of VCAM-1 (an endothelial adhesion molecule)
    - PGs (prostaglandins)
    - PAF (platelet activating factor)
    - Leukotrienes
  - Ischemia
  - AV shunting in gut (plus ischemia → GI bleeding)
  - Possible reperfusion injury

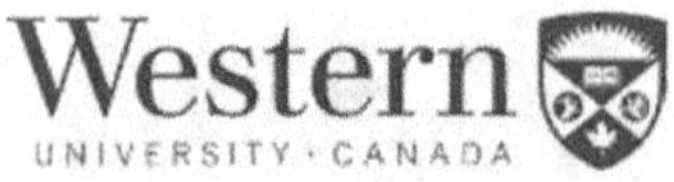

- o Immune changes
  - Activation of complement and release of C5a
  - Recruitments of PMNs and macrophages
  - ↑ proinflammatory cytokines
  - ↑ mediators of inflammation
    - Arachidonic acid metabolites
    - NO (nitric oxide)
    - Reactive oxygen metabolites
- o Failure of anti-autodigestion mechanisms

- Give the four main mechanisms that have been suggested to **prevent autodigestion**.
  - o Separation of zymogen granules and lysosomes within the acinar cell
  - o Trypsin inhibitors (SPINK) within the acinar cells and the pancreatic duct
  - o The digestive enzymes secreted as precursors
  - o Activation of trypsin actually occurs OUTSIDE the pancreas by duodenally secreted enterokinases (pepsinogen activated kinase)

Adapted from: Hirota M, et al. *J Gastroenterol* 2006;41(9):832-6.

- Give the mechanisms by which the activity of trypsin is switched on and off.
  - o Activation of trypsin
    - TAP (trypsinogen activation peptide)
    - The trypsin plus TAP peptides form the inactive trypsinogen enzyme.
    - The TAP is cleared from trypsinogen to form the active trypsin.

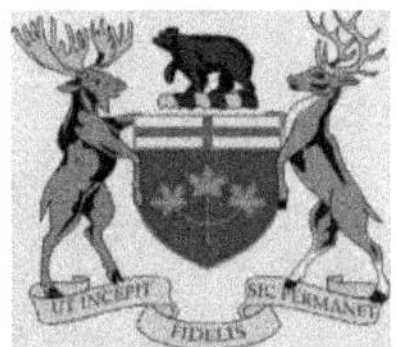

- The activation of the cleavage of TAP results from enterocyte brush border membrane enterokinase, or by other molecules of trypsin.
- This activation of trypsin by trypsin is called "autoactivation".
- Trypsin is activated by ↑ Ca^{2+} (↑ Ca^{2+} blocks trypsin degradation), and is inactivated (degraded) in the acinar cell by ↓ Ca^{2+} (↓ Ca^{2+} blocks activation).
- Degradation of trypsin also results from CTRC (chymotrypsin-C)

o Dereactivation (autolysis) of trypsin
- Trypsin may autolyse itself ("trypsin-mediated autolysis") by acting at its own connecting chain.
- CTRC (chymotrypsin C, aka enzyme Y) degrades the connecting chain calcium and
- Calcium binding pockets ("switch" sites)
  - The local concentration of Ca^{2+} will either modify trypsin by exposing or blocking the separate sites for exposing of the activation site (↑ activation), or the autolysis (↑ deactivation site).

o Calcium
- The local concentration of Ca^{2+} will activate or deactivate trypsin, either by exposing the activation site or the blocking site (autolysis).
- The intra-acinar (autoreaction) concentration of Ca^{2+} is detected ("sensed") by the G-protein coupled receptor CASR (calcium-sensing receptor).
- Low Ca^{2+} favours autolysis, and high Ca^{2+} favours autoreaction.
- Intra acinar cell Ca^{2+} concentrations may increase as a result of numerous factors:
  - ↑ extracellular Ca^{2+}
  - ↑ Ca^{2+} entry

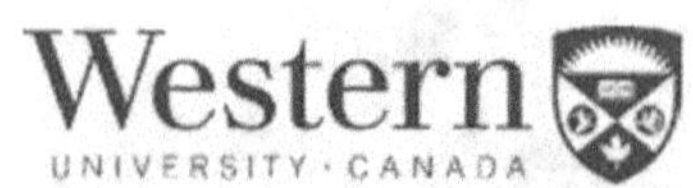

- Opening of Ca^{2+}
  - Channels
  - Tunnels
  - Bile reflux

➢ Types

- Give the types of acute pancreatitis.
  - Interstitial (edematous) pancreatitis
    - Mild disease on CT/MRI
    - No extrahepatic organ dysfunction
  - Severe (necrotizing) pancreatitis
    - Atlanta criteria
      - Pseudocyst
    - Organ failure
      - SBP < 90 mm Hg
      - Pa $O_2 \leq 60$ mm Hg
      - Serum creatinine > 2 mg/dL
      - GIB > 500 mL/24 hr
    - Local complications (sterile or infected)
      - Abscess (not all guidelines use this term; infected pancreatic necrosis)
      - Peripancreatic necrosis
    - Adverse early prognostic signs
      - Ranson's signs (3 or more criteria for non-gallstone pancreatitis)
      - APACHE – II (> 8 points)

Abbreviations: GIB, gastrointestinal bleeding; SBP, systolic blood pressure

➢ Clinical

- Perform a focused physical examination for acute pancreatitis.
  - Abdomen
    - Centre (periumbilical), Cullen sign
    - 1 or both flanks Grey, Turner sign hepatomegaly

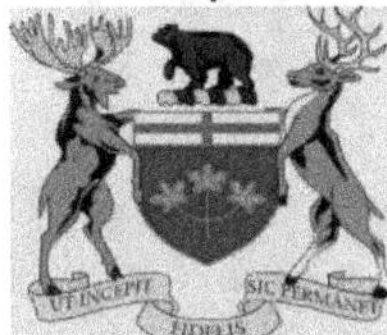

- Lung
  - Tachypnea
  - Shallow breathing signs of effusions, atelectasis
- CNS
  - Confusion
  - Agitation
  - Hallucinations
  - Coma
- Eyes
  - Jaundice
  - Band keratopathy
  - Lipemia retinalis
  - Purtsher retinopathy
- Salivary glands
  - Parotid glands large and tender
- Skin
  - Subcutaneous fat necrosis
    - Tender, red nodules
    - Distal extremities
    - Scalp, trunk, buttocks
    - Eruptive xanthomas
    - Thrombophlebitis
- MSK
  - Polyarteritis

SO YOU WANT TO BE A GASTROENTEROLOGIST!

- In the context of Acute Pancreatitis, give the meaning of **Purtsher Retinopathy**.
  - In the patient with acute pancreatitis, there may be micro-embolization to the choroidal and retinal arteries.
  - This arterial embolization causes flame-shaped retinal hemorrhage, with cotton spots
  - These retinal lesions cause sudden blindness in the affected eye
  - Purtsher retinopathy is the development of sudden blindness in the persons with pancreatitis due to microembolization to the choroidal and retinal arteries, causing hemorrhages and cotton spots.

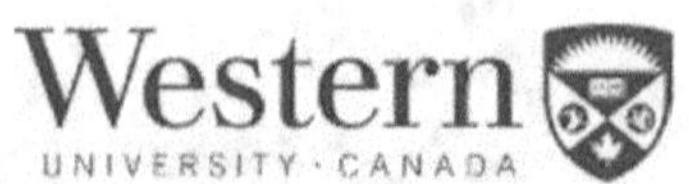

- Complications

- Give 20 complications of acute pancreatitis.
  - Local
    - Sterile necrosis
    - Infected necrosis
    - Abscess
    - Pseudocyst
    - Gastrointestinal bleeding
  - Pancreatitis-related:
    - Splenic artery rupture or splenic artery pseudoaneurysm rupture
    - Splenic vein rupture
    - Portal vein rupture
    - Splenic/portal vein thrombosis, leading to gastroesophageal varices with rupture
    - Pseudocyst or abscess hemorrhage
    - Postnecrosectomy bleeding
  - Non-pancreatitis-related:
    - Mallory-Weiss tear
    - Alcoholic gastropathy
    - Stress-related mucosal gastropathy
  - Splenic injury
    - Infarction
    - Rupture
    - Hematoma

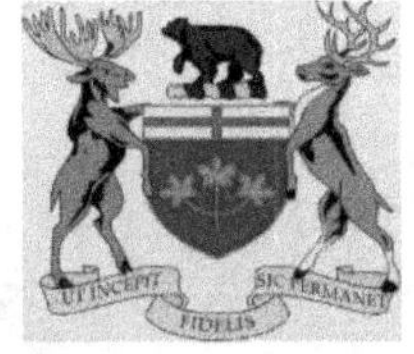

- Fistulization to or obstruction of small or large bowel
- Right-sided hydronephrosis
- Systemic (systemic cytokine response, aka "cytokine" storm)
  - CNS
    - Retinopathy
    - Psychosis
  - Heart
    - Shock (circulatory failure)
    - Death
  - Lung
    - Respiratory failure
  - GI
    - Bleeding
    - Pseudocyst
    - Abscess (infected pancreatic necrosis)
  - Endocrine
    - Hyperglycemia
    - Hypoglycemia
    - Hypocalcemia
    - Hypomagnesemia
    - Subcutaneous nodules due to fat necrosis
  - Nutrition
    - Malnutrition
  - Blood
    - Disseminated intravascular coagulation (DIC)
  - Kidney
    - Acute renal failure

Adapted from: Keller J, et al. *Best Practice & Research Clinical Gastroenterology* 2007; 21(3): pg. 524.

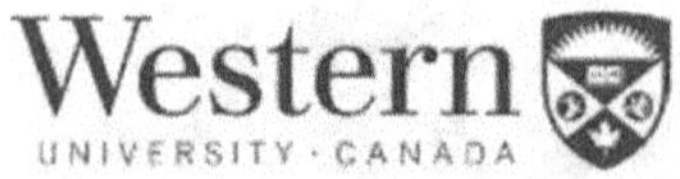

SO YOU WANT TO BE A GASTROENTEROLOGIST!

A patient with acute pancreatitis develops an UGIB (**upper GI bleeding**).

- Give 5 causes of the UGIB, which are related to the underlying acute pancreatitis.
  - Splenic artery – Rupture
  - Portal vein – Rupture
  - Splenic vein – Rupture
    – Gastric varices +/- esophageal varices
  - Pseudocysts – Pseudoaneurysms
    – Rupture of pseudoaneurysm (mortality rate, 40%)
    – Bleeding from wall of pseudocyst
  - Surgery, drainage – Necrotizing pancreatitis, WOPN, pseudocyst

Abbreviations: WOPN, walled-off pancreatic necrosis

- Give the anatomical basis for the development of gastric varices arising from splenic vein thrombosis in a patient with chronic pancreatitis.
  - Obstruction of splenic vein → ↑ flow in short gastric veins → coronary vein → development of variceal channels in gastric cardia/fundus.

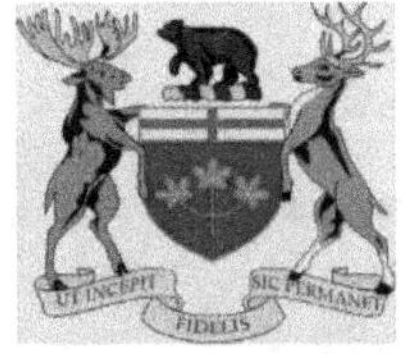

- Risk stratification

There are numerous ways to predict the severity of pancreatitis, including clinical profile, scoring systems, organ failure, or anatomic complications.

- Give 5 methods used to estimate the severity of acute pancreatitis.

- Clinical
  - Apache II > 8
  - Apache 0 >10
  - Ranson ≥ 3
  - Glasgow scope ≥ 3
  - Evidence of systemic complications

- Laboratory
  - Hematocrit ≥ 44
  - ↑ BUN (blood urea nitrogen)
  - ↑ CRP (C reactive protein)

- CT scan
  - CT ≥ 30% pancreatic necrosis

Source: Vege Santhi Swaroop, and Baron Todd H. *Mayo Clinical Gastroenterology and Heptalogy Board Review*: page 461.

  - Time-sensitive scoring systems for severity or complications of acute pancreatitis useful in
    - First 24 hours
      - Apache II

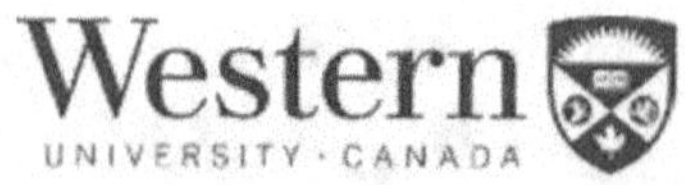

- BISAP (bedside index for severity in acute pancreatitis)
- BUN (blood urea nitrogen), or Hct (hematocrit), especially when measured serially; also useful at 48 hours

- First 48 hours
  - Ranson score (most useful to exclude severe pancreatitis)
  - Glasgow score
  - Hct (hematocrit)

➢ Really simple assessment of severe pancreatitis on admission

- ↑ Age
- ↑ BMI (body mass index)
- Lung
  - Pleural effusions
  - Infiltrates
- SIRS ≥ 2 of the following
  - RR > 20 / min, or pCO_2 < 32 mm Hg
    - PR > 90 bpm
    - RT 36 °C > 38 °C, or
    - WBC < 4,000 or > 12,000 / mm^2
- ↑ Hct (hematocrit) or BUN (blood urea nitrogen)

Abbreviations: BMI, body mass index; BUN, blood urea nitrogen Hct, hematocrit; PR, pulse rate; RR, respiratory rate; RT, rectal temperature; SIRS, systemic inflammatory response syndrome

---

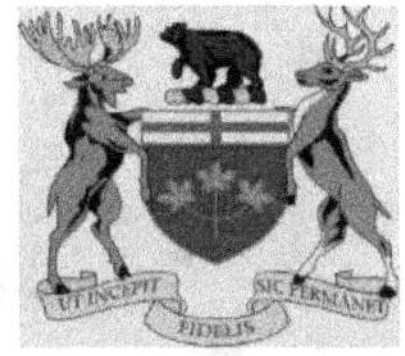

ACUTE PANCREATITIS

- Give the risk stratification and management of the patient with acute pancreatitis.
    - Clinical criteria-based scoring systems: Ranson, Glasgow, Apache (not accurate until 48 hours)
    - Atlanta symposium criteria: Pancreatic necrosis (seen in 20% of acute pancreatitis)
    - SIRS (systemic inflammatory response syndrome) leading to organ failure: cardiovascular, pulmonary, renal, GI bleeding
    - Laboratory
        - ↑ Hematocrit
        - ↑ Urinary TAP (trypsinogen activation peptide
        - ↑ BUN
        - ↑ CRP
    - Diagnostic imaging: CT, MR – sensitive for necrosis (note: the amount of necrosis does not correlate with the development of organ failure; necrosis may not develop for 24-48 hours, so CT may be negative for detectable early necrosis

Trivia

- Patients with acute pancreatitis and who are found within 24 hours of admission to have pleural effusion and/or infiltrate on chest X-ray are more likely to have a worse prognosis.
- These complications are more likely to develop if the necrotizing pancreatitis was treated with necrosectomy.

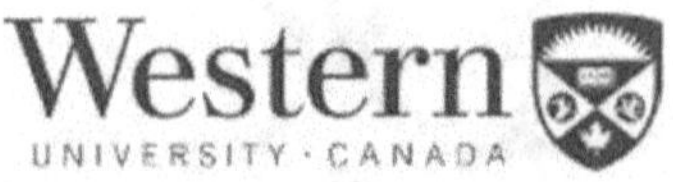

MCQ Alert

- In a patient with acute pancreatitis, suspect severe pancreatitis (necrosis), if the stem provides
  - History / signs
    - Mention of cytokines / leukotrienes
    - Fever, hypotension, tachycardia, dyspnea, oliguria
    - Abdominal guarding, rebound tenderness, ileus
    - Hemorrhage
    - Persisting /non-responsive pain
  - Abnormal blood tests
  - Abnormal CT scan

Non-enhancing areas of large portions (> 50%) of pancreas

- The patient has experienced repeated episodes of severe abdominal pain radiating to the back, in associating with high levels of alcohol ingestion. On the occasion she/ he had similar pain and alcohol abuse, and the serum amylase or lipase is normal. You are offered several plausible MCQ choices, as well as acute pancreatitis. Chronic pancreatitis is the answer
  - Caution: normal serum amylase or lipase do not R/O chronic pancreatitis.

- In the patient with acute pancreatitis, suspect biliary tract gallstones if
  - Bilirubin > 4 mg/dL
  - ALT, AST > 1000 U/mL

- If the patient with acute pancreatitis has also been drinking alcohol recently, the ALT, AST may be > 1000 U/mL, and the bilirubin may be increased (true, often > 15 mg/dL). But, alcoholics have an ↑ risk of having gallstones, so beware of gallstone pancreatitis in the alcoholic.

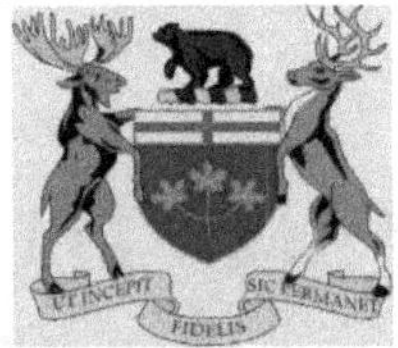

- Give the performance characteristics of 4 predictors of severity of acute pancreatitis.

	Sensitivity	Specificity	PPV	NPV
o Ranson (cut off, 3 signs)				
– At 48 hours	40% to 88%	43% to 90%	50%	90%
o Apache-II				
– At admission	34% to 70%	76% to 98%		
– At 48 hours	< 50%	90% to 100%		
o Hematocrit > 44%				
– At admission	72%			
– At 24 hours	94%			96%
o C-reactive protein	60% to 100%	75% to 100%		
o Fluid on peritoneal lavage	36% to 72%	80% to 100%		
o Procalcitonin	86%	95%		

Abbreviations: NPV, negative predictive value; PPV, positive predictive value

Note: it is the NPV of Ranson criteria and hematocrit which are most helpful clinically, in terms of predicting who will not have severe acute pancreatitis.

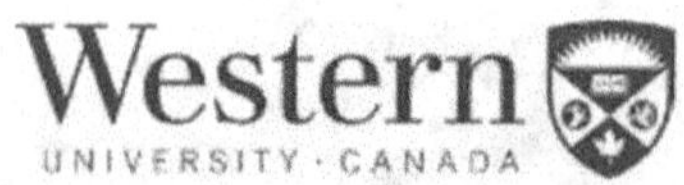

ACUTE PANCREATITIS

- Give the specific predictions made from 4 scoring systems of acute pancreatitis.
  - Ranson score
    - Pancreatic necrosis
    - Infected necrosis
    - Systemic complications
    - Death
  - Apache-II score
    - Severity of pancreatitis
    - Death
  - Hematocrit
    - Pancreatic necrosis
  - C-reactive protein
    - Severity of pancreatitis
  - Peritoneal lavage
    - Death
  - Procalcitonin
    - Organ failure
  - BISAP
    - Complications
    - Death
  - CT grading scores
    - Local complications (pseudocyst, abscess)

- Give the **Ranson** prognostic criteria for acute pancreatitis.
  - On admission

Age (years)	>55	>70
White blood cell count (cells/mm^3)	>16, 000	>18, 000
Blood glucose (mg/dL)	>200	>220
Lactate dehydrogenase (IU/L)	>350	>400
Aspartate aminotransferase (IU/L)	>250	>250

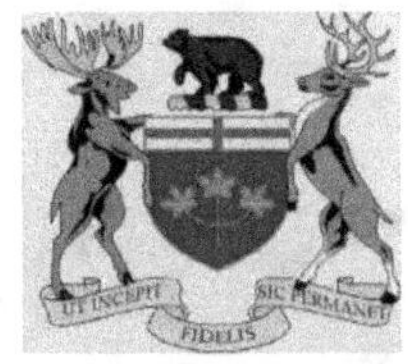

o During Initial 48 hours		
– Decrease in hematocrit (%)	>10	>10
– Increase in blood urea nitrogen (mg/dL)	>5	>2
– Calcium (mg/dL)	<8	<8
– pO_2 (mm Hg)	<60	NA
– Base deficit (mEq/L)	>4	>5
– Estimated fluid sequestration (L)	>6	>4

Source:Quoted from original paper in Steinberg, William M. *Sleisenger & Fordtran's Gastrointesintal and Liver Disease: Pathophysiology/ Diagnosis/Management* 2006: 1241-1270.

- Give the components, which comprise the **Marshall scoring system** for the diagnosis of **Multisystem Organ Failure (MOF).**
    - 2 or more falling on same day
    - Mortality rate ~ 50%
  - o Heart
    - Myocardial infarction
    - Dysrhythmias
    - Pericardial effusions
  - o Lung
    - Pleural effusion
    - Pneumonia
    - Atelectasis
    - Elevated diaphragm
    - ARDS

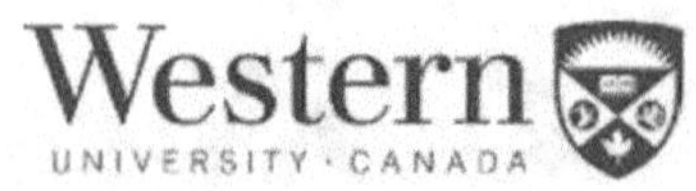

ACUTE PANCREATITIS

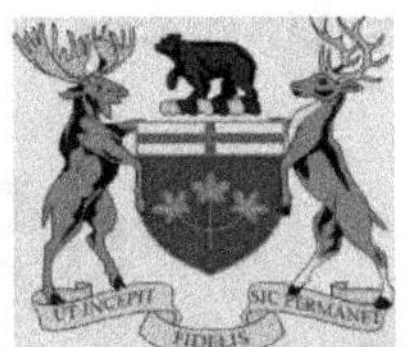

- Kidney
  - Hypovolemia
  - Hypotension
  - Acute tubular necrosis
  - Shock
- CT Grading System (Balthazar) and CT Severity Index
  - Extent of fluid collection and necrosis

- In the context of the patient with chronic pancreatitis and upper GI bleeding, give the meaning of
  - "hemosuccus pancreaticus".
  - Hemosuccus pancreaticus is bleeding from the wall of the pseudocyst into the pancreatic duct.

- Laboratory
  - PAP (pancreatitis-associated protein) and PSP (pancreatic-specific protein) have the same accuracy as serum amylase for diagnosing acute pancreatitis.
  - The most laboratory tests used to predict the severity of acute pancreatitis are surrogate markers of local inflammation.
  - Urinary TAP (trypsinogen activation peptide) is a marker for
    - Pancreatic necrosis
    - Systemic inflammatory response (sepsis)
  - The extent of elevation of serum amylase or lipase do not correlate with the severity of pancreatitis.
  - Performance in acute pancreatitis

  - Elevated serum amylase or lipase concentrations are only ~85% sensitive, and their specificity, especially for values of < 3x ULN, is only ~50%.

- Give 6 causes of an elevated serum amylase/lipase.
  - Salivary glands
    - Salivary gland disease, e.g. mumps
  - Stomach
    - Peptic ulcer disease with penetration
  - Small bowel
    - Intestinal ischemia
    - Small bowel obstruction
    - Bowel perforation
    - Celiac disease
  - Pancreas
    - Pancreatitis
    - Pancreatic cancer
  - Colon, appendix
    - Appendicitis
  - Biliary tree
    - Cholecystitis
  - In a patient with acute pancreatitis, the best management steps are
    - Large volume IV infusion
    - Risk stratification for necrotizing pancreatitis
    - Evaluation for cause
      - Alcohol
      - Gallstones
      - Drugs
      - ↑ TG (> 1000 mg/dL)
      - ↑ Ca^{2+}
      - Post ERCP

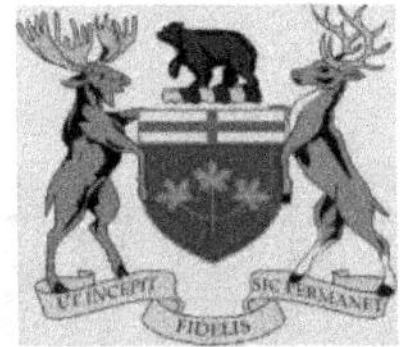

CLINICAL GEM

- Give the reason why **serial serum ionized Ca^{2+}** must be measured in the patient with acute pancreatitis.
    - Hypocalcemia may occur in acute pancreatitis.
    - Correct any associated hypomagnesemia
    - Cautious use of IV calcium gluconate to prevent dysrhythmia (IV Ca^{2+} increases binding of Ca^{2+} to myocardial receptors; ↑ Ca^{2+} on myocardial receptors displaces K^{+} from the myocardial receptors, leading to dysrhythmia)

Please see Feldman M, et al. Sleisenger and Fordtran's Gastrointestinal and Liver Disease. 9th Edition. Saunders/Elsevier 2010, Table 58.8, for Table of Complications of Acute Pancreatitis

- Give 3 causes of **falsely negative serum amylase** in acute pancreatitis.
    - Blood sampled too late after onset of symptoms (T1/2, 10 hrs)
    - Not correlated with severity of pancreatitis (may be normal with fatal disease, or with mild disease)
    - Acute on chronic pancreatitis
    - Hypertriglyceridemia-associated pancreatitis (↑ triglyceride in serum may produce an inhibitor of amylase, resulting in falsely low serum amylase concentrations)

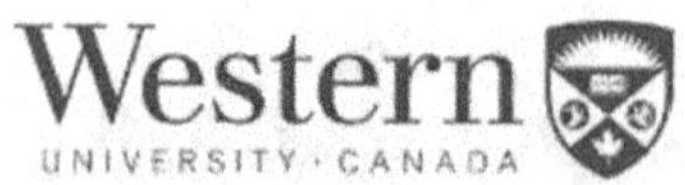

- Give 6 causes of falsely **positive serum amylase**.
    - Macroamylasemia (amylase binds to immunoglobulin in serum, and is not filtered / excreted by kidney)
    - Disease of
        - Salivary glands
        - Fallopian tubes
        - Ovary
            - Cyst
            - Cystadenoma
    - Kidney
        - Renal failure - ↓ clearance of amylase
        - Hemodialysis (> peritoneal dialysis)
    - Psychiatric disorders
        - Munchausen syndrome

Recurrent attacks of acute pancreatitis may be caused by alcohol abuse or by gallstones. In the patient with both alcohol use and known gallstones, the finding of an ↑ ALT (> 3x ULN) is often used clinically as a reliable indicator of biliary pancreatitis.

- Give a comment on the use of an elevated serum ALT as a test to support the diagnosis of gallstone pancreatitis by giving its performance characteristics.
    - An elevated (> 3x ULN) is often serum ALT to differentiate biliary pancreatitis from alcoholic pancreatitis, has a specificity of 96%, but a sensitivity of only 48%, yielding a positive predictive value of 95%.
    - Thus, a normal ALT does not exclude gallstone pancreatitis, but an ↑ ALT does suggest gallstone pancreatitis.

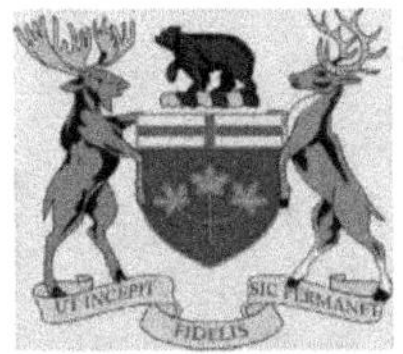

SO YOU WANT TO BE A GASTROENTEROLOGIST!

- In the context of an elevated serum amylase, give the rational for measuring **UACR** (a urinary amylase-to-creatinine ratio), and **urinary salivary amylase**.
    - ↓ UACR
        - In macroamylasemia, where amylase is bound to immunoglobulin and persists in the blood because of lack of renal excretion, the UACR may be low
        - UACR may also be low with renal insufficiency
        - UACR may be high when contaminated with salivary amylase
    - ↑ urinary salivary amylase
        - Saliva contains amylase, and if the patient spits into the urine collection, the total amylase level will be increased, and the UACR will also rise.
        - Persons with Munchausen Syndrome may spit into urine sample, so that the urine total amylase and UACR are increased.
- Give the advantage of measuring serum lipase rather than amylase to diagnose acute pancreatitis.
    - Serum lipase concentrations are not elevated in disorders of salivary glands, fallopian tubes or ovary with Munchausen syndrome or macroamylasemia.
    - Measurement of the serum lipase concentration has greater sensitivity, and especially better specificity.

➢ Diagnostic imaging

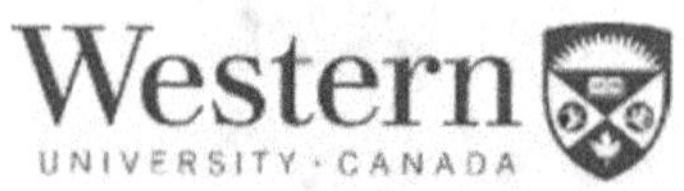

- Abdominal ultrasound may be hypoechoic in acute pancreatitis, but its usefulness may be limited by overlying bowel gas (in ~ 1/3), its poor sensitivity to detect CBD stones, and the challenge to differentiate hypoechoic areas from acute versus chronic pancreatitis, a malignancy.
- Sensitivity of detecting CBD stones EUS = ERCP = MRCP > US or CT
- In the patient with suspected necrotizing pancreatitis, EUS is superior to ERCP because of the lack of risk of introducing infection.
- Abdominal ultrasound not sensitive to detect cholelithiasis / choledochalithiasis in acute pancreatitis; use MRI or EUS

- Give the way to distinguish on diagnostic imaging the possibilities of alcoholic pancreatitis versus biliary tract stones.
    - Abdominal ultrasound
        - Not sensitive for bile duct (BD) stones
        - May show indirect evidence of
            - Stones
                - Dilated BD or cystic duct
            - Cholecystitis
                - Gallbladder wall > 4 mm
                - ↑ pericholecystic fluid

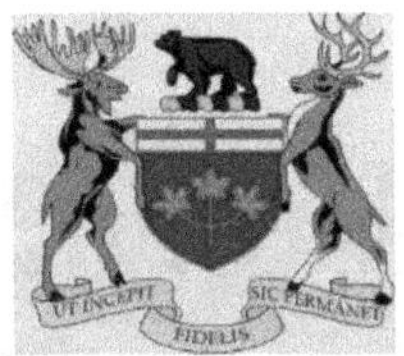

ACUTE PANCREATITIS

The abdominal plain film (APF) is useful to support the diagnosis of acute pancreatitis.

- Give findings on the APF (abdominal plain film), which suggest acute pancreatitis, and distinguish between the "sentinel loop" and the "colon cut-off" signs.

  - Stomach
    - Anterior displacement
    - Separation of the contours of the stomach and transverse colon
  - Duodenum
    - Descending portion displaced and stretched by head of enlarged pancreas
  - Jejunum / Ileum
    - "sentinel loop" (localized dilated segment of small bowel)
    - Ileus
  - Colon
    - "colon cut-off" sign
      - Spasm of colon with
        - Proximal dilation
        - Distal lack of gas
    - Irregular haustral pattern
  - Gallbladder
    - Calcified stones
  - Pancreas
    - Stones
    - Calcification
    - Ascites
    - Retroperitoneal air (abscess)
      - Gas-forming organism
      - Microperforation of gut
      - Adjacent pseudocyst

➢ Treatment

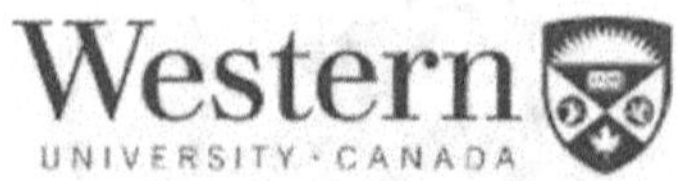

- Pain control
- Risk stratification
- IV fluids, 200-250 cc/hr (3 cc/kg per hr) for 24 hr (may start with 1L bolus infusion)
  - Then reassess for rate / volume depending upon clinical status
- NG/NJ tube feeding (no difference in outcome, NG = NJ feeding)
- Antibiotics
  - Only if infected necrosis suspected (usually after day 10)
  - Do not give prophylactically since only 1/3 of patients with necrosis can develop infected necrosis
- Early ERCP for
  - Gallstone pancreatitis (ALT 3XULN, PPV- 95%; ↑bilirubin on day

  Sphincterotomy and stone extraction
- CT-guided FNA for culture of necrotic pancreatic material
- Debridement
  - By surgery, endoscopy, radiology

Abbreviation: EUS, endoscopic ultrasound; FNA, fine needle aspiration; NG/NJ, nasogastric/ nasojejunal; ULN, upper limit of normal; US, ultrasound

Adapted from: Forsmark CE, and Baillie J. *Gastroenterology* 2007;132(5):2022-44.

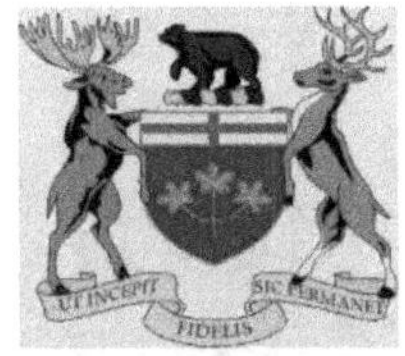

- Complications
  - Pseudocyst "…..is a fluid collection that persists for 4 to weeks and becomes encapsulated by a wall of fibrous or granulation tissue (Feldman M., et al. Sleisenger and Fordtran's Gastrointestinal and Liver Disease. 9th Edition. Saunders/Elsevier, Philadelphia, 2010, page 941).
  - Usually or adjacent to the pancreas, but occasionally seen in pelvis or chest
  - Conceptually, fluid filled sacs, sometimes with necrotic pancreatic debris
  - Pseudocyst plus liquefied necrotic debris after 5 to 6 weeks may be termed WOPN (walled off pancreatic necrosis)
  - When there is infection, may be called infected pseudocyst or infected necrosis, rather than an "abscess"
  - Bleeding into a pseudocyst is usually from a pseudoaneurysm.
  - Pancreatic abscess is "….a circumscribed intra-abdominal collection of pus occurring after an episode of acute pancreatitis or pancreatic trauma" (Feldman M., et al. Sleisenger and Fordtran's Gastrointestinal and Liver Disease. 9th Edition. Saunders/Elsevier, Philadelphia, 2010, page 961).
    - Preferred terms:
      - Infected pseudocyst (always contains liquid)
      - Infected necrosis (liquid plus debris with the debris becoming liquefied after 5 to 6 weeks)

Suggested in-depth background reading Re Acute Pancreatitis

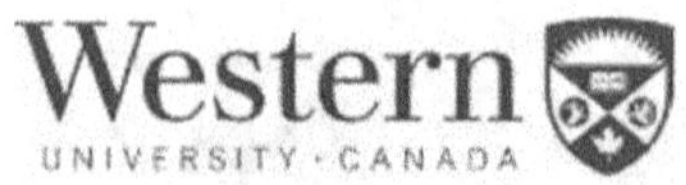

Feldman M., et al. Sleisenger and Fordtran's Gastrointestinal and Liver Disease. 9th Edition. Saunders/Elsevier, Philadelphia, 2010:

Table 58.2 Ranson's prognostic criteria, page 960

Table 58.3Conditions that predispose to acute pancreatitis, page 963

Table 58.4 Drugs associated with acute pancreatitis, page 965

Table 58.5 Complications of acute pancreatitis, page 975

Table 58.7 Computed tomography (CT) severity index (CTSI), page 980

Alcoholic Pancreatitis

- Pathology
  - "About 60% of ……persons who present with their first attack of acute alcoholic pancreatitis have already developed histologic chronic pancreatitis" (Feldman M., et al. Sleisenger and Fordtran's Gastrointestinal and Liver Disease. 9th Edition. *Saunders/Elsevier*, Philadelphia, 2010, page 989).
  - In persons with acute alcoholic pancreatitis who have not yet developed obvious chronic pancreatitis, stopping alcohol.
    ↓ rate of progression to chronic pancreatic insufficiency
    Does not alter the frequency of recurrent attacks of acute pancreatitis
- Pathophysiology

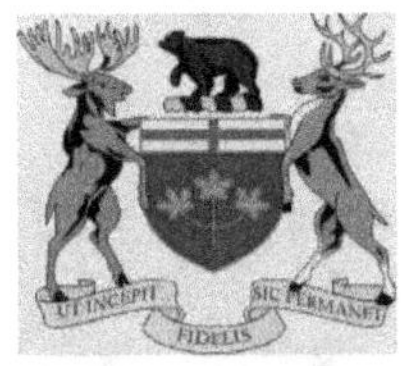

- Give the pathophysiology of alcohol-associated damage to the pancreas.

- Acute
  - Direct effect of alcohol and its "toxic" metabolites on pancreatic acinar cells.
  - ↑ lithogenicity of pancreatic fluid (alcohol-related ↑ secretion and viscosity of pancreatic juice → precipitation of protein (such as GP-2) → formation of pancreatic stones (crystals of calcium carbonate, polysaccharides, fibrillar proteins, and a gel-like matrix)
  - Acute and sometimes subclinical pancreatitis → scaring of preductular area → stasis of ductules → progression to fibrosis
  - Acute pancreatitis activates trypsin → ↑ inflammation → ↑ cytokines → activates pancreatic stellate cells → fibrosis

Direct injury by alcohol or a metabolite	– Liver ▪ Acetaldehyde – Pancreas ▪ FAEs (fatty acid esters) → ↑ Ca_i^{2+}
Oxidative stress	– Production of free radicals – ↑ peroxidation of membrane lipids

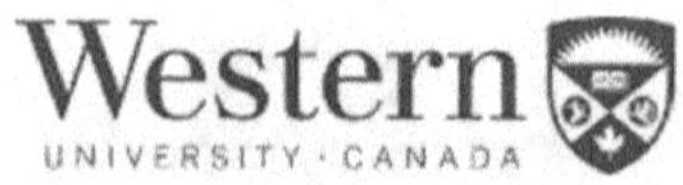

ACUTE PANCREATITIS

- CCK
  - Alcohol-associated ↑ sensitivity of acinar cells to CCK
  - Redirection of CCK-mediation zymogen granule exocytosis from apical to basolateral membrane of acinar cell.
- Genes / enzymes
  - Alcohol-associated
    - Altered expression of genes responsive to physiologic stress
  - Over
    - ↑ expression / activity of necrosis / apoptosis
- Stellate cells
  - ↑ activity of pancreatic acinar cells associated stellate (myofibroblastic) cells
    - ↑ extracellular matrix → ↑ fibrosis → ischemia
    - ↑ proliferation
    - Phagocytosis
  - Alcohol / alcohol metabolites
  - Cytokines (from necrosis of cells)
  - Growth factors (PDGF, TGF-B1)
  - Transcription factors
  - Angiotensin II
  - Autocrine factors
- Protein precipitation (plugs)
  - Alcohol stimulates pancreatic secretion of fluid with ↑ protein, ↓ volume and HCO_3^-

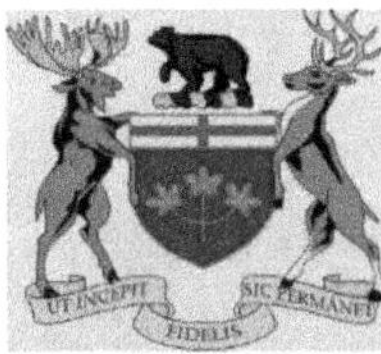

- Gain of function gene mutation, leading to SAPE
  - CFTR (cystic fibrosis transmembrane conductance regulator gene)
  - PRSS1 (cationic trypsinogen gene)
  - SPINK1 (a trypsin inhibitor)
  - These genetic mutations are hypothesized to lead to repeated episodes of acute pancreatitis, which set in motion a process that leads to chronic pancreatitis (SAPE, sentinel acute pancreatitis event)

Abbreviations: Ca_i^{2+}, intracellular Ca^{2+}; CCK, cholecystokinin; PDGF, platelet-derived growth factor; SAPE, sentinel acute pancreatic event; TGF, transforming growth factor

- Give the mechanism of the ↑ risk of complications in obesity in acute pancreatitis.
  - ↑ unsaturated fatty acids (UFAs) from the breakdown of visceral adipocyte triglycerides are proinflammatory and induce
    - Necrotic death
    - Necrosis of pancreas
    - Intrapancreatic necrosis in obesity
    - Multisystem organ failure (including respiratory and renal failure).

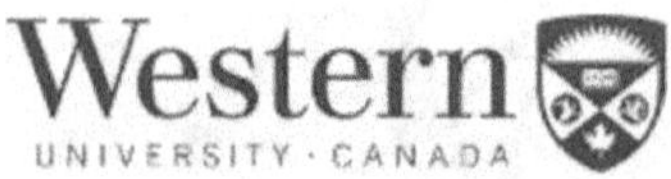

In the context of acute pancreatitis, ↑ **BMI is a risk factor** for "severe" disease.

- Give characteristics of acute pancreatitis which are more prominent in obesity (↑ BMI).
    - In the obese patient with acute pancreatitis, there are increased
        - ↑ local complications
        - Multisystem organ failure (MOF)
            - Respiratory failure
            - Renal failure
        - Sterile pancreatic necrosis
        - Death

ERCP-Associated Acute Pancreatitis

➢ Definition

- Pain + > 3x ↑ amylase within 24 hours requiring admission > 48 hrs
- Use prophylactic stents in high risk patients

- Give 10 **risk factors** associated with the development of post-ERCP pancreatitis.
    - Operator related
        - Lower ERCP volume
    - Patient related
        - Younger age
        - Female sex (possible)
        - Suspected sphincter of Oddi dysfunction (SOD)
        - Normal bilirubin
        - History of pancreatitis, recurrent of post-ERCP pancreatitis
        - Prior post-ERCP pancreatitis

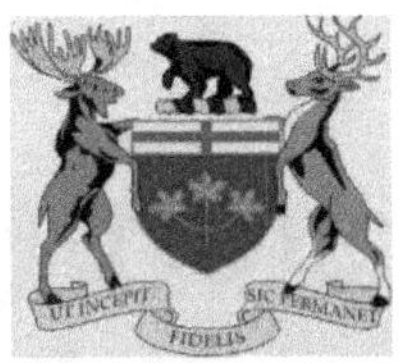

- o Procedure-related factors
  - Difficult or multiple cannulation attempts
  - Multiple pancreatic contrast injections
  - Pancreatic acinerization
  - Precut sphincterotomy
  - Endoscopic papillary balloon dilation
  - Sphincter of Oddi manometry
  - Distal common bile duct diameter ≤ 10 mm
  - Procedures not involving stone removal

Abbreviation: CCK, cholecystokinin; ERCP, endoscopic retrograde cholangiopancreatography

Printed with permission: Blero D, et al. Endoscopic complications--avoidance and management. Nat Rev Gastroenterol Hepatol. 2012;9(3):162-72. Box 1.

The placement of temporary prophylactic pancreatic duct stents is suggested for high risk patients following ERCP.

- Give 3 features giving a high risk of post-ERCP pancreatitis and 3 features giving a low risk.

High	Low
o Recent biliary sphincterotomy	o Young
o Ampullectomy	o Female
o Sphincter of Oddi dysfunction	o Non-dilated bile ducts
o Prior episode of post-ERCP pancreatitis	o Trainee participation in procedure

Adapted from: Elta GH. *Gastrointest Endosc* 2008;67(2):262-64.; and Freeman ML, et al. *Gastrointest Endosc* 2001;54(4):425-434.

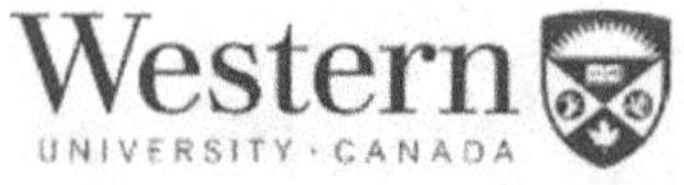

Indications for prophylactic pancreatic stent placement during ERCP

- Prophylaxis (in high risk patient)
  - Pre-ERCP indomethacine suppository
    - Use guideline for canulation
    - Stenting

Necrotizing Pancreatitis and Abscess

- Pathological types
  - Walled-off pancreatic necrosis (WOPN)
    - Several weeks after pancreatic necrosis and duct disruption, the cystic area contains liquid as well as solid material (non-enhancing pancreatic parenchyma on contrast-enhanced CT scan).
  - Pancreatic abscess
    - ".....infected pseudocyst or infected liquefied collections without significant solid debris (pancreatic necrosis" (Feldman M., et al. Sleisenger and Fordtran's Gastrointestinal and Liver Disease. 9th Edition. *Saunders/Elsevier*, Philadelphia, 2010, page 1038).
    - Strictly speaking, a pancreatic pseudocyst is not a cyst, because although there may be cystic spaces filled with pancreatic secretion fluid from a duct which has been disrupted by obstruction or inflammation, the cystic space does not have an epithelial lining, and so is actually not a true cyst.
    - Cytology of fluid in pseudocysts may show histocytes.

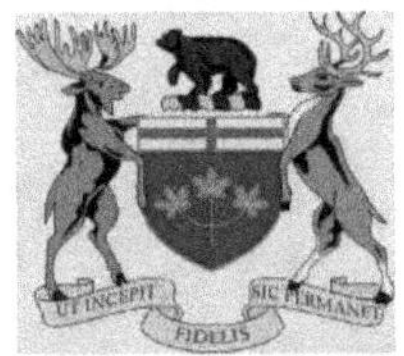

- ERCP / MRCP – shows communication with pancreatic duct

- Pathophysiology

SO YOU WANT TO BE A GASTROENTEROLOGIST!

- Give the pathophysiology of the failure of 3 organs in necrotizing pancreatitis.

- Heart
  - SIRS (systemic inflammatory response syndrome)
    - Activation of
      - Trypsin
      - Phospholipase
      - Elastase

- Lung
  - ARDS (acute respiratory distress syndrome)
    - Breakdown of surface from
      - ↑ activity of phospholipase A

- Kidney
  - ↓ SBP (hypotension) ↓ blood volume (hypovolemia) → ATN

- GI tract
  - Microcirculatory changes e.g. vasoconstriction → ischemia, AV shunting in gut

- Liver
  - Release into portal circulation of TNF, PAS
    - Activation of hepatic Kupffer cells
    - ↑ CRP (C-reactive protein)
    - ↑ IL-6

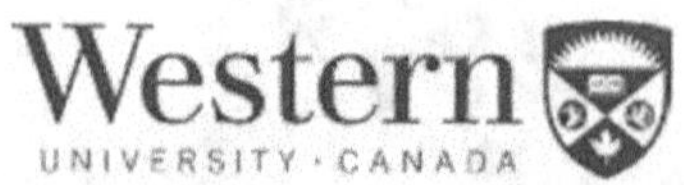

MINI UPDATE

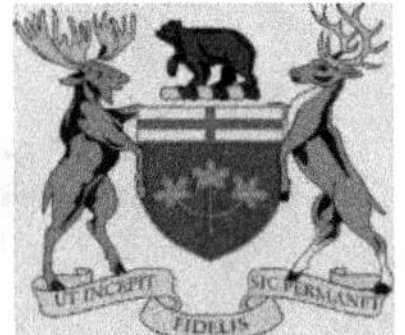

NUTRITION

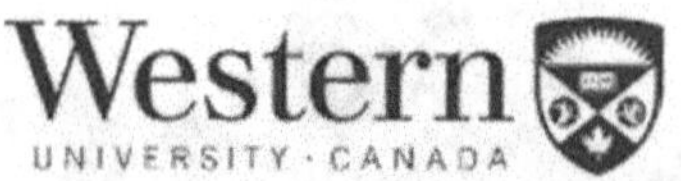

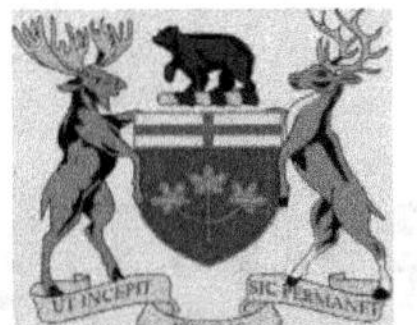
UT INCEPIT
FIDELIS
SIC PERMANET

Fat, Protein, Carbohydrate and Vitamin Absorption

Mahmoud Mosli

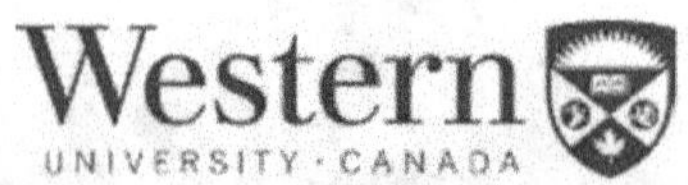

FAT, PROTEIN, CARBOHYDRATE AND VITAMIN ABSORPTION

Introduction

- In humans, most nutrients are absorbed with remarkable efficiency.
- Only less than 5% of ingested carbohydrate, fat, and protein is usually excreted in the stool of adults who consume a normal "balanced" diet.

Digestion Overview

- Generally, digestion occurs in 3 Phases:
  - Intraluminal digestion
  - Mucosal absorption.
  - Delivery into the portal/lymphatic system.

Some factors that delay gastric emptying. Food particles larger than 2 mm in diameter are rejected by the antrum. Receptors for pH, osmolarity, fatty acids, and other nutrients in the duodenum signal gastric delay by means of neurohumoral mechanisms. Nutrients in the ileum and colon also influence gastric emptying by the so-called ileal brake mechanism, which may involve peptide tyrosine-tyrosine (PYY) and glucagon-like peptides GLP-1 and GLP-2.

Digestion in Stomach

- In the stomach: acid is secreted by gastric mucosa
- Pepsinogen release from chief cells
  Stimulated by gastrin, histamine, cholinergic
- Rate of digestion depends
  - Rate of gastric emptying,
  - pH of intra-gastric contents
  - Types of protein ingested

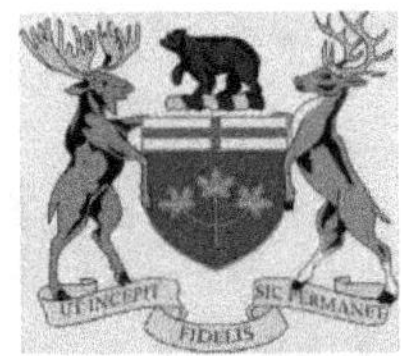

FAT, PROTEIN, CARBOHYDRATE AND VITAMIN ABSORPTION

Digestion

- Presence of nutrients in the duodenal lumen stimulates CCK and Secretin release into the portal circulation by APUD cells of the duodenum, causing the gallbladder to contract and the pancreas to secrete their digestive enzymes respectively.
- The simultaneous release of bile salts, pancreatic enzymes, and bicarbonate provides optimal conditions (milieu) for further nutrient digestion.
- Digestion of carbohydrate and protein depends on the combined actions of intra-luminal secreted enzymes and then brush border and mucosal cytosolic enzymes.

Pancreatic Enzymes

- Proteases (acinar cells):
    - Trypsinogen (converted to active form trypsin after cleaved by brush border enzyme enterokinase)
    - Chemotrypsinogen (converted to active form chemotrypsin by trypsin)
    - Proelastase (converted to active form elastase by trypsin)
    - Procarboxypeptidase A/B (converted to active forms carboxypeptidase A/B by trypsin)
    - Ribonuclease (secreted in active form).

FAT, PROTEIN, CARBOHYDRATE AND VITAMIN ABSORPTION

- Other enzymes:
  - Prophospholipase A (converted to active form phospholipase A by trypsin)
  - Amylase (secreted in active form)
  - Lipase (secreted in active form).

Enzyme	Action	Products
Trypsin	– Endopeptidase; cleaves internal bonds at lysine or arginine residues; cleaves other pancreatic proenzymes	Oligopeptides and proteolytic enzymes
Chymotrypsin	– Endopeptidase; cleaves bonds at aromatic or neutral amino acid residues	Oligopeptides
Elastase	– Endopeptidase; cleaves bonds at aliphatic amino acid residues	Oligopeptides
Carboxy-peptidase A	– Exopeptidase; cleaves aromatic amino acids from C-terminal end of proteins and peptides	Aromatic amino acids and peptides
Carboxy-peptidase B	– Exopeptidase; cleaves arginine or lysine from C-terminal end of proteins and peptides	Arginine, lysine, and peptides

FAT, PROTEIN, CARBOHYDRATE AND VITAMIN ABSORPTION

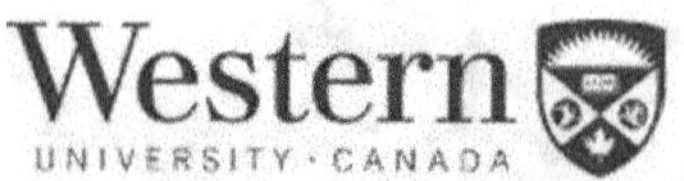

Pancreatic Proteases

- Each of the pancreatic proteases is secreted as a proenzyme
  - Must be activated within the lumen
  - Endo- vs exo- peptidase
- Enterokinase (enteropeptidase)
  - Liberated from its superficial position in the brush border membrane by the action of bile acids

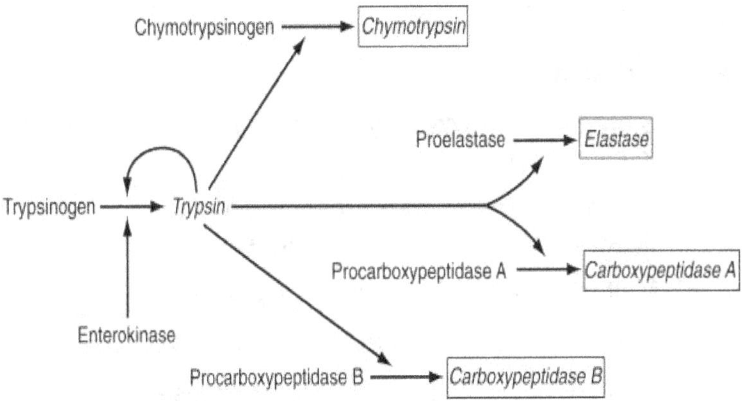

Activation of pancreatic proteolytic enzymes

Amylase

- Salivary and pancreatic amylases
  - Endoenzymes that cleave oligosaccharides with maltotriose and maltose

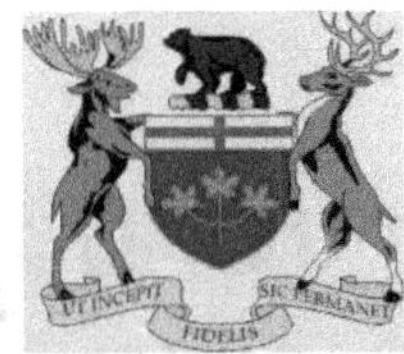

2. Salivary amylase:
    - Depends on its proximity to the ingested starches and the time they spend within the mouth
    - Inactivated rapidly by gastric acid
3. Pancreatic amylase:
    - Found within the intestinal lumen (brush border membrane)
    - Concentration is limiting only if level is reduced to below 10% of normal

Carbohydrates

- Starch is hydrolyzed by salivary/pancreatic amylase to oligo/disaccharides.
- Brush border enzymes digest oligo and disaccharides to monosaccharides:
- Maltose (maltase) to glucose + glucose.
- Sucrose (sucrase) to fructose + glucose
- Lactose (lactase) to galactose + glucose
- Trehalose (trehalase) to glucose.

	Enzyme	Substrate	Product(s)
o	Lactase	Lactose	Glucose Galactose
o	Maltase (glucoamylase)	α-1,4-Linked oligosaccharides; up to 9 residues	Glucose

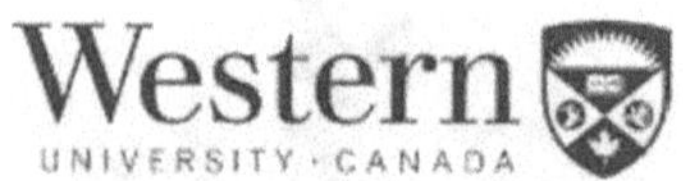

	Enzyme	Substrate	Product(s)
o	Sucrase-isomaltase (sucrose α-dextrinase)		
o	Sucrase	Sucrose	Glucose Fructose
o	Isomaltase	α-Limit dextrin α-1,6 Link	Glucose
o	Both enzymes	α-Limit dextrin α-1,4 Link at non-reducing end	Glucose
o	Trehalase	Trehalose	Glucose

Actions of brush border membrane hydrolases

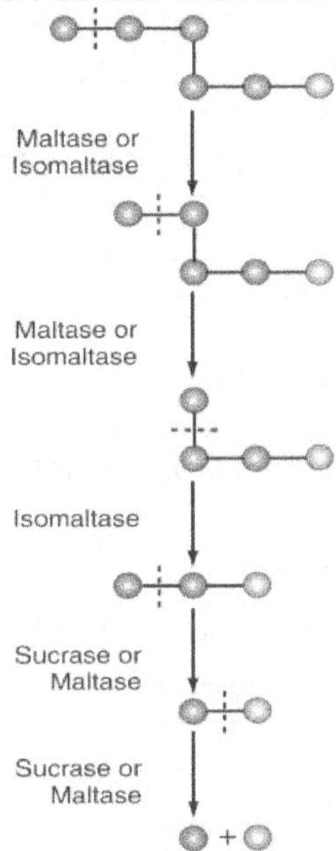

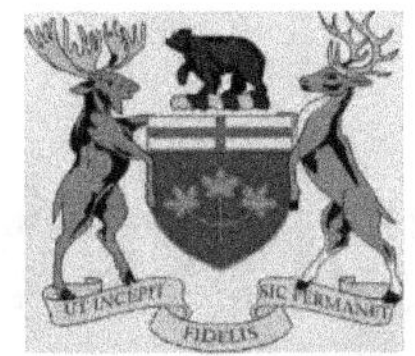

- The combined actions of maltase, isomaltase, and sucrase yield glucose molecules from α-limit dextrins.
- Isomaltase is necessary to split the α1-6 link, glucose units; reducing glucose units.

Carbohydrate Absorption

- Provides approximately 45% of total energy; about 180 g per day
- All ingested glucose and galactose is absorbed normally, but the capacity to absorb fructose (>50g) is limited
- Common CHO
  - Starch (amylose and amylopectin)
  - Lactose (milk)
  - Fructose, glucose, sucrose (the cells of fruit and vegetables)
  - Sucrose (purified from cane or beet sources).
- Monosaccharides are absorbed into the enterocytes by transporters:
  - Glucose and galactose enter via co-transporter SGLT1 (Na-glucose co-transporter or secondary active transport).
  - Fructose enter via GLUT5 (facilitated diffusion).
- Monosaccharides are exported out of the enterocytes into the portal venous system via transporter:
  - Glucose and galactose via GLUT2
  - Fructose via GLUT5

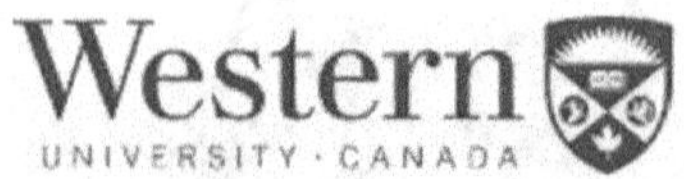

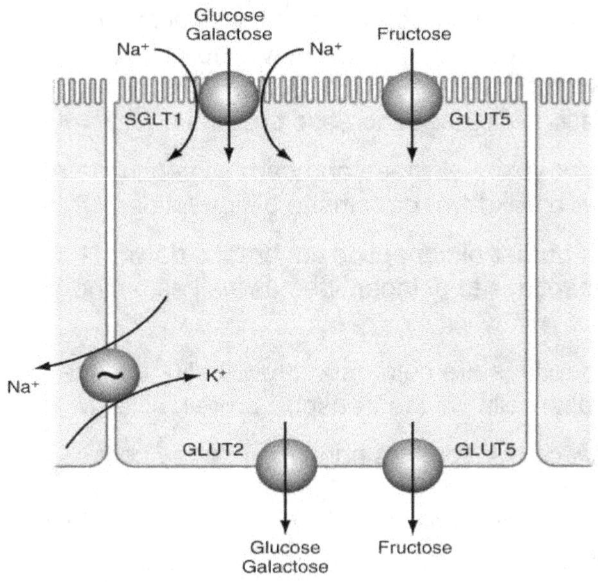

Protein Digestion

- Products of intraluminal digestion :
  - Cooperative activity of endo- and exo-peptidases
  - End result is neutral and basic amino acids and/or peptides of 2 to 6 amino acids in length
- pH < 4 activates pepsinogen (secreted by gastric chief cells) to pepsin breaking down proteins to oligo-peptides.
- Acid along with protein and fat in the duodenum stimulates secretin and CCK release, which stimulates the exocrine pancreas to secrete HCO3 to increase the alkalinity of the duodenum (pancreatic enzymes work best at higher pH).

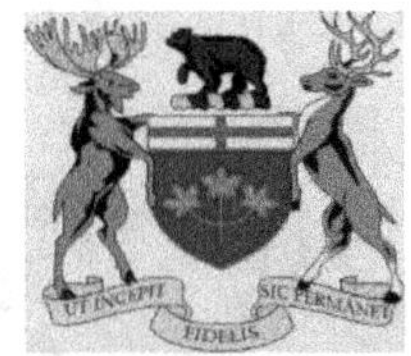

FAT, PROTEIN, CARBOHYDRATE AND VITAMIN ABSORPTION

- In the duodenum, activation of the pancreatic enzyme trypsinogen to its cleaved form trypsin (converted by enterokinase) leads to further activation of other pancreatic enzymes.
- Chemotrypsin, elastase and carboxypeptidase A/B further breakdown proteins to oligopeptides.
- Brush border oligopeptidases breaks down oligopeptides to di/tripeptides as well as amino acids.
- Di/tripeptides are cotransported with H+ into the epithelial cells via the transport protein hPep1.
- Na-AA co-transporters bring AA into the cells

• Brush Border Membrane Peptidases		Action	Products
o Amino-oligopeptidases (at least two types)	-	Cleave amino acids from C terminal end of 3 to 8 amino acid peptides	Amino acids and dipeptides
o Aminopeptidase A	-	Cleaves dipeptides with acidic amino acids at N terminal end	Amino acids
o Dipeptidase I	-	Cleaves dipeptides containing methionine	Amino acids
o Dipeptidase III	-	Cleaves glycine-containing dipeptides	Amino acids
o Dipeptidyl aminopeptidase IV	-	Cleaves proline-containing peptides with free a-amino groups	Peptides and amino acids

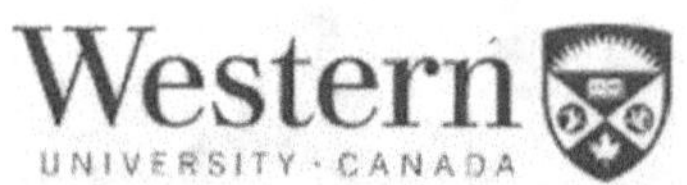

FAT, PROTEIN, CARBOHYDRATE AND VITAMIN ABSORPTION

• Brush Border Membrane Peptidases		Action	Products
○ Carboxypeptidase P	-	Cleaves proline-containing peptides with free C terminal end	Peptides and amino acids
○ Gamma glutamyl transpeptidase	-	Cleaves gamma-glutamyl bonds and transfers glutamine to amino acid or peptide acceptors	Gamma-glutamyl amino acid or peptide
○ Folate conjugase	-	Cleaves pteroyl polyglutamates	Mono-glutamate

• Cytoplasmic Peptidase		Action	Products
○ Dipeptidases (several types)	-	Cleave most dipeptides	▪ Amino acids
○ Aminotripeptidase	-	Cleaves tripeptides	▪ Amino acids
○ Proline dipeptidase	-	Cleaves proline-containing dipeptides	▪ Proline and amino acids

Absorption of protein and amino acids

- Dietary proteins are the major source of amino acids; 10% to 15% of energy intake.
- At least 70 g of protein per day
- Variety of types of animal and plant proteins
  - Plant proteins are less digestible than those derived from animals

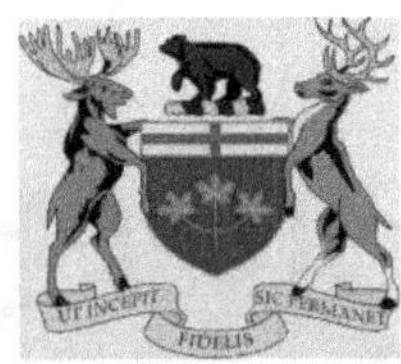

FAT, PROTEIN, CARBOHYDRATE AND VITAMIN ABSORPTION

- Proteins rich in essential amino acids are "high quality"

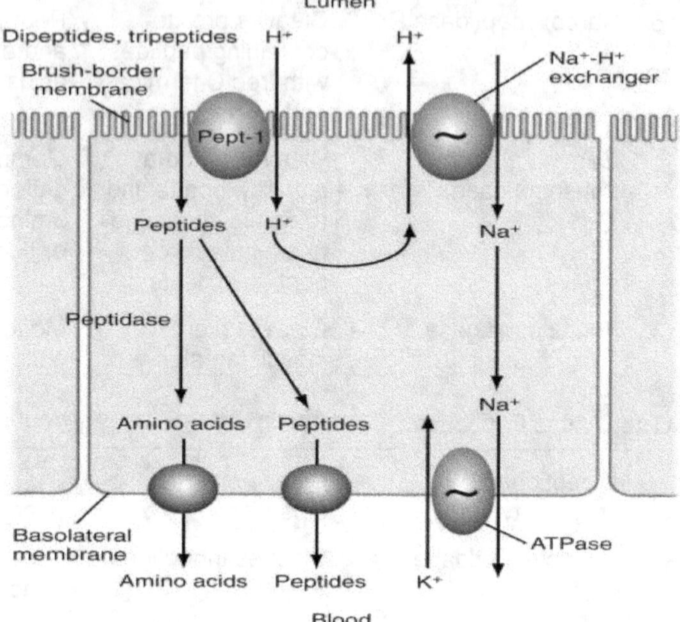

- Amino acids are transported across the brushborder membrane (BBM) and the basolateral membrane (BLM)
- The transport is partially carrier-mediated (active, and fascilitated) as well as by diffusion
- There are several groupings of the numerous transporters
- Most of the absorbed products are in the form of single amino acids.
- Digestion of protein continues into the ileum (up to 40% of protein)

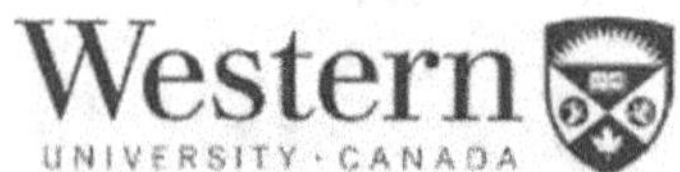

FAT, PROTEIN, CARBOHYDRATE AND VITAMIN ABSORPTION

Fat Digestion/Absorption

- Approximately 40% of adult energy requirements is supplied by lipids, of which triglycerides account for a major portion.
- Most dietary lipid is absorbed in the upper two thirds of jejunum.
- Gastric contractions and gastric lipases converts fat in the stomach to fine emulsions.
- Food in the duodenum stimulates the release of the GI peptides CCK and secretin
- CCK stimulates
  - Release pancreatic digestive enzymes
  - Contraction of the gallbladder, with release into the duodenum of bile stored in the gallbladder during fasting
- In the duodenum, pancreatic lipases (alkaline PH) hydrolyze TG to FFA and monoglycerides.
- Bile acids helps create miscelles consisting of FFA and MG, which are absorbed into the enterocytes.
- Lipolysis
  - The initial step in lipolysis is to increase the stability of the fatty emulsion.
  - Gastric lipase acts to yield fatty acids (FA) and diglyceride (DG); the latter enhances emulsification.
  - This step is further enhanced in the duodenum by bile salts (BS) and phospholipid (PL), which enable lipase, in the presence of colipase, to act at the surface of the emulsion droplet, bringing it close to the triglyceride molecule and resulting in the release of monoglyceride (MG) and fatty acids.

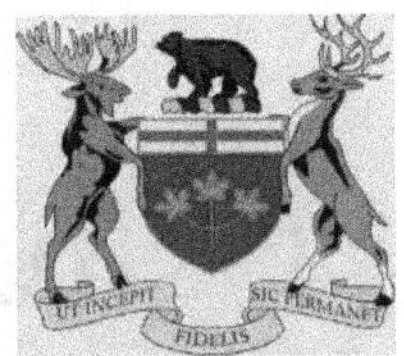

FAT, PROTEIN, CARBOHYDRATE AND VITAMIN ABSORPTION

- Lipolysis in the duodenum yields two fatty acid molecules and a monoglyceride molecule and occurs in a rapid and efficient manner at nearly neutral pH.
- Bile salt molecules oriented at an oil-water interface with a hydrophobic sterol backbone in oil phase and its hydrophilic hydroxyl and either taurine or glycine conjugates in aqueous phase.
- The products of lipolysis are dispersed into lamellae at the surface of the oil phase, each about 4 to 5 nm thick, with water spacings up to 8 nm, and from there into vesicles approximately 20 to 130 nm in diameter.
- Fatty acids and monoglyceride within the vesicles pass on into mixed micelles.
- At concentrations above critical micellar concentration (CMC), bile salts aggregate as simple micelles in water with their hydrophilic groups facing into the water.

Enterohepatic circulation of bile salts. Active transport in the ileum retrieves most bile salts, and the small fraction lost into the colon is compensated for by fresh hepatic synthesis.

- Triglyceride and phospholipid are synthesized in the smooth endoplasmic reticulum (SER) and accumulate there as dense droplets.
- Apolipoproteins, synthesized in the rough endoplasmic reticulum (RER), assist in the formation of chylomicrons in the tubular endoplasmic reticulum and Golgi apparatus. 3) These lipoproteins finally are released across the basolateral membrane by exocytosis.

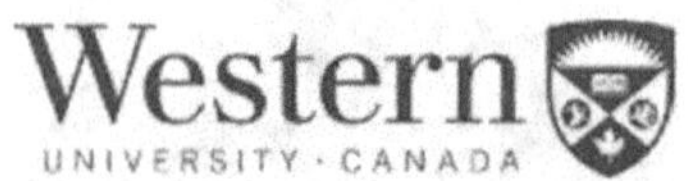

- Once intestinal *chyme* leaves the ileum and enters the colon, most nutrients have been digested and absorbed.
- Colonic function serves largely to dehydrate luminal contents by absorbing salt and water and to store the residuum.
- Dietary fiber may be digested by bacteria, with release of short-chain fatty acids

Vitamins

- Sources
  - Vitamin A (retinol)
    - Milk and milk products, egg yolk, and fish
  - Vitamin B
    - Sequence of steps leading to the binding of vitamin B12 to intrinsic factor (IF). Food-bound B12 is released by gastric acid and pepsin and binds preferentially by salivary R protein in the stomach.
    - Proteolysis of R protein by trypsin releases B12 for binding to IF.
    - Binding and uptake of the IF-B12 complex occurs through a specific receptor-mediated process on the brush border membrane of ileal enterocytes.
    - Vitamin B12 is released at an intracellular site, transported across the basolateral membrane, and taken up by transcobalamin II for transport to the portal circulation.

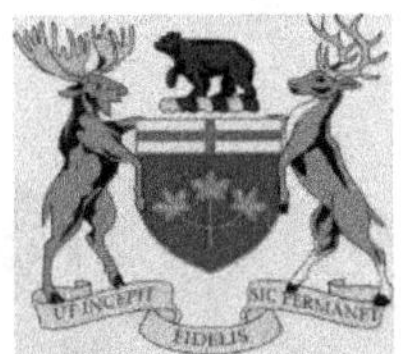

FAT, PROTEIN, CARBOHYDRATE AND VITAMIN ABSORPTION

- Vitamin D
  - Vitamins D2 (ergocalciferol) and D3 (cholecalciferol)
  - Vitamin D3 is found in a restricted range of foods, predominantly the oils of fatty fish
  - Synthesized with sunlight

- Vitamin E
  - Distributed widely in the diet
  - Vegetable oils, cereals, eggs, and fruit are good sources

- Vitamin K is found in two forms
  - K1, derived largely from plants, is phytomenadione
    - Mainly vegetables, beef liver
  - Absorption of K1 from the small intestine is dependent on luminal bile salts
  - K2 comprises a group of bacteria-produced compounds, the multiprenyl mena-quinones.

- Water Soluble Vitamins:
  - Ascorbic Acid
  - B-complex

- Fat Soluble Vitamins:
  - A,D,K, E

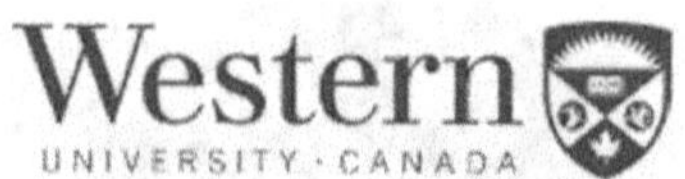

FAT, PROTEIN, CARBOHYDRATE AND VITAMIN ABSORPTION

Vitamin	Reference Nutrient Intake	Transport Mechanism
○ Ascorbic acid	40 mg/day	- Active; sodium-dependent process at BBM
○ Folic acid	200 mg/day	- Hydrolysis of dietary polyglutamates by folate conjugase at BBM; sodium-dependent active transport or facilitated diffusion of monoglutamate at BBM
○ Cobalamin (vitamin B_{12})	1.5 µg/day	- Intrinsic factor binding; uptake of intrinsic factor–B_{12} complex at BBM by a specific receptor
○ Thiamine	1 mg/day	- Sodium-dependent active transport; absorption includes hydrolytic and phosphorylation steps
○ Riboflavin	1.3 mg/day	- Absorption includes hydrolytic and phosphorylation steps
○ Pantothenic acid	3-7 mg/day[†]	?
○ Biotin	10-200 µg/day[†]	?

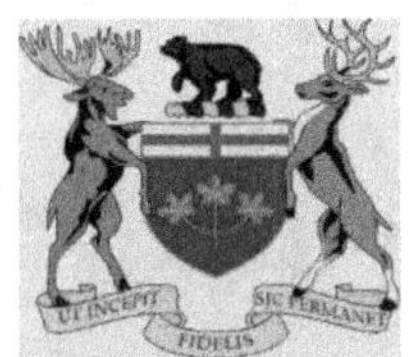

FAT, PROTEIN, CARBOHYDRATE AND VITAMIN ABSORPTION

Vitamin	Reference Nutrient Intake	Transport Mechanism
○ Pyridoxine	1.5 mg/day	- Simple diffusion
○ Niacin	18 mg/day	?
• Fat soluble		
○ Vitamin A (retinol)	700 µg/day	Passive diffusion
○ Vitamin D (cholecalciferol)	10 µg/day	Passive diffusion
○ Vitamin E (a-tocopherol)	>4 mg/day	Passive diffusion
○ Vitamin K	1 µg/kg/day	
- Phytomenadione (K_1)		Carrier-mediated uptake
- Menaquinones (K_2)		Passive diffusion

> "The price of greatness is responsibility."
>
> Winston Churchill

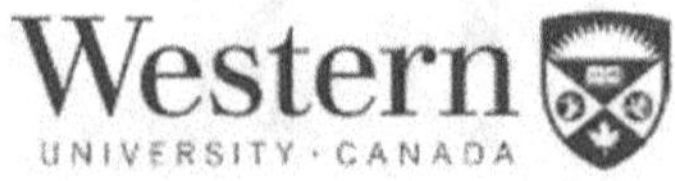

MINI UPDATE

Protein Losing Gastroenteropathy

Keith McIntosh

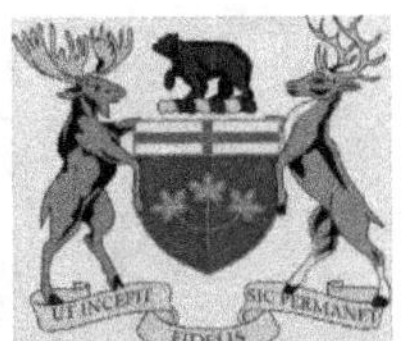

Protein Losing Gastroenteropathy (PLG)

- Definition
  - Diverse group of disorders resulting in excessive loss of serum proteins into the gastrointestinal tract
  - Syndrome resulting in
    - Hypoproteinemia
    - Edema
    - Sometimes associated with pleural and pericardial effusions.

- Pathophysiology

- Give the pathophysiology of PLG (protein losing gastroenteropathy).
  - In healthy subjects, GI tract protein losses play only a minor role in total protein metabolism
  - Daily enteric loss of serum proteins accounts for less than 1-2% of the total serum protein pool
  - Most proteins found in the lumen of the GI tract come from sloughed enterocytes and pancreatic and biliary secretions
  - These are metabolized by existing proteases much like other peptides into constituent amino acids and then resorbed
  - In protein losing enteropathy however, as much as 60% of the total pool of albumin can be lost through the GI tract
  - There are 3 major mechanisms by which this occurs:
    - Diseases associated with Mucosal Erosions or Ulcerations

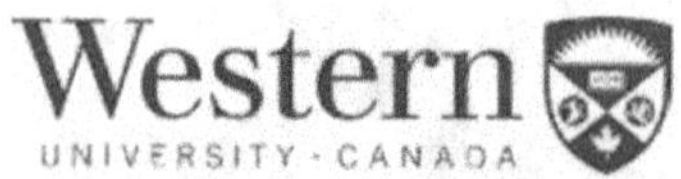

PROTEIN LOSING GASTROENTEROPATHY

- Diseases without Mucosal Erosions or Ulcerations
- Diseases with Lymphatic Obstruction or Increased Lymphatic Pressure

- The loss of serum proteins is independent of molecular weight (in contrast to nephrotic syndrome where low MW albumin is lost preferentially)
- When the rate of protein loss exceeds the body's capacity to synthesize new protein, hypoproteinemia develops
- Albumin production for example is normally 0.15 g/kg day, which in healthy subjects will equal the rate of elimination
- In protein losing enteropathy, as albumin is lost, albumin synthesis can be increased up to 25%, but once this threshold is exceeded by losses, hypoproteinemia will occur
- In addition to hypoproteinemia, protein losing gastroenteropathy can result in loss of other serum components as well:
  - Lipids
  - Fe
  - Trace metals
- Lymphatic obstruction can also result in lymphocytopenia, with resultant alterations in cellular immunity
- Simple approach to pathophysiology: disease associated with
  - Mucosal erosions or ulcerations
  - No mucosal erosions or ulcerations
  - Lymphatic obstruction or ↑ lymphatic pressure

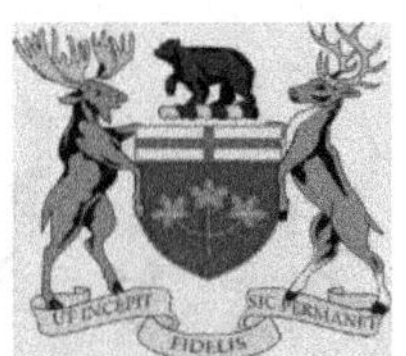

PROTEIN LOSING GASTROENTEROPATHY

Proteins preferentially Lost	Proteins generally spared (due to rapid turnover and synthesis)
o Albumin	o Insulin
o Immunoglobulins – IgG – IgA – IgM	o Clotting factors o IgE o Prealbumin
o Fibrinogen	
o Lipoproteins	
o A1AT	
o Transferrin	
o Ceruloplasmin	

➢ Causes / associations

- Give 20 causes of protein losing gastroenteropathy (PLG).

- Diseases with Mucosal Erosions or Ulcerations
  - Amyloidosis
  - Behcet Disease
  - Carcinoid Syndrome
  - Crohn Disease / Ulcerative Colitis
  - Duodenitis
  - Erosive Gastritis
  - H. Pylori Gastritis
  - Infectious Diarhea (eg. C. difficile)

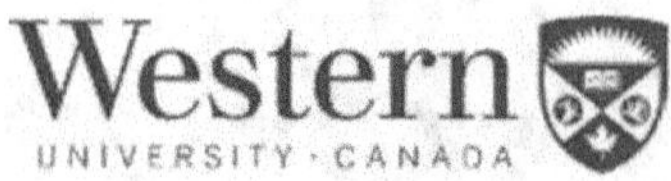

  - Ischemic Colitis
  - Lymphoma
  - NSAID induced enteropathy
  - Sarcoidosis
  - Waldenstrom Macroglobulinemia

- Diseases without Mucosal Erosions or Ulcerations
  - AIDS gastroenteropathy
  - Bacterial Overgrowth
  - Celiac Disease
  - Collagenous colitis
  - Giant hypertrophic gastropathy (Menetrier's disease)
  - H. Pylori gastritis
  - Intestinal Parasitosis
  - Lymphocytic colitis
  - SLE
  - Tropical Sprue
  - Viral gastroenteritis
  - Whipple disease

- Diseases with Lymphatic Obstruction or ↑ Lymphatic Pressure
  - Cardiac disease
    - Heart failure
    - Constrictive pericarditis
    - Fontan procedure
  - Crohn Disease
  - Intestinal Lymphangiectasia

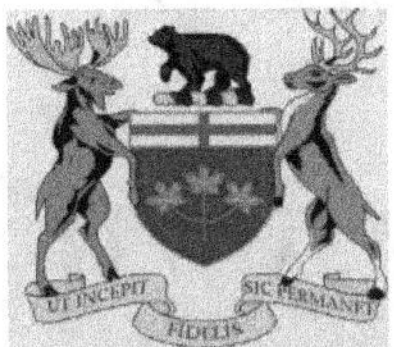

- Mesenteric Venous thrombosis
- Neoplastic disease involving mesenteric lymphatics (eg. Lymphoma)
- Portal hypertensive gastroenteropathy
- Retroperitoneal Fibrosis
- SLE (systemic lupus erythematosis)
- Superior vena cava thrombosis
- Whipple disease

Examples of Luminal Causes of PLG

Menetrier Disease

- Definition
  - Giant hypertrophic gastropathy is the most common gastric lesion causing severe protein loss
  - ↑ risk of carcinoma (~15% of patients)
- Clinical
  - Symptoms: dyspepsia, postprandial nausea, emesis, edema and weight loss
- Pathology
  - Prominent, thick gastric folds with substantial mucus and protein rich exudates are seen
  - Normal gastric glands are replaced by mucous secreting cells, reducing the number of parietal cells resulting in hypochlorydia
  - Tight junctions between cells are wider than normal, resulting in increased intercellular permeability to protein loss

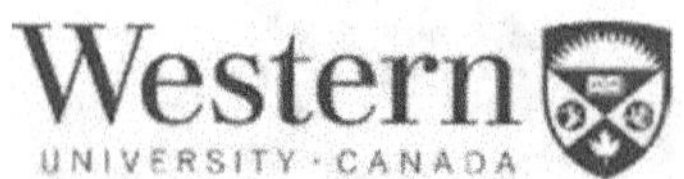

- May be self-limited and completely resolve in patients younger than 10 years of age (thought to be associated with CMV infection)

➤ Treatment

- Treat associated
  - CMV
  - H. pylori
- Anti-secretory Rx
  - PPI
  - Octreotide
- Surgery
  - Partial or total gastrectomy

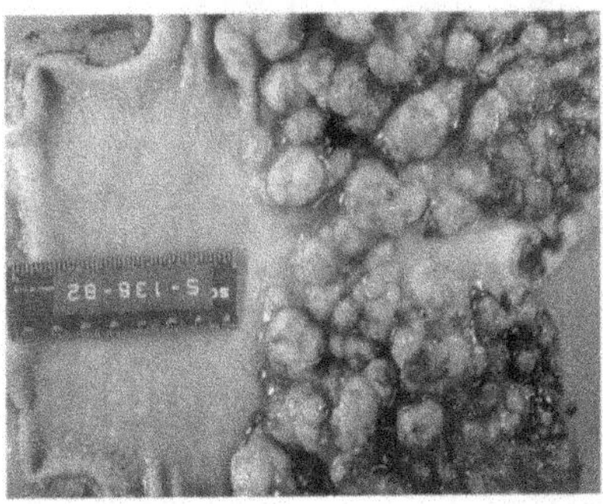
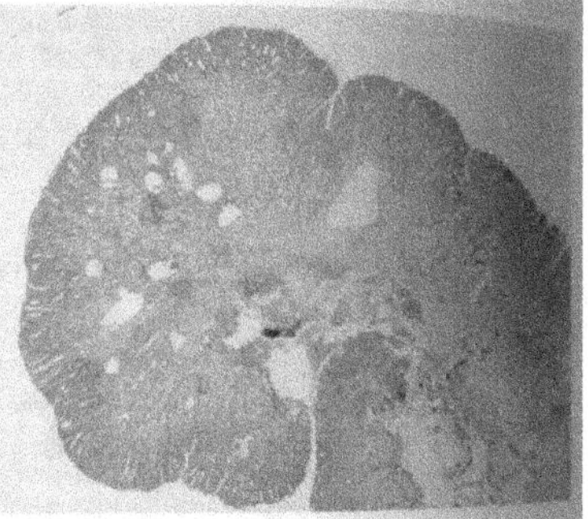

H. Pylori Gastritis

- H. Pylori gastritis has been associated with protein losing gastropathy
- Some patients may have mucosal erosions or ulcerations leading to loss although this is not a necessary requirement for protein loss
- Successful treatment and eradication of H. Pylori results in improvement of protein loss

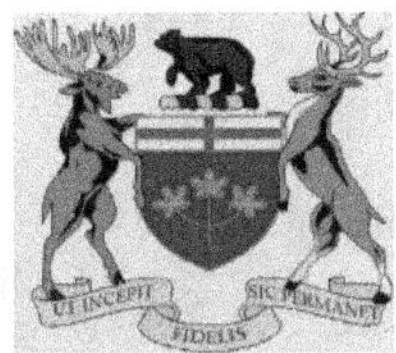

Allergic Eosinophilic Gastroenteritis

- Mostly in childhood but can be in adults as well
- Common symptoms include abdominal pain, vomiting, diarrhea
- Findings include hypoproteinemia, iron deficiency anemia, and peripheral eosinophilia
- Small bowel biopsy shows a marked increase in number of eosinophils
- Charcot Leyden crystals (collections of eosinophilic granules) may be found on stool examination
- Treatment: identification and avoidance of food allergies, elemental diets, steroids

Systemic Lupus Erythematosus (SLE)

- Commonly associated with protein losing enteropathy
- Mesenteric vasculitis can result in intestinal ischemia, edema & altered intestinal vascular permeability
- Gastritis and mucosal ulcerations also can contribute to protein loss
- Treatment with steroids and immunomodulator agents can lead to remission of protein-losing enteropathy

Inflammatory Bowel Disease (IBD)

- Both Crohn's and UC can result in severe protein loss
- Secondary to
  - Mucosal erosions and ulcerations
  - Mesenteric lymphatic obstruction

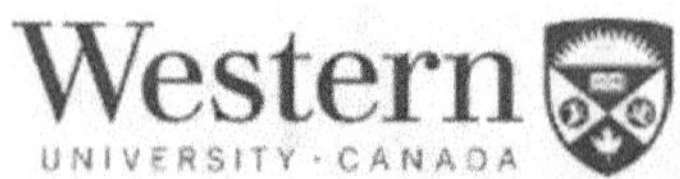

- Treatment with steroids and immunomodulators generally improves PLG

Primary Intestinal Lymphangiectasias

- Generally present by 30 years of age with edema, hypoproteinemia, diarrhea, and lymphocytopenia
- Diagnosis: abnormal dilation of lymphatic channels on biopsy, lymphangiography
- Dietary restriction is the mainstay of treatment
- High Protein, Low fat diet with medium chain triglycerides (do not require lymphatic transport)
- Intestinal resection is sometimes required for refractory disease

➢ Clinical Features

- Edema
  - Predominantly dependent edema
  - Anasarca is rare
  - Unilateral, Upper extremity, Facial & macular edema can be seen in lymphangiectasia
- Most of the rest of the manifestations are due to the underlying disease state and not the protein loss itself
  - Diarrhea
  - Fat & Fat soluble vitamin malabsorption
  - Carbohydrate malabsorption
  - Lymphocytopenia (in lymphangiectasia)
- Note:
  - Despite decreased Ig levels, increased susceptibility to infection is uncommon
  - Coagulation status is typically unaffected

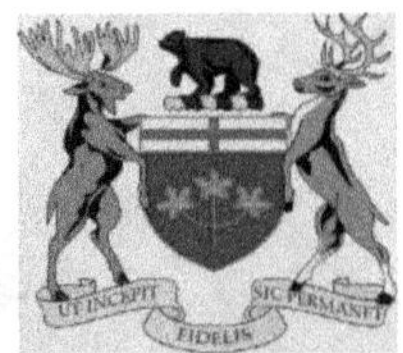

- Diagnostic tests

- Give the laboratory abnormalities in PLG, and give one method to quantify GI protein loss.

- Laboratory Abnormalities
  - Hypoproteinemia
  - Hypoalbuminemia
  - Decreased Serum gamma globulins (IgG, IgA, IgM)
  - Decreased Serum proteins:
    - Ceruloplasmin
    - A1AT
    - Transferrin
    - Fibrinogen
  - +/- Lymphocytopenia

- GI Protein Loss
  - A1AT plasma clearance
  - Similar sized protein to albumin that is neither actively absorbed or secreted and is resistant to luminal proteolysis
  - Measurement of A1AT clearance from the plasma by performing a 72 hour stool collection can quantify enteric protein loss

$$\text{A1AT plasma clearance} = \frac{(\text{stool volume})\,(\text{stool A1AT})}{(\text{serum A1AT})}$$

- A1AT Plasma Clearance
  - Normal < 24 ml / day
  - Caveats:
    - Diarrhea will significantly increase A1AT clearance, so in patients with diarrhea > 56 ml/day is abnormal

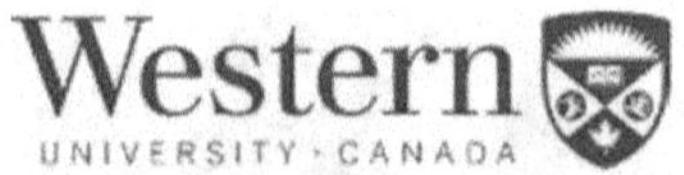

- There is inverse correlation between albumin and A1AT, thus with albumin below 30 g/L, A1AT clearance can exceed 180 ml/day
- A1AT is degraded by pepsin at a gastric pH < 3. A PPI is often used to overcome this limitation
- GI bleeding will increase A1AT and so stool for FOBT should be checked
- Limited availability of the test

- Other Methods to Quantify GI Protein Loss
  - Nuclear Medicine Scans:
    - Technetium labeled albumin
    - Technetium labeled human immunoglobulin
    - Indium labeled transferrin
  - Caveats
    - May help quantify and localize site of GI protein loss
    - Not widely available

- Give 8 diagnostic tests used for establishing the cause of PLG, and for each test give the condition for which the information is useful.

Investigation (clinically indicated)	Looking for:
EGD	H. Pylori, Menetrier, Celiac, Whipple
Colon	IBD, Microscopic Colitis
Stool Cultures	C. difficile, Parasitosis
ESR/CRP	IBD, systemic lupus erythematosis (SLE), or connective tissue diseases (CTD)

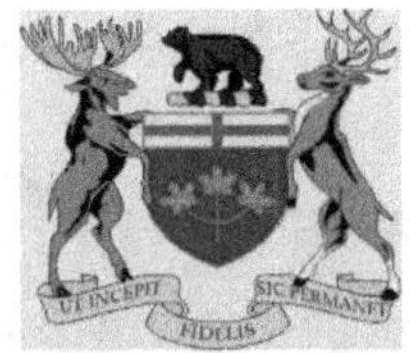

PROTEIN LOSING GASTROENTEROPATHY

Investigation (clinically indicated)	Looking for:
o ANA, RF	- SLE, CTD
o ECG, Echo	- CHF, Constrictive Pericariditis
o SPEP/UPEP	- Amyloidosis, Waldenstrom macroglobulinemia
o Ca, CXR	- Sarcoidosis
o HIV testing	- HIV
o Lymphangiogram	- Lymphangiectasia
o CT abdo/Pelvis	- Malignancy

➤ Treatment

- Give the treatment of protein losing gastroenteropathy.
  - Directed at identifying the cause of protein loss and correction of the underlying disease
  - Most etiologies of protein losing disorders are easily detectable and treatable and many can be cured
  - Rule out non-GI luminal causes of hypoproteinemia:
    - Proteinuria / Nephrotic Syndrome
    - Liver Disease / Cirrhosis
    - Malnutrition
    - Eating Disorders / Diuretic / Laxative Abuse
    - Malignancy
  - General supportive measures include:
    - High Protein, Low Fat diet
    - Octreotide may be useful in some to decrease fluid and protein exudation from the bowel
    - +/- diuretics
    - Compression stockings
    - Meticulous skin care
    - Encourage exercise and ambulation
    - Antibiotics for H. Pylori, bacterial overgrowth, Whipple disease, infectious colitis

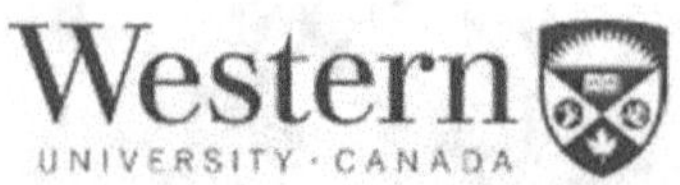

REFERENCES AND SUGGESTED READING

Barrett esophagus and GERD

Ajumobi A, et al. Surveillance in Barrett esophagus: an audit of practice. *Dig Dis Sci.* 2010;55(6):1615-1621.

American Gastroenterological Association et al. American Gastroenterological Association medical position statement on the management of Barrett esophagus. *Gastroenterology.* 2011;140:1084-1091.

Badreddine RJ, et al. Barrett esophagus: an update. *Nat Rev Gastroenterol Hepatol* 2010;7(7):369-378.

Badreddine RJ, et al. Prevalence and predictors of recurrent neoplasia after ablation of Barrett esophagus. *Gastrointest Endos* 2010;71(4):697-703.

Balasubramanian G, et al. Prevalence and predictors of columnar lined esophagus in gastroesophageal reflux disease (GERD) patients undergoing upper endoscopy. *Am J Gastroenterol.* 2012;107(11):1655-1661.

Barbiere JM, et al. Cost effectiveness of endoscopic screening followed by surveillance for Barrett esophagus: A review. *Gastroenterology* 2009;137:1869-1876.

Bulsiewicz WJ and Shaheen NJ. The role of radiofrequency ablation in the management of Barrett esophagus. *Gastrointest Endos Clin North Am* 2011;21(1):95-109.

Canto MI. Endomicroscopy of Barrett Esophagus. *Gastroenterol Clin North Am.* 2010;39(4):759-69.

Chen AM, and Pasricha PJ, Cryotherapy for Barrett Esophagus: Who, How, and Why? *Gastrointest Endos Clin* 2011;21:111-118.

Cobb MJ, et al. Imaging of subsquamous Barrett epithelium with ultrahigh-resolution optical coherence tomography: a histologic correlation study. *Gastrointest Endos* 2010;71(2):223-30.

Coleman HG, et al. Tobacco smoking increases the risk of high-grade dysplasia and cancer among patients with Barrett esophagus. *Gastroenterology.* 2012;142(2):233-240.

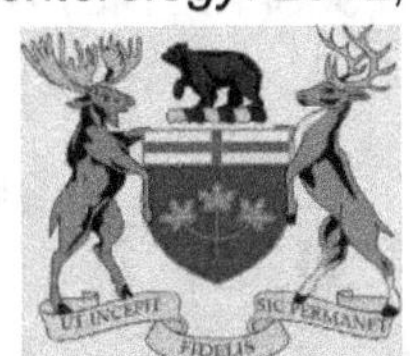

REFERENCES AND SUGGESTED READING

Crockett SD, et al. Overutilization of endoscopic surveillance in nondysplastic Barrett esophagus: a multicenter study. *Gastrointest Endosc.* 2012;75(1):23-31.

Curvers WL, et al. Endoscopic tri-modal imaging is more effective than standard endoscopy in identifying early-stage neoplasia in Barrett esophagus. *Gastroenterology.* 2010;139(4):1106-1114.

Curvers WL, et al. Low-grade dysplasia in Barrett esophagus: overdiagnosed and underestimated. *Am J Gastroenterol.* 2010;105(7):1523-1530.

de Jonge PJ, et al. Risk of malignant progression in patients with Barrett oesophagus: a Dutch nationwide cohort study. *Gut.* 2010;59(8):1030-1036.

Deprez P.H., et al. Current practice with endoscopic submucosal dissection in Europe: position statement from a panel of experts. *Endoscopy* 2010;42:853-858.

Dunbar KB, et al. The risk of lymph-node metastases in patients with high-grade dysplasia or intramucosal carcinoma in Barrett esophagus: a systematic review. *Am J Gastroenterol.* 2012;107(6):850-862.

Fleischer DE, et al. Endoscopic radiofrequency ablation for Barrett esophagus: 5-year outcomes from a prospective multicenter trial. *Endoscopy.* 2010;42(10):781-789.

Herrero LA, et al. Autofluorescence and narrow band imaging in Barrett esophagus. *Gastroenterol Clin North Am* 2010;39:747-758.

Hvid-Jensen F, et al. Incidence of adenocarcinoma among patients with Barrett esophagus. *N Engl J Med.* 2011;365(15):1375-1383.

Jung KW, et al. Epidemiology and natural history of intestinal metaplasia of the gastroesophageal junction and Barrett esophagus: a population-based study. *Am J Gastroenterol* 2011;106(8):1447-1455.

Kahrilas PJ. The problems with surveillance of Barrett esophagus. *N Engl J Med* 2011;13;365(15):1437-1438.

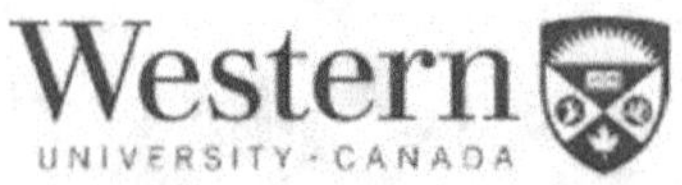

Konda VJ, et al. Endotherapy for Barrett esophagus. *Am J Gastroenterol.* 2012;107(6):827-833.

Kusunoki M, et al. The incidence of deep vein thrombosis in Japanese patients undergoing endoscopic submucosal dissection. *Gastrointest Endos* 2011;74(4):798-804.

Mannath JJ, et al. Narrow band imaging for characterization of high grade dysplasia and specialized intestinal metaplasia in Barrett esophagus: a meta-analysis. *Endoscopy.* 2010;42(5):351-359

Nguyen DM, et al Medication usage and the risk of neoplasia in patients with Barrett esophagus. *Clin Gastroenterol Hepatol* 2009;7:1299-1304.

Nicholson AM, et al. Barrett metaplasia glands are clonal, contain multiple stem cells and share a common squamous progenitor. *Gut* 2012;61(10): 1380-1389

Omer ZB, et al. Aspirin protects against Barrett esophagus in a multivariate logistic regression analysis. *Clin Gastroenterol Hepatol.* 2012;10(7):722-727.

Paterson WG. Canadian Association of Gastroenterology practice guidelines: management of noncardiac chest pain. *Can J Gastroenterol* 1998; 12:401-407.

Pauw RE, et al. Efficacy of radiofrequency ablation combined with endoscopic resection for Barrett esophagus with early neoplasia. *Clin Gastroenterol Hepatol.* 2010;8:233-239.

Pech O, et al. Comparison between endoscopic and surgical resection of mucosal esophageal adenocarcinoma in Barrett esophagus at two high-volume centers. *Ann Surg.* 2011;254(1):67-72.

Playford RJ. Barrett oesophagus guidelines for the diagnosis and management of New British Society of Gastroenterology (BSG). *Gut* 2006; 55:442-449.

Pouw RE, et al. Efficacy of radiofrequency ablation combined with endoscopic resection for Barrett esophagus with early neoplasia. *Clin Gastroenterol Hepatol.* 2010;8(1):23-29.

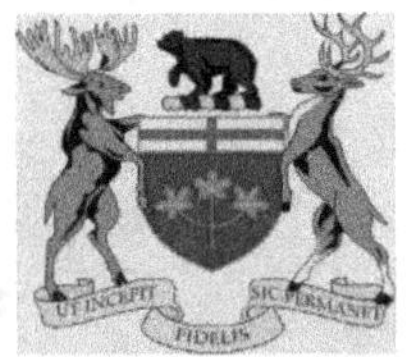

Pouw RE, et al. Stepwise radical endoscopic resection for eradication of Barrett oesophagus with early neoplasia in a cohort of 169 patients. *Gut.* 2010;59(9):1169-1177.

Prasad GA, et al. Endoscopic and surgical treatment of mucosal (T1a) esophageal adenocarcinoma in Barrett esophagus. *Gastroenterology.* 2009;137(3):815-823.

Reid BJ, et al. Otimizing endoscopic biopsy detection of early cancers in Barrett high-grade dysplasia in 380 lesions. *Am J Gastroenterol* 2000; 95:3089-3096.

Repaka A, et al. Endoscopic management of Barrett esophagus. *Nat Rev Gastroenterol Hepatol* 2011;8:582-591.

Sachin W, et al. Risk Factors for Progression of Low-Grade Dysplasia in Patients With Barrett Esophagus. *Gastroenterology* 2011;141:1179-1186.

Schlemper M, et al. The Vienna Classification of gastrointestinal epithelial neoplasia. *Gut* 2000; 47:251-255.

Shaheen NJ, et al. Durability of radiofrequency ablation in Barrett esophagus with dysplasia. *Gastroenterology* 2011;141(2):460-468.

Shaheen NJ, et al. Radiofrequency ablation in Barrett esophagus with dysplasia. *N Engl J Med* 2009;360(22):2277-88.

Sharma P, et al. The development and validation of an endoscopic grading system for Barrett esophagus: the Prague C & M criteria. *Gastroenterology* 2006; 131: 1392-1399.

Sharma P. A Critical Review of the Diagnosis and Management of Barrett Esophagus: The AGA Chicago Workshop. *Gastroenterology* 2004;127:310-330.

Sikkema M, et al. Predictors for neoplastic progression in patients with Barrett Esophagus: a prospective cohort study. *Am J Gastroenterol.* 2011;106(7):1231-8.

Spechler SJ, Barrett esophagus without dysplasia: wait or ablate? *Dig Dis Sci.*2011;56:1962-1928.

Spechler SJ. Epidemiology, clinical manifestations and diagnosis of Barrett Esophagus. *UpToDate*. www.uptodate.com

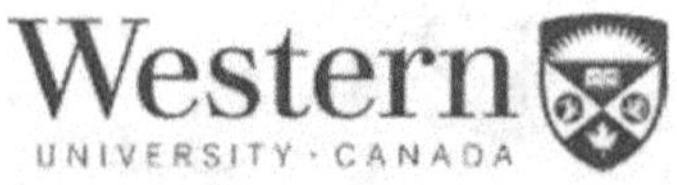

Spechler SJ. Pathogenesis of Barrett esophagus and its malignant transformation. *UpToDate*. www.uptodate.com

Sudarshan RK, et al. Acceptability and accuracy of a non-endoscopic screening test for Barrett oesophagus in primary care: cohort study. *BMJ*. 2010; 341: c4372.

Thomas T, et al. High-resolution endoscopy and endoscopic ultrasound for evaluation of early neoplasia in Barrett esophagus. *Surg Endos* 2010;24(5):1110-1116.

van Vilsteren FG, et al. Stepwise radical endoscopic resection versus radiofrequency ablation for Barrett oesophagus with high-grade dysplasia or early cancer: a multicentre randomised trial. *Gut*. 2011 ;60(6):765-773.

Varghese S, et al. Identification and clinical implementation of biomarkers for Barrett esophagus. *Gastroenterology* 2012;142(3):435-441.

Vassiliou MC, et al. Treatment of ultralong-segment Barrett using focal and balloon-based radiofrequency ablation. *Surg Endos* 2010;24:786-791.

Wallace MB, et al. Preliminary accuracy and interobserver agreement for the detection of intraepithelial neoplasia in Barrett esophagus with probe-based confocal laser endomicroscopy. *Gastrointest Endos* 2010;72(1):19-24.

Wani S, et al. Endoscopic eradication of Barrett esophagus. *Gastrointest Endos* 2010;71(1):147-166.

Wani S, et al. Esophageal adenocarcinoma in Barrett esophagus after endoscopic ablative therapy: a meta-analysis and systematic review. *Am J Gastroenterol*. 2009;104:502-513.

Wani S, et al. Greater interobserver agreement by endoscopic mucosal resection than biopsy samples in Barrett dysplasia. *Clin Gastroenterol Hepatol*. 2010;8(9):783-738.

Wani S, et al. Patients with non-dysplastic Barrett esophagus have low risks for developing dysplasia or esophageal adenocarcinoma. *Clin Gastroenterol Hepatol* 2011;9(3):220-227.

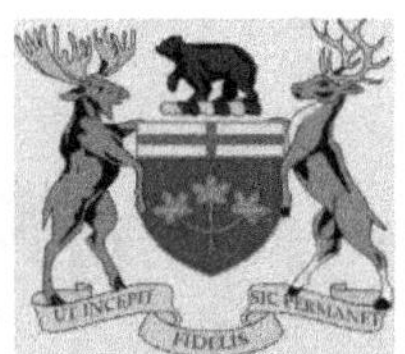

Wani S, et al. Risk factors for progression of low-grade dysplasia in patients with Barrett esophagus. *Gastroenterology* 2011;141(4):1179-1186.

Xian W, et al. Cellular origin of Barrett esophagus: controversy and therapeutic implications. *Gastroenterology*. 2012;142(7):1424-1430.

Yachimski P, et al. Subsquamous intestinal metaplasia: implications for endoscopic management of Barrett esophagus. *Clin Gastroenterol Hepatol* 2012;10(3):220-224.

Eosinophilic Esophagitis

Alexander JA, et al. Swallowed fluticasone improves histologic but not symptomatic response of adults with eosinophilic esophagitis. *Clin Gastroenterol Hepatol*. 2012;10(7):742-749.

Atkins D, et al. Eosinophilic esophagitis: the newest esophageal inflammatory disease. *Nat Rev Gastroentol Hepatol* 2009;6(5):267-278.

Dellon ES, et al. Diagnostic utility of major basic protein, eotaxin-3, and leukotriene enzyme staining in eosinophilic esophagitis. *Am J Gastroenterol*. 2012;107(10):1503-1511.

Dellon ES, et al. Inter- and intraobserver reliability and validation of a new method for determination of eosinophil counts in patients with esophageal eosinophilia. *Dig Dis Sci* 2010;55(7):1940-1949.

Dellon ES, et al. Inverse association of esophageal eosinophilia with Helicobacter pylori based on analysis of a US pathology database. *Gastroenterology* 2011;141(5):1586-1592.

Dellon ES, et al. Viscous topical is more effective than nebulized steroid therapy for patients with eosinophilic esophagitis. *Gastroenterology*. 2012;143(2):321-324.

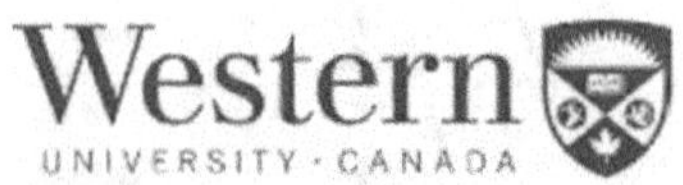

Dellon ES. Diagnosis and management of eosinophilic esophagitis. *Clin Gastroenterol Hepatol.* 2012;10(10):1066-1078.

Dohil R, et al. Oral viscous budesonide is effective in children with eosinophilic esophagitis in a randomized, placebo-controlled trial. *Gastroenterology* 2010;139(2):418-429.

Furuta GT, et al. First International Gastrointestinal Eosinophil Research Symposium (FIGERS) Subcommittees. Eosinophilic esophagitis in children and adults: A systemic review and consensus recommendation for diagnosis and treatment.*Gastroenterology* 2007;133:1342.

Gonsalves N, et al. Elimination diet effectively treats eosinophilic esophagitis in adults; food reintroduction identifies causative factors. *Gastroenterology*. 2012;142(7):1451-1459.

Helou EF, et al. Three year follow-up of topical corticosteroid treatment for eosinophilic esophagitis in adults. *Am J Gastroenterol* 2008;103:2194-2199.

Henderson CJ, et al. Comparative dietary therapy effectiveness in remission of pediatric eosinophilic esophagitis. *J Allergy Clin Immunol.* 2012;129(6):1570-1578.

Hurrell JM, et al. Prevalence of esophageal eosinophilia varies by climate zone in the United States. *Am J Gastroenterol*. 2012;107(5):698-706.

Lee J, et al. Esophageal diameter is decreased in some patients with eosinophilic esophagitis and might increase with topical corticosteroid therapy. *Clin Gastroenterol Hepatol.* 2012;10(5):481-486.

Liacouras CA, et al. Eosinophilic esophagitis: updated consensus recommendations for children and adults. *J Allergy Clin Immunol.* 2011;128(1):3-20.

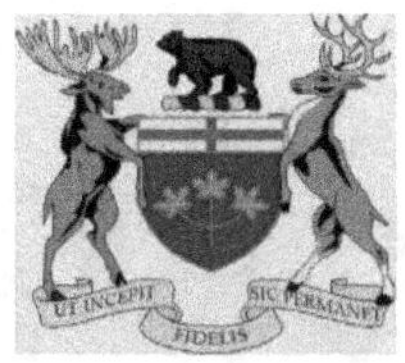

Sharma HP, et al. disparities in the presentation of pediatric eosinophilic esophagitis. Journal Allergy Clin Immunol 2011; 127(2): AB110.

Sperry SL, et al. Toward uniformity in the diagnosis of eosinophilic esophagitis (EoE): the effect of guidelines on variability of diagnostic criteria for EoE. *Am J Gastroenterol* 2011;106(5):824-832.

Straumann A, et al. Therapeutic concepts in adult and paediatric eosinophilic oesophagitis. *Nat Rev Gastroenterol Hepatol*. 2012;9(12):697-704.

Dyspepsia

Bektas M, et al. The effect of Helicobacter pylori eradication on dyspeptic symptoms, acid reflux and quality of life in patients with functional dyspepsia. *Eur J Intern Med* 2009;20(4):419-423.

Canadian Agency for Drugs and Technologies in Health. Evidence for PPI use in gastroesophageal reflux disease, dyspepsia and peptic ulcer disease: scientific report. *Compus.* 2007;1(2):1-178.

Ford AC, et al. Effect of dyspepsia on survival: a longitudinal 10-year follow-up study. *Am J Gastroenterol*. 2012;107(6):912-921.

Ford AC, et al. Managing dyspepsia. *Curr Gastroenterol Rep*. 2009;11(4):288-294.

Ford AC, et al. Systematic review and meta-analysis of the prevalence of irritable bowel syndrome in individuals with dyspepsia. *Clin Gastroenterol Hepatol* 2010; 8:401-409.

Ford AC, et al. What is the prevalence of clinically significant endoscopic findings in subjects with dyspepsia? Systematic review and meta-analysis. *Clin Gastroenterol Hepatol* 2010; 8:830-837.

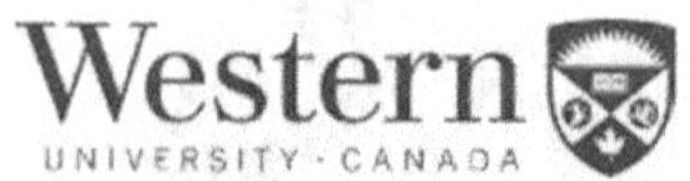

Graham DY, et al. Clinical practice: diagnosis and evaluation of dyspepsia. *J Clin Gastroenterol.* 2010;44(3):167-172.

Hiyama T et al. Meta-analysis of the effects of prokinetic agents in patients with functional dyspepsia. *J Gastroenterol Hepatol.* 2007;22(3):304-310.

Mazzoleni LE, et al. Helicobacter pylori eradication in functional dyspepsia: HEROES trial. *Arch Intern Med.* 2011;171(21):1929-1936.

McColl KE. Clinical practice. Helicobacter pylori infection. *N Engl J Med.* 2010;362(17):1597-1604.

Saad RJ. Review article: current and emerging therapies for functional dyspepsia. *Aliment Pharmacol Ther* 2006;24(3):475-492.

Tack J, et al. Efficacy of buspirone, a fundus-relaxing drug, in patients with functional dyspepsia. *Clin Gastroenterol Hepatol.* 2012;10(11):1239-1245.

Talley NJ, American Gastroenterological Association. American Gastroenterological Association medical position statement: evaluation of dyspepsia. *Gastroenterology* 2005; 129:1753-1755.

Talley NJ, et al. American gastroenterological association technical review on the evaluation of dyspepsia. *Gastroenterology* 2005; 129:1756-1780.

Talley NJ, et al. Guidelines for the management of dyspepsia. *Am J Gastroenterol* 2005; 100:2324-2337.

Defecation Disorder and Constipation

Belsey J, et al. Systematic review: impact of constipation on quality of life in adults and children. *Aliment Pharmacol Ther* 2010;31(9):938-949.

Bharucha AE, et al. Obstetric trauma, pelvic floor injury and fecal incontinence: a population-based case-

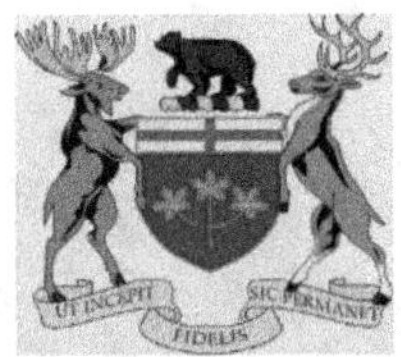

control study. *Am J Gastroenterol* 2012;107(6):902-911.

Camilleri M, et al. Clinical trial: the efficacy of open-label prucalopride treatment in patients with chronic constipation - follow-up of patients from the pivotal studies. *Aliment Pharmacol Ther* 2010;32(9):1113-1123.

Camilleri M, et al. Prucalopride for constipation. *Expert Opin Pharmacother* 2010;11(3):451-461.

Coyne KS, et al. The prevalence of chronic constipation and faecal incontinence among men and women with symptoms of overactive bladder. *BJU Int* 2011;107(2):254-261.

Deibert P, et al. Methylnaltrexone: the evidence for its use in the management of opioid-induced constipation. *Core Evid* 2010;4:247-258.

Ford AC and Suares NC. Effect of laxatives and pharmacological therapies in chronic idiopathic constipation: systematic review and meta-analysis. *Gut* 2011;60(2):209-218.

Gallegos-Orozco JF, et al. Chronic constipation in the elderly. *Am J Gastroenterol* 2012;107(1):18-25.

Goldberg M, et al. Clinical trial: the efficacy and tolerability of velusetrag, a selective 5-HT4 agonist with high intrinsic activity, in chronic idiopathic constipation - a 4-week, randomized, double-blind, placebo-controlled, dose-response study. *Aliment Pharmacol Ther* 2010;32(9):1102-1112.

Lembo AJ, et al. Efficacy of linaclotide for patients with chronic constipation. *Gastroenterology* 2010;138(3):886-895.

Lembo AJ, et al. Two randomized trials of linaclotide for chronic constipation. *N Engl J Med* 2011;365(6):527-536.

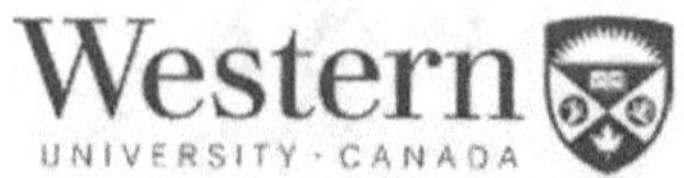

Leroi AM, et al. Transcutaneous electrical tibial nerve stimulation in the treatment of fecal incontinence: a randomized trial (CONSORT 1a). *Am J Gastroenterol* 2012;107(12):1888-1896.

Noelting J, et al. Normal values for high-resolution anorectal manometry in healthy women: effects of age and significance of rectoanal gradient. *Am J Gastroenterol* 2012;107(10):1530-1536.

Schey R, et al. Medical and surgical management of pelvic floor disorders affecting defecation. *Am J Gastroenterol* 2012;107(11):1624-1633.

Shah BJ, et al. *Fecal incontinence in the elderly: FAQ. Am J Gastroenterol* 2012;107(11):1635-1646.

Tack J and Müller-Lissner S. Treatment of chronic constipation: current pharmacologic approaches and future directions. *Clin Gastroenterol Hepatol* 2009;7(5):502-508.

Colorectal Cancer

Atkin WS, et al. (Department of Surgery and Cancer, Imperial College of London, St. Mary's Campus, UK). Once-only flexible sigmoidoscopy screening in prevention of colorectal cancer: a multi-centre randomised controlled trial. *Lancet* 2010;375:1624-1633.

Audisio RA and Papamichael D. Treatment of colorectal cancer in older patients. *Nat Rev Gastroenterol Hepatol* 2012;9(12):716-725.

Aune D, et al. Nonlinear reduction in risk for colorectal cancer by fruit and vegetable intake based on meta-analysis of prospective studies. *Gastroenterology* 2011;141:106-118.

Baca B, et al. Surveillance after colorectal cancer resection: a systematic review. *Dis Colon Rectum* 2011;54:1036-1048.

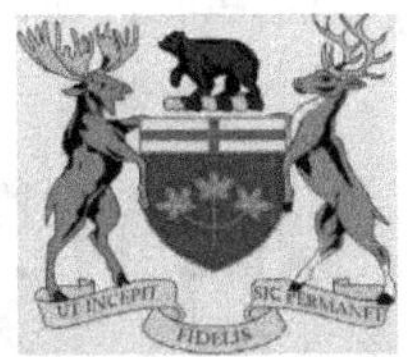

Bardelli A. and Siena S. Molecular mechanisms of resistance to cetuximab and panitumumab in colorectal cancer. *J Clin Oncol* 2010;28:1254-1261.

Baxter NN, et al. Association of colonoscopy and death from colorectal cancer. *Ann Intern Med* 2009;150:1-8.

Ben Q, et al. Body mass index increases risk for colorectal adenomas based on meta-analysis. *Gastroenterology* 2012;142(4):762-772.

Berg M and Søreide K. Genetic and epigenetic traits as biomarkers in colorectal cancer. *Int J Mol Sci* 2011;12(12):9426-9439.

Boparai KS, et al. Increased colorectal cancer risk during follow-up in patients with hyperplastic polyposis syndrome: a multicentre cohort study. *Gut* 2010;59:1094-1100.

Botma A, et al. Body mass index increases risk of colorectal adenomas in men with Lynch syndrome: the GEOLynch cohort study. *J Clin Oncol* 2010;28:4346-4353.

Brenner H, et al. Long-term risk of colorectal cancer after negative colonoscopy. *J Clin Oncol* 2011;29(28):3761-3767.

Brenner H, et al. Protection from colorectal cancer after colonoscopy. *Ann Intern Med* 2011;154:22-30.

Brenner H, et al. Protection from right- and left-sided colorectal neoplasms after colonoscopy: population-based study. *J Natl Cancer Inst* 2010;102:89-98.

Bretthauer M. Evidence for colorectal cancer screening. *Best Pract Res Clin Gastroenterol* 2010;24:417-425.

Buchner AM, et al. High-definition colonoscopy detects colorectal polyps at a higher rate than standard white-light colonoscopy. *Clin Gastroenterol Hepatol* 2010;8:364-370.

Burn J, et al. Long-term effect of aspirin on cancer risk in carriers of hereditary colorectal cancer: an analysis from

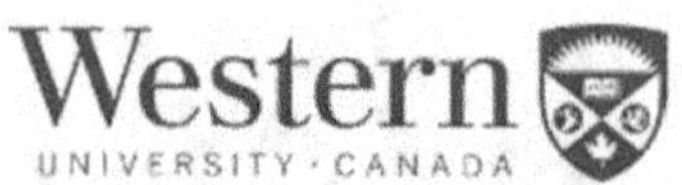

the CAPP2 randomised controlled trial. *Lancet* 2011;378(9809):2081-2087.

Cairns SR, et al. Guidelines for colorectal cancer screening and surveillance in moderate and high risk groups (update from 2002). *Gut* 2010; 59:666-889.

Chaput U, et al. Risk factors for advanced adenomas amongst small and diminutive colorectal polyps: A prospective monocenter study. *Dig Liver Dis.* 2011; 43(8): 609-612.

Choong MK and Tsafnat G. Genetic and epigenetic biomarkers of colorectal cancer. *Clin Gastroenterol Hepatol* 2012;10(1):9-15.

Chung SJ, et al. Efficacy of computed virtual chromoendoscopy on colorectal cancer screening: a prospective, randomized, back-to-back trial of Fuji Intelligent Color Enhancement versus conventional colonoscopy to compare adenoma miss rates. *Gastrointest Endos* 2010;72:136-142.

Cole BF, et al. Aspirin for the chemoprevention of colorectal adenomas: meta-analysis of the randomized trials. *J Natl Cancer Inst* 2009;101:256-266.

Crotta S, et al. High rate of advanced adenoma detection in 4 rounds of colorectal cancer screening with the fecal immunochemical test. *Clin Gastroenterol Hepatol* 2012;10(6):633-638.

Dahabreh IJ, et al. Systematic review: Anti epidermal growth factor receptor treatment effect modication by KRAS mutations in advanced colorectal cancer. *Ann Intern Med* 2011;154:37-49.

Dahm CC, et al. Dietary fiber and colorectal cancer risk: a nested case-control study using food diaries. *J Natl Cancer Inst* 2010;102:614-626.

Dahm CC, et al. Dietary fiber and colorectal cancer risk: a nested case-control study using food diaries. *Am J Clin Nutr* 2010;92:1429-1435.

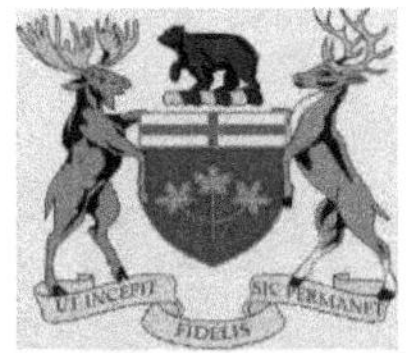

Dan YY, et al. Screening based on risk for colorectal cancer is the most cost-effective approach. *Clin Gastroenterol Hepatol* 2012;10(3):266-271.

Day LW, et al. Colorectal cancer screening and surveillance in the elderly patient. *Am J Gastroenterol* 2011;106:1197-1206.

Diaz LA Jr, et al. The molecular evolution of acquired resistance to targeted EGFR blockade in colorectal cancers. *Nature* 2012;486(7404):537-540.

Duffy MJ, et al. Use of faecal markers in screening for colorectal neoplasia: a European group on tumor markers position paper. *Int J Cancer* 2011;128(1):3-11.

Farraye FA, et al. AGA medical position statement on the diagnosis and management of colorectal neoplasia in inflammatory bowel disease. *Gastroenterology* 2010;138:738-745.

Farraye FA, et al. AGA technical review on the diagnosis and management of colorectal neoplasia in inflammatory bowel disease. *Gastroenterology* 2010;138:746-774.

Ferlitsch M, et al. Sex-specific prevalence of adenomas, advanced adenomas, and colorectal cancer in individuals undergoing screening colonoscopy. *JAMA* 2011;306(12):1352-1358.

Fornaro L, et al. Palliative treatment of unresectable metastatic colorectal cancer. *Expert Opinion on Pharmacotherapy* 2010;11:63-77.

Fung TT. The Mediterranean and Dietary Approaches to Stop Hypertension(DASH) diets and colorectal cancer. *Am J Clin Nutr* 2010;92:1429-1435.

Goel A and Boland CR. Epigenetics of colorectal cancer. *Gastroenterology* 2012;143(6):1442-1460.

Goetz M, et al. In vivo molecular imaging of colorectal cancer with confocal endomicroscopy by targeting

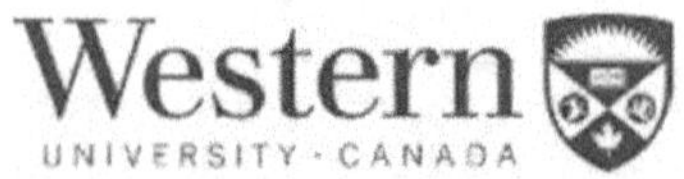

epidermal growth factor receptor. *Gastroenterology* 2010;138(2):435-446.

Grazzini G, et al. Influence of seasonal variations in ambient temperatures on performance of immunochemical faecal occult blood test for colorectal cancer screening: observational study from the Florence district. *Gut* 2010;59(11):1511-1515.

Grothey A. EGFR antibodies in colorectal cancer: where do they belong? *Journal of Clinical Oncology* 2010;28:4668-4670.

Gupta S, et al. Polyps with advanced neoplasia are smaller in the right than in the left colon: implications for colorectal cancer screening. *Clin Gastroenterol Hepatol* 2012;10(12):1395-1401.

Gustafsson UO, et al. Adherence to the enhanced recovery after surgery protocol and outcomes after colorectal cancer surgery. *Arch Surg* 2011;146:571-577.

Hassan C, et al. Meta-analysis: adherence to colorectal cancer screening and the detection rate for advanced neoplasia, according to the type of screening test. *Aliment Pharmacol Ther.* 2012;36(10):929-940.

Hetzel JT, et al. Variation in the detection of serrated polyps in an average risk colorectal cancer screening cohort. *Am J Gastroenterol* 2010;105(12):2656-64.

Hiraoka S, et al. The Presence of Large Serrated Polyps Increases Risk for Colorectal Cancer. *Gastroenterology* 2010;139:1503-1510.

Hlavaty T, et al. Colorectal cancer screening in patients with ulcerative and Crohn colitis with use of colonoscopy, chromoendoscopy and confocal endomicroscopy. *Eur J Gastroenterol Hepatol* 2011;23:680-689.

Hoff G, et al. Contrasting US and European approaches to colorectal cancer screening: which is best? *Gut* 2010;59(3):407-414.

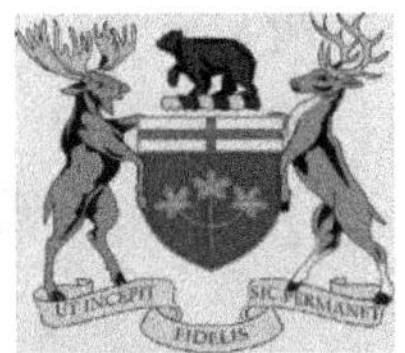

Hoffman A, et al. High definition colonoscopy combined with i-Scan is superior in the detection of colorectal neoplasias compared with standard video colonoscopy: a prospective randomized controlled trial. *Endoscopy* 2010;42:827-833.

Hoffman RM, et al. Colorectal cancer screening adherence is higher with fecal immunochemical tests than guaiac-based fecal occult blood tests: a randomized, controlled trial. *Prev Med* 2010;50(5-6):297-299.

Hoffmeister M, et al. Male sex and smoking have a larger impact on the prevalence of colorectal neoplasia than family history of colorectal cancer. *Clin Gastroenterol Hepatol* 2010;8:870-876.

Hol L, et al. Screening for colorectal cancer: randomised trial comparing guaiac-based and immunochemical faecal occult blood testing and flexible sigmoidoscopy. *Gut* 2010;59(1):62-68.

Hundt S, et al. Comparative evaluation of immunochemical fecal occult blood tests for colorectal adenoma detection. *Annals of Internal Medicine* 2009;150:162-169.

Jenab M, et al. Association between pre-diagnostic circulating vitamin D concentration and risk of colorectal cancer in European populations: A nested case-control study. *BMJ* 2010;340:b5500.

Jess T, et al. Decreasing risk of colorectal cancer in patients with inflammatory bowel disease over 30 years. *Gastroenterology* 2012;143(2):375-381.

Jess T, et al. Risk of colorectal cancer in patients with ulcerative colitis: a meta-analysis of population-based cohort studies. *Clin Gastroenterol Hepatol* 2012;10(6):639-645.

Jiang Y, et al. Assessment of K-ras mutation: A step toward personalized medicine for patients with colorectal cancer. *Cancer* 2009;115(16):3609-3617.

Johnson CC, et al. Non-Steroidal Anti-Inflammatory Drug Use and Colorectal Polyps in the Prostate, Lung,

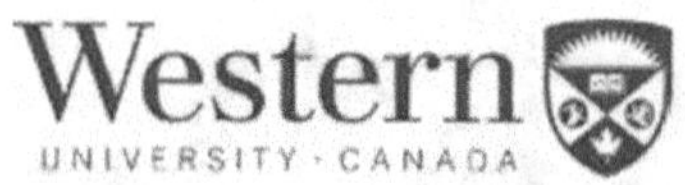

Colorectal, and Ovarian Cancer Screening Trial. *Am J Gastroenterol* 2010;10:2646-2655.

Jover R, et al. 5-Fluorouracil adjuvant chemotherapy does not increase survival in patients with CpG island methylator phenotype colorectal cancer. *Gastroenterology* 2011;140(4):1174-1181.

Kimura T, et al. A novel pit pattern identifies the precursor of colorectal cancer derived from sessile serrated adenoma. *Am J Gastroenterol* 2012;107(3):460-469.

Kirkegaard H, et al. Association of adherence to life style recommendations and risk of colorectal cancer: A prospective Danish cohort study. *BMJ* 2010;341:c5504

Laiyemo AO, et al. Race and colorectal cancer disparities: health-care utilization vs different cancer susceptibilities. *J Natl Cancer Inst* 2010;102:538-546.

Lane JM, et al. Interval fecal immunochemical testing in a colonoscopic surveillance program speeds detection of colorectal neoplasia. *Gastroenterology* 2010;139:1918-1926.

Lansdorp-Vogelaar I, et al. Stool DNA testing to screen for colorectal cancer in the Medicare population: a cost-effectiveness analysis. *Ann Inter Med* 2010;153:368-377.

Lao VV, et al. Epigenetics and colorectal cancer. *Nat Rev Gastroenterol Hepatol* 2011;8(12):686-700.

Levin B, et al. Screening and surveillance for the early detection of colorectal cancer and adenomatous polyps, 2008: a joint guideline from the American Cancer Society, the US Multi-Society Task Force in Colorectal Cancer, and the American College of Radiology. *Gastroenterology* 2008;134(5):1570-95.

Levin TR, et al. Organized colorectal cancer screening in integrated health care systems. *Epidemiol Rev* 2011;33(1):101-10.

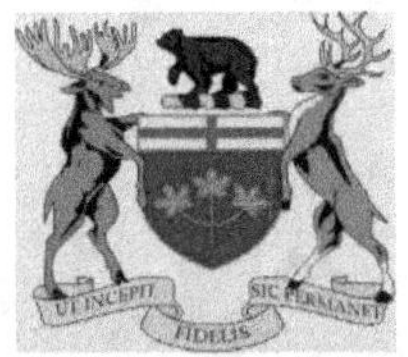

Li D, et al. Association of large serrated polyps with synchronous advanced colorectal neoplasia. *Am J Gastroenterol* 2009;104:695-702.

Limsui D, et al. Postmenopausal hormone therapy and colorectal cancer risk by molecularly defined subtypes among older women. *Gut* 2012; 61(9):1299-1305.

Liu Z, et al. Randomised clinical trial: the effects of perioperative probiotic treatment on barrier function and post-operative infectious complications in colorectal cancer surgery – a double-blind study. *Aliment Pharmacol Ther* 2011;33:50-63.

McCutchen AS, et al. Lower albumin levels in African Americans at colon cancer diagnosis; a potential explanation for outcome disparities between groups? *Int J Colorect Dis* 2011;26:469-472.

Misale S, et al. Emergence of KRAS mutations and acquired resistance to anti-EGFR therapy in colorectal cancer. *Nature* 2012;486(7404):532-536.

Murff HJ, et al. Dietary intake of PUFAs and colorectal polyp risk. *Am J Clin Nutr* 2012;95(3):703-712.

Naishadham D, et al. State disparities in colorectal cancer mortality patterns in the United States. *Cancer Epidemiol Biomarkers Prev* 2011;20(7):1296-1302.

Niimi K, et al. Long-term outcomes of endoscopic submucosal dissection for colorectal epithelial neoplasms. *Endoscopy* 2010;42:723-729.

Ollberding NJ, et al. Racial/ethnic differences in colorectal cancer risk: the multiethnic cohort study. *International Journal of Cancer* 2011 March 25.

Pan MH, et al. Molecular mechanisms for chemoprevention of colorectal cancer by natural dietary compounds. *Molecular Nutrition Food and Research* 2011;55:32-45.

Pander J, et al. Correlation of FCGR3A and EGFR germline polymorphisms with the efficacy of cetuximab

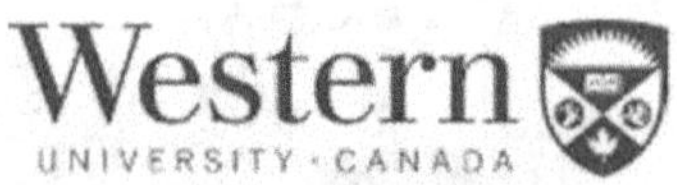

in KRAS wild-type metastatic colorectal cancer. *European Journal of Cancer*. 2010;46:1829-1834.

Park DI, et al. Comparison of guaiac-based and quantitative immunochemical fecal occult blood testing in a population at average risk undergoing colorectal cancer screening. *Am J Gastroenterol* 2010;105(9):2017-2025.

Parsche B, et al. Constitutively decreased TGFBR1 allelic expression is a common finding in colorectal cancer and is associated with three TGFBR1 SNPs. *J Exp Clin Cancer Res* 2010;29:57.

Pohl H, et al. Colorectal cancers detected after colonoscopy frequently result from missed lesions. *Clin Gastroenterol Hepatol* 2010;8:858-864.

Qaseem A, et al. Screening for colorectal cancer: a guidance statement from the American College of Physicians. *Ann Intern Med* 2012;156(5):378-386.

Rabeneck L, et al. Association between colonoscopy rates and colorectal cancer mortality. *Am J Gastroenterol* 2010;105:1627.

Rennert G. et al. Colorectal cancer screening: will global warming affect the accuracy of FIT testing? *Gut* 2010;59(11):1451-1452.

Rex DK, et al. American College of Gastroenterology guidelines for colorectal cancer screening 2008. *Am J Gastroenterol* 2009;104:739-750.

Rex DK, et al. Guidelines for colonoscopy surveillance after cancer resection: A consensus update by the American Cancer Society and the U.S Multi Society Task Force on Colorectal Cancer. *Gastroenterology* 2006;130:1865-1871.

Rothwell PM, et al. Long-term effect of aspirin on colorectal cancer incidence and mortality: 20-year follow-up of five randomized trials. *Lancet* 2010;376:1741-1750.

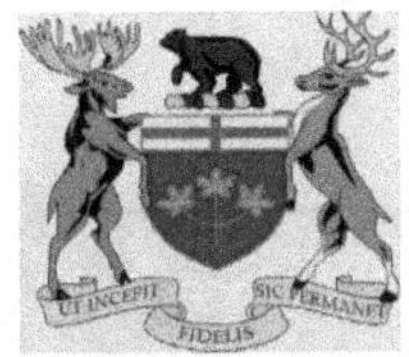

Rotondano G., et al. Endocytoscopic classification of preneoplastic lesions in the colorectum. *Int J Colorect Dis* 2010;25:1111-1116.

Saito Y., et al. A prospective, multicenter study of 1111 colorectal endoscopic submucosal dissections (with video). *Gastrointestinal Endoscopy* 2010;72:1217-1225.

Sandler RS. Colonoscopy and colorectal cancer mortality: Strong beliefs or strong facts? *Am J Gastroenterol* 2010;105:1633.

Sanduleanu S., et al. In vivo diagnosis and classification of colorectal neoplasia by chromoendoscopy-guided confocal laser endomicroscopy. *Clin Gastroenterol Hepatol* 2010;8:371-378.

Shahid MW, et al. Diagnostic accuracy of probe-based confocal laser endomicroscopy and narrow band imaging for small colorectal polyps: a feasibility study. *Am J Gastroenterol* 2012;107(2):231-239.

Shen Z, et al. Clinical study on the correlation between metabolic syndrome and colorectal carcinoma. *ANZ J Surg* 2010;80(5):331-336.

Sheth RA, et al. Optical molecular imaging and its emerging role in colorectal cancer. *American Journal of Physiology Gastrointestinal and Liver Physiology* 2010;299:G807-G820.

Singh H, et al. Rate and Predictors of Early/Missed Colorectal Cancers After Colonoscopy in Manitoba: A Population-Based Study. *Am J Gastroenterol* 2010;105:2588-2596.

Singh H, et al. The reduction in colorectal cancer mortality after colonoscopy varies by site of the cancer. *Gastroenterology* 2010;139:1128-1137.

Stallmach A., et al. An unmet medical need: advances in endoscopic imaging of colorectal neoplasia. *Journal of Biophotonics* 2011;4:482-489.

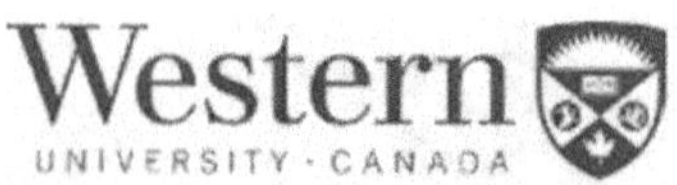

Steckelberg A., et al. Effect of evidence based risk information on “informed choice” in colorectal cancer screening: randomized controlled trial. *BMJ* 2011;342:d3193.

Stoffel EM, et al. Genetic Testing for Hereditary Colorectal Cancer: Challenges in Identifying, Counseling, and Managing High-Risk Patients. *Gastroenterology* 2010;139:1436-1443.

Stoop EM, et al. Participation and yield of colonoscopy versus non-cathartic CT colonography in population-based screening for colorectal cancer: a randomised controlled trial. *Lancet Oncol* 2012;13(1):55-64.

Söderlund S, et al. Decreasing time-trends of colorectal cancer in a large cohort of patients with inflammatory bowel disease. *Gastroenterology* 2009;136:1561-1567

Tribonias G., et al. Comparison of standard vs. high-definition, wide-angle colonoscopy for polyp detection: a randomized controlled trial. *Colorectal Disease* 2010;12:e260-e266.

U.S. Preventive Services Task Force. Screening for colorectal cancer: U.S. Preventive Services Task Force recommendation statement. *Ann Intern Med* 2008;149(9):627-637.

van Roon AH, et al. Are fecal immunochemical test characteristics influenced by sample return time? A population-based colorectal cancer screening trial. *Am J Gastroenterol* 2012;107(1):99-107.

Vasen HFA, et al. One to 2-year surveillance intervals reduce risk of colorectal cancer in families with Lynch syndrome. *Gastroenterology* 2010;138:2300.

Wallace MB, et al. Advances in endoscopic imaging of colorectal neoplasia. *Gastroenterology* 2010;138:2140-2150.

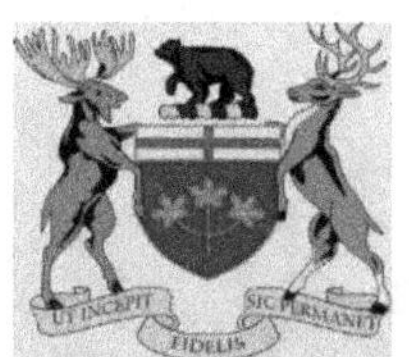

Wallace MB, et al. The safety of intravenous fluorescein for confocal laser endomicroscopy in the gastrointestinal tract. *Aliment Pharmacol Ther* 2010;31:548-552.

Walter LC, et al. Impact of age and comorbidity on colorectal cancer screening among older veterans. *Ann Intern Med* 2009;150(7):465-473.

Whynes DK, et al. Analysis of deaths occurring within the Nottingham trial of faecal occult blood screening for colorectal cancer. *Gut* 2010;59:1088-1093.

Winawer SJ, et al. Guidelines for colonoscopy surveillance after polypectomy: A consensus update by the US Multi-Society Task Force on colorectal cancer and the American Cancer Society. *Gastroenterology* 2006;130:1872-1885.

Zauber AG, et al. Colonoscopic polypectomy and long-term prevention of colorectal-cancer deaths. *N Engl J Med* 2012;366(8):687-696.

Irritable Bowel Syndrome

Bertram S et al. The patient's perspective of irritable bowel syndrome. J Fam Pract 2001; 50:521-5.

Dixon-Woods M et al. Medical and lay views of irritable bowel syndrome. Fam Pract 2000; 17:108-13.

Hu WHC, et al. Anxiety but not depression determines health care-seeking behaviour in Chinese patients with dyspepsia and irritable bowel syndrome: A population-based study. Aliment Pharmacol Ther 2002; 16:2081-8.

Koloski N, et al. Predictors of health care seeking for irritable bowel syndrome and nonulcer dyspepsia: A critical review of the literature on symptom and psychosocial factors. Am J Gastroenterol 2001; 96:1340-9.

Owens DM et al. The irritable bowel syndrome: Long-term prognosis and the physician-patient interaction. Ann Intern Med 1985; 122:107-112.

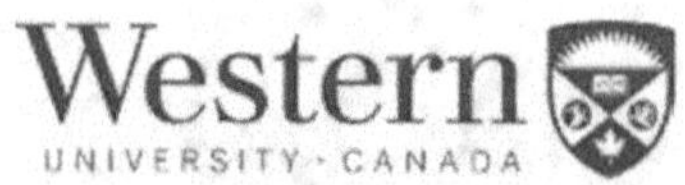

Smith RC, et al. Psychosocial factors are associated with health care seeking rather than diagnosis in irritable bowel syndrome. Gastroenterology 1990; 98:293-301.

Wells M, et al. Sleep disruption secondary to overnight call shifts is associated with irritable bowel syndrome in residents: A cross-sectional study. *Am J Gastro* 2012; 107(8):1151-6.

Vascular Diseases of the Liver

Bittencourt PL, et . Portal vein thrombosis and Budd-Chiari syndrome. *Clinical Liver Disease* 2009; 13(1):127-144.

DeLeve LD, et al. Vascular disorders of the liver. *Hepatology* 2009;49(5):1729-1764.

Delgado MG, et al. Efficacy and safety of anticoagulation on patients with cirrhosis and portal vein thrombosis. *Clin Gastroenterol Hepatol.* 2012; 10(7):776-783.

Helmy A. Review article: updates in the pathogenesis and therapy of hepatic sinusoidal obstruction syndrome. *Alimentary Pharmacology & Therapeutics* 2006;23(1):11-25

Herve P, et al. Pulmonary vascular abnormalities in cirrhosis. *Best Practice & Research Clinical Gastroenterology* 2007; 21(1):141-159.

Kamath, et al. Vascular diseases of the liver. *Mayo Clinic Gastroenterology and Hepatology Board Review, Third Edition* 2008; 337-343.

Primignani M. Portal vein thrombosis, revisited. *Digestive and Liver Disease* 2009;42(3):163-170.

Rebours V, et al. Extrahepatic portal venous system thrombosis in recurrent acute and chronic alcoholic pancreatitis is caused by local inflammation and not thrombophilia. *Am J Gastroenterol.* 2012; 107(10):1579-1585.

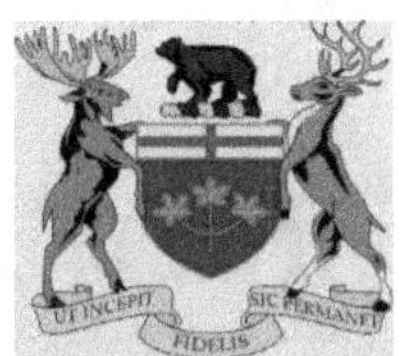

Sabbà C, et al. Review article: The hepatic manifestations of hereditary haemorrhagic telangiectasia. *Alimentary Pharmacology and Therapeutics* 2008; 28(5):523-533.

Spaander VM, et al. Review article: the management of non-cirrhotic non-malignant portal vein thrombosis and concurrent portal hypertension in adults. *Alimentary Pharmacology and Therapeutics* 2007;26 Suppl 2:203-209.

Tsochatzis EA, et al. Systematic review: portal vein thrombosis in cirrhosis. *Alimentary Pharmacology & Therapeutics* 2010;31(3):366-374.

Villa E, et al. Enoxaparin prevents portal vein thrombosis and liver decompensation in patients with advanced cirrhosis. *Gastroenterology*. 2012;143(5):1253-1260.

NAFLD and Alcoholic Liver Disease

Alisi A, et al. Pediatric nonalcoholic fatty liver disease: a multidisciplinary approach. *Nat Rev Gastroenterol Hepatol*. 2012;9(3):152-161.

Bhala N, et al. The natural history of nonalcoholic fatty liver disease with advanced fibrosis or cirrhosis: an international collaborative study. *Hepatology* 2011;54(4):1208-1216.

Birerdinc A, et al. Caffeine is protective in patients with non-alcoholic fatty liver disease. *Aliment Pharmacol Ther* 2012;35(1):76-82.

Carter-Kent C, et al. Cytokines in the pathogenesis of Fatty Liver and Disease progression to steatohepatitis: Implications for treatment. *The American Journal of Gastroenterology* 2008;103:1036-1042.

Cassiman D, et al. NASH may be trash. *Gut* 2008;57(2):141-144.

Chalasani N, et al. The diagnosis and management of non-alcoholic fatty liver disease: Practice guideline by the American Association for the Study of Liver Diseases,

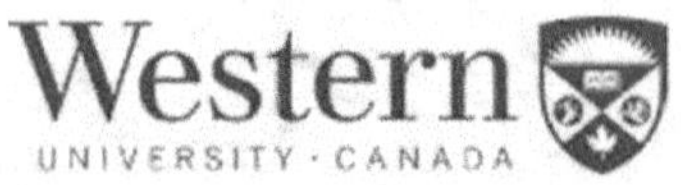

American College of Gastroenterology, and the American Gastroenterological Association. *Am J Gastroenterol.* 2012;107(6):811-826.

Cheung O, et al. Abnormalities of lipid metabolism in nonalcoholic fatty liver disease. *Seminars in Liver Disease* 2008;28:351-359.

Cheung O, et al. Recent advances in nonalcoholic fatty liver disease. *Current Opinion in Gastroenterology* 2009;25:230-237.

Choi K, et al. Molecular mechanism of insulin resistance in obesity and type 2 diabetes. *Korean Journal of Internal Medicine* 2010;25:119-129.

Corey KE, et al. Non-high-density lipoprotein cholesterol as a biomarker for nonalcoholic steatohepatitis. *Clin Gastroenterol Hepatol.* 2012;10(6):651-656.

Cusi K. Role of obesity and lipotoxicity in the development of nonalcoholic steatohepatitis: pathophysiology and clinical implications. *Gastroenterology.* 2012;142(4):711-725.

Dunn W, et al. The interaction of rs738409, obesity, and alcohol: a population-based autopsy study. *Am J Gastroenterol.* 2012;107(11):1668-7164.

Foster T, et al. Atorvastatin and antioxidants for the treatment of non-alcoholic fatty liver disease: The St Francis Heart Study randomised clinical trial. *The American Journal of Gastroenterology* 2011;106:71-77.

Francque SM, et al. Noninvasive assessment of nonalcoholic fatty liver disease in obese or overweight patients. *Clin Gastroenterol Hepatol.* 2012;10(10):1162-1168.

Greenfield V, et al. Recent advances in non-alcoholic fatty liver disease. *Current Opinion in Gastroenterology* 2008;24(3):320-7.

Henao-Mejia J, et al. Inflammasome-mediated dysbiosis regulates progression of NAFLD and obesity. *Nature* 2012;482(7384):179-185.

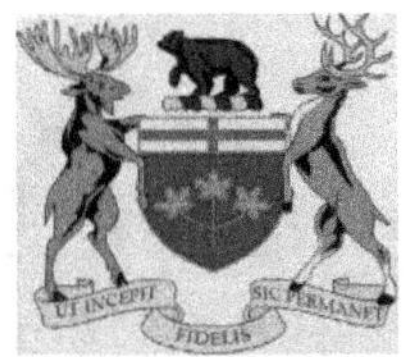

Jou J, et al. Mechanisms of disease progression in nonalcoholic fatty liver disease. *Seminars in Liver Disease* 2008;28: 370-379.

Kilpeläinen TO, et al. Physical activity attenuates the influence of FTO variants on obesity risk: a meta-analysis of 218,166 adults and 19,268 children. *PLoS Med* 2011;8(11):e1001116.

Kistler KD, et al. Physical activity recommendations, exercise intensity, and histological severity of nonalcoholic fatty liver disease. *Am J Gastroenterol* 2011;106(3):460-468.

Kistler KD, et al. Physical activity recommendations, exercise intensity, and histological severity of nonalcoholic fatty liver disease. *Am J Gastroenterol*. 2011;106(3):460-468.

Kwon YM, et al. Association of nonalcoholic fatty liver disease with components of metabolic syndrome according to body mass index in Korean adults. *Am J Gastroenterol*. 2012;107(12):1852-1858.

Lefkowitch JH. Steatosis, steatohepatitis and related conditions. In: Lefkowitch JH, ed. Scheuer's Liver Biopsy Interpretation. 8th ed. New York. *Saunders-Elsevier* 2010: 93-114.

Leuschner UF, et al. High-dose ursodeoxycholic acid therapy for nonalcoholic steatohepatitis: a double-blind, randomized, placebo-controlled trial. *Hepatology*. 2010;52(2):472-479.

Mendes FD, et al. Prevalence and indicators of portal hypertension in patients with nonalcoholic fatty liver disease. *Clin Gastroenterol Hepatol*. 2012;10(9):1028-1033.

Molloy JW, et al. Association of coffee and caffeine consumption with fatty liver disease, nonalcoholic steatohepatitis, and degree of hepatic fibrosis. *Hepatology*. 2012;55(2):429-436.

Musso G, et al. A meta-analysis of randomized trials for the treatment of nonalcoholic fatty liver disease. *Hepatology* 2010;52:79-104.

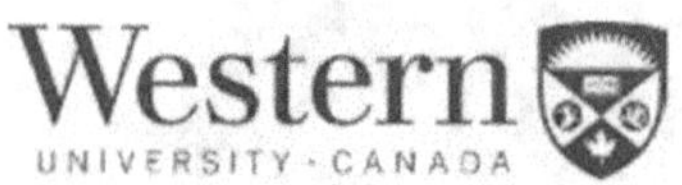

Rakoski MO, et al. Meta analysis: insulin sensitizers for the treatment of non-alcoholic steatohepatitis. *Alimentary Pharmacology and Therapeutics* 2010;32:1211-1221.

Ratziu V, et al. A randomized controlled trial of high-dose ursodesoxycholic acid for nonalcoholic steatohepatitis. *J Hepatol.* 2011;54(5):1011-1019.

Ratziu V, et al. Therapeutic trials in nonalcoholic steatohepatitis: insulin sensitizers and related methodological issues. *Hepatology* 2010;52:2206-2215.

Rodriguez B, et al. Physical activity: an essential component of lifestyle modification in NAFLD. *Nat Rev Gastroenterol Hepatol.* 2012;9(12):726-731.

Rotman Y, et al. The association of genetic variability in patatin-like phospholipase domain-containing protein 3 (PNPLA3) with histological severity of nonalcoholic fatty liver disease. *Hepatology* 2010;52:894-903.

Sanyal AJ, et al. Pioglitazone, vitamin E, or placebo for nonalcoholic steatohepatitis. *The New England Journal of Medicine* 2010;362:1675-1685.

Serino M, et al. Intestinal microflora and metabolic diseases. *Diabetes & Metabolism* 2009;35:262-272.

Sheth SG. Nonalcoholic steatohepatitis. *UpToDate online journal.* www.uptodate.com

Sinn DH, et al. Ultrasonographically detected non-alcoholic fatty liver disease is an independent predictor for identifying patients with insulin resistance in non-obese, non-diabetic middle-aged Asian adults. *Am J Gastroenterol* 2012;107(4):561-567.

Socha P, et al. Pharmacological interventions for nonalcoholic fatty liver disease in adults and in children: A systematic review. *Journal of Pediatric Gastroenterology and Nutrition* 2009; 48:587-596.

Stepanova M and Younossi ZM. Independent association between nonalcoholic fatty liver disease and

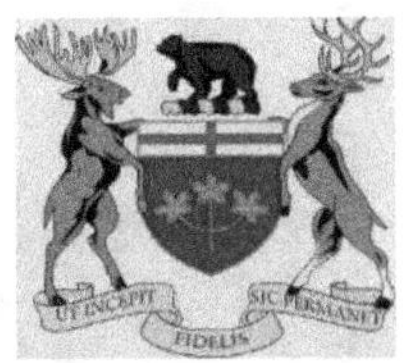

cardiovascular disease in the US population. *Clin Gastroenterol Hepatol.* 2012;10(6):646-650.

Suzuki A, et al. Association between puberty and features of nonalcoholic fatty liver disease. *Clin Gastroenterol Hepatol.* 2012;10(7):786-794.

Targher G, et al. Risk of cardiovascular disease in patients with non-alcoholic fatty liver disease. *The New England Journal of Medicine* 2010;363:1341-50.

Tendler DA. Pathogenesis of non-alcoholic fatty liver disease. *UpToDate.* www.uptodate.com

Vuppalanchi R, et al. Nonalcoholic fatty liver disease and nonalcoholic steatohepatitis: Selected practical issues in their evaluation and management. *Hepatology* 2009;49:306-317.

White DL, et al. Association between nonalcoholic fatty liver disease and risk for hepatocellular cancer, based on systematic review. *Clin Gastroenterol Hepatol.* 2012;10(12):1342-1359.

Williams CD, et al. Prevalence of non-alcoholic fatty liver disease and non-alcoholic steatohepatitis among a largely middle aged population utilizing ultrasound and liver biopsy: A prospective study. *Gastroenterology* 2011;140:124-131.

Wong VW, et al. Coronary artery disease and cardiovascular outcomes in patients with non-alcoholic fatty liver disease. *Gut* 2011;60(12):1721-1727.

Wong VW, et al. Liver stiffness measurement using XL probe in patients with nonalcoholic fatty liver disease. *Am J Gastroenterol.* 2012;107(12):1862-1871.

Zein CO, et al. Pentoxifylline improves nonalcoholic steatohepatitis: a randomized placebo-controlled trial. *Hepatology* 2011;54(5):1610-1619.

Complications of Portal Hypertension

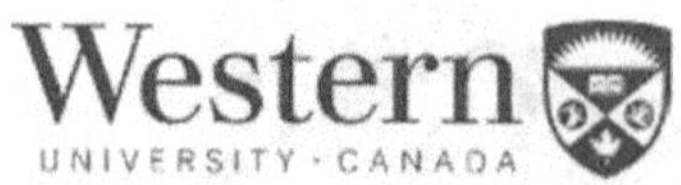

REFERENCES AND SUGGESTED READING

Angeli P, et al. Combined versus sequential diuretic treatment of ascites in non-azotemic patients with cirrhosis: results of an open randomized clinical trial. *Gut* 2010; 59:1-10.

Cárdenas, et al. Management of ascites and hepatic hydrothorax. *Best Practice & Research Clinical Gastroenterology* 2007; 21(1): 55-75.

Gines P, et al. EASL clinical practice guidelines on the management of ascites, spontaneous bacterial peritonitis, and hepatorenal syndrome in cirrhosis. *Journal of Hepatology* 2010;53:397-417.

Hernández-Gea V, et al. Development of ascites in compensated cirrhosis with severe portal hypertension treated with β-blockers. *Am J Gastroenterol* 2012;107(3):418-27.

Kuiper JJ, et al. Management of ascites and associated complications in patients with cirrhosis. *Alimentary Pharmacology and Therapeutics* 2007;26 Suppl 2:183-93.

Moore KP, et al. Guidelines on the management of ascites in cirrhosis. *Gut* 2006; 55:1-12.

Moore KP, et al. The management of ascites – Report on the consensus conference of the International Ascites Club. *Hepatology* 2003;38:258-266.

Runyon B. AASLD Practice Guidelines-Management of adult patients with ascites due to cirrhosis: an update. *Hepatology* 2009;49:2087-2107.

Runyon BA. Management of adult patients with ascites due to cirrhosis: an update. *Hepatology* 2009; 49:2087-2107.

Runyon, Bruce A. Ascites and spontaneous bacterial peritonitis. *Sleisenger & Fordtran's gastrointestinal and liver disease: Pathophysiology/ Diagnosis/ Management* 2006: pg. 1946.

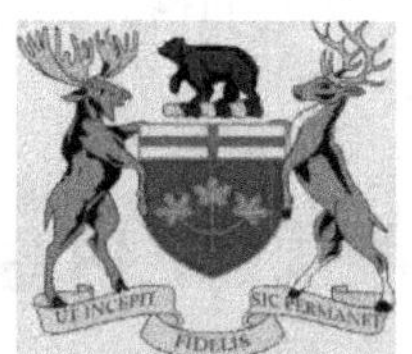

HBV and HCV Infection

Ahlenstiel G, et al. Early Changes in Natural Killer Cell Function Indicate Virologic Response to Interferon Therapy for Hepatitis C. *Gastroenterology* 2011;141:1231-1239.

Ahlenstiel G, et al. Natural killer cells are polarized toward cytotoxicity in chronic hepatitis C in an interferon-alfa-dependent manner. *Gastroenterology* 2010;138:325-335.

Alter G., et al. Reduced frequencies of NKp30+NKp46+, CD161+, and NKG2D+ NK cells in acute HCV infection may predict viral clearance. *Journal of Hepatology* 2010;55:278-288.

Amadei B., et al. Activation of natural killer cells during acute infection with hepatitis C virus. *Gastroenterology* 2010;138:1536-1545.

Arora S, et al. Outcomes of treatment for hepatitis C virus infection by primary care providers. *The New England Journal of Medecine* 2011;364:2199-2207.

Bacon BR, et al. Boceprevir for previously treated chronic HCV genotype 1 infection. *N Engl J Med.* 2011;364(13):1207-1217.

Balagopal A, et al. *IL28B* and the control of Hepatitis C virus infection. *Gastroenterology* 2010;139:1865-1876.

Barnes E, et al. Novel adenovirus-based vaccines induce broad and sustained T cell responses to HCV in man. *Sci Transl Med* 2012;4(115):115ra1.

Behairy BE, et al. Serum cystatin C correlates negatively with viral load in treatment-naïve children with chronic hepatitis C. *J Pediatr Gastroenterol Nutr* 2012;54(3):364-368.

Carrion AF and Martin P. Viral hepatitis in the elderly. *Am J Gastroenterol.* 2012;107(5):691-697.

Carrion AF and Martin P. Viral hepatitis in the elderly. *Am J Gastroenterol.* 2012;107(5):691-697.

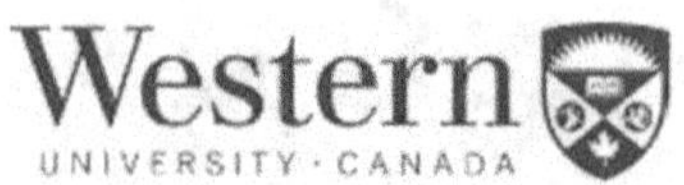

Chan HL, et al. A longitudinal study on the natural history of serum hepatitis B surface antigen changes in chronic hepatitis B. *Hepatology* 2010;52(4):1232-1241.

Chang TT, et al. Entecavir treatment for up to 5 years in patients with hepatitis B e antigen positive chronic hepatitis B. *Hepatology* 2010;51(2):422-30.

Chaves SS, et al. Improved anamnestic response among adolescents boosted with a higher dose of the hepatitis B vaccine. *Vaccine* 2010;28(16):2860-2864.

Cheent K. and Khakoo SI. Natural killer cells and hepatitis C: action and reaction. *International Journal of Gastroenterology and Hepatology* 2011;60:268-278.

Chen CF, et al. Changes in serum levels of HBV DNA and alanine aminotransferase determine risk for hepatocellular carcinoma. *Gastroenterology* 2011;141(4):1240-1248.

Chen HL, et al. Effects of maternal screening and universal immunization to prevent mother-to-infant transmission of HBV. *Gastroenterology* 2012;142(4):773-781.

Chen YC, et al. Decreasing levels of HBsAg predict HBsAg seroclearance in patients with inactive chronic hepatitis B virus infection. *Clin Gastroenterol Hepatol* 2012;10(3):297-302.

Chevaliez S, et al. New virologic tools for management of chronic hepatitis B and C. *Gastroenterology*. 2012;142(6):1303-1313.

Cholongitas E, et al. Novel therapeutic options for chronic hepatitis C. *Alimentary Pharmacology and Therapeutics* 2008;27(10):866-884.

Chopra S. Clinical features and natural history of hepatitis C virus infection. *UpToDate online journal*. www.uptodate.com

Chuen-Fei C, et al. Changes in Serum Levels of HBV DNA and Alanine Aminotransferase Determine Risk for

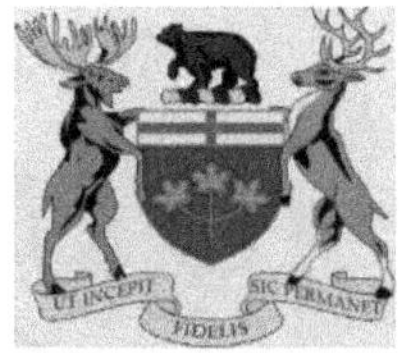

Hepatocellular Carcinoma. Gastroenterology 2011;141:1240-1248.

Ciesek S. and Manns M.P. Hepatitis in 2010: the dawn of a new era in HCV therapy. *Nature Reviews Gastroenterology and Hepatology* 2011;8:69-71.

Crespo G, et al. Viral hepatitis in liver transplantation. *Gastroenterology*. 2012;142(6):1373-1383.

Crotta S, et al. Hepatitis C virions subvert natural killer cell activation to generate a cytokine environment permissive for infection. *Journal of Hepatology* 2010;52:183-190.

De Vries-Sluijs TEMS, et al. Long-term therapy with Tenofovir is effective for patients co-infected with human immunodeficiency virus and Hepatitis B virus. *Gastroenterology* 2010;139:1934-1941.

Degertekin B, et al. Impact of virologic breakthrough and HBIG regimen on hepatitis B recurrence after liver transplantation. *American Journal of Transplantation* 2010;10:1823-1833.

Dessouki O, et al. Chronic hepatitis C viral infection reduces NK cell frequency and suppresses cytokine secretion: reversion by anti-viral treatment. *Biochemical and Biophysical Research Communications* 2010;393:331-337.

Di Bisceglie AM, et al. Excess mortality in patients with advanced chronic hepatitis C treated with long-term peginterferon. *Hepatology* 2011;53:1100-1108.

Dring MM, et al. Innate immune genes synergize to predict increased risk of chronic disease in hepatitis C virus infection. *Proceedings of the National Academy of Sciences of the United States* 2011;108:5736-5741.

Dusheiko G, et al. Current Treatment of Hepatitis B. *Gut* 2008;57:105-124.

Eurich D, et al. Role of IL28B polymorphism in the development of hepatitis C virus-induced hepatocellular

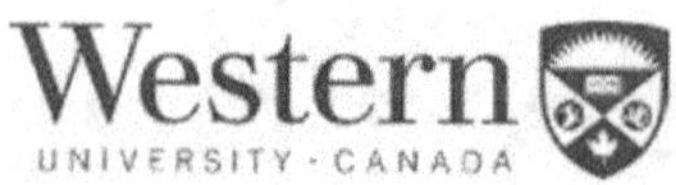

carcinoma, graft fibrosis, and posttransplant antiviral therapy. *Transplantation* 2012;93(6):644-649.

European Association for the Study of the liver. EASL Clinical practice guidelines: Management of chronic hepatitis B. *Journal of Hepatology* 2009;50(2): 227-42.

European Association for the Study of the Liver. EASL clinical practice guidelines: management of hepatitis C virus infection. *Journal of Hepatology* 2011;55:245-264.

Everhart JE, et al. Weight-related effects on disease progression in the hepatitis C antiviral long-term treatment against cirrhosis trial. *Gastroenterology* 2009;137:549-557.

Farnik H, et al. Meta-analysis Shows Extended Therapy Improves Response of Patients With Chronic Hepatitis C Virus Genotype 1 Infection. *Clinical Gastroenterology and Hepatology* 2010;8:884-890.

Feld JJ, et al. S-adenosyl methionine improves early viral responses and interferon-stimulated gene induction in hepatitis C nonresponders. *Gastroenterology* 2011;140:830-839.

Fernandez-Rodriguez CM, et al. Peginterferon plus ribavirin and sustained virological response in HCV-related cirrhosis: outcomes and factors predicting response. *The American Journal of Gastroenterology* 2010;105:2164-2172.

Fletcher NF, et al. Hepatitis C virus infects the endothelial cells of the blood-brain barrier. *Gastroenterology* 2012;142(3):634-643.

Foster G, et al. Subanalysis of the telaprevir lead-in arm in the REALIZE study: Response at week 4 is not a substitute for prior null response categorization. *Journal of Hepatology* 2011;54(suppl 1):S3-S4.

Fred P, et al. Boceprevir for Untreated Chronic HCV Genotype 1 Infection. *The New England Journal of Medicine* 2011; 364:1195-1206.

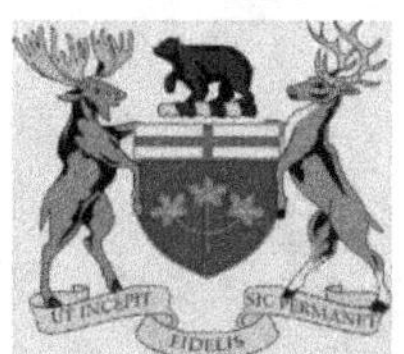

Freedman ND, et al. Silymarin use and liver disease progression in the Hepatitis C Antiviral Long-Term Treatment against Cirrhosis trial. *Alimentary Pharmacology and Therapeutics* 2011;33:127-137.

Gane EJ, et al. Oral combination therapy with a nucleoside polymerase inhibitor (RG7128) and danoprevir for chronic hepatitis C genotype 1 infection (INFORM 1): a randomised, double blind, placebo controlled, dose escalation trial. *The Lancet* 2010;376:1467-1475.

Garcia-Tsao G, et al. Management and treatment of patients with cirrhosis and portal hypertension: recommendations from the Department of Veterans Affairs Hepatitis C Resource Center Program and the National Hepatitis C Program. *The American Journal of Gastroenterology* 2009;104(7):1802-1829.

Ghany MG, et al. Predicting clinical and histologic outcomes based on standard laboratory tests in advanced chronic hepatitis C. *Gastroenterology* 2010;138:136-146.

Ghany MG., et al. Diagnosis, management, and treatment of hepatitis C: An update. *Hepatology* 2009; 49(4): 1335–1374.

Gisbert JP, et al. Efficacy of hepatitis B vaccination and revaccination and factors impacting on response in patients with inflammatory bowel disease. *Am J Gastroenterol*. 2012;107(10):1460-1466.

Harrison RJ, et al. Association of NKG2A with treatment treatment for chronic hepatitis C virus infection. *Clinical and Experimental Immunology* 2010;161:306-314.

Hayes CN, et al. Genetics of IL28B and HCV--response to infection and treatment. *Nat Rev Gastroenterol Hepatol*. 2012;9(7):406-417.

Heathcote EJ, et al. Three year efficacy and safety of tenofovir disoproxil fumarate treatment for chronic hepatitis B. *Gastroenterology* 2011;140:132-143.

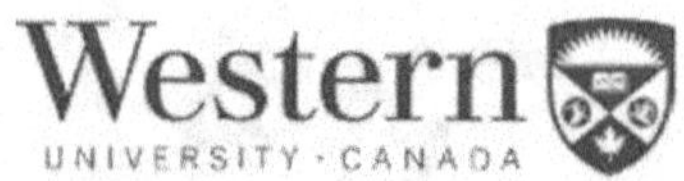

Hezode C, et al. Telaprevir and peginterferon with or without ribavirin for chronic HCV infection. *The New England Journal of Medicine* 2009;360:1839-1850.

Holness G, et al. Hepatitis B therapies and antiviral resistance detection and management. *Expert Rev Gastroenterol Hepatol.* 2009;3(6):693-699.

Hosel M, et al. Not interferon, but interleukin-6 controls early gene expression in hepatitis B virus infection. *Hepatology* 2009;50:1773-1782.

Jacobson IM, et al. Manifestations of Chronic Hepatitis C Virus Infection Beyond the Liver. *Clinical Gastroenterology and Hepatology* 2010;8:1017-1029.

Jacobson IM, et al. Telaprevir for previously untreated chronic hepatitis C virus infection. *N Engl J Med* 2011;364(25):2405-2416.

James F, et al. Entecavir Monotherapy Is Effective in Suppressing Hepatitis B Virus After Liver Transplantation. *Gastroenterology* 2011;141:1212-1219.

Jimenez-Perez M., et al. Efficacy and safety of entecavir and/or tenofovir for prophylaxis and treatment of hepatitis B recurrence post-liver transplant. *Transplantation Proceedings* 2010;42:3167-3168.

Kallwitz ER, et al. Ethnicity and body mass index are associated with hepatitis C presentation and progession. *Clinical Gastroenterology and Hepatology* 2010;8:72-78.

Kamal SM. Acute Hepatitis C: a systematic review. *The American Journal of Gastroenterology* 2008;103:1283-1297.

Kanda T, et al. Efficacy of lamivudine or entecavir on acute exacerbation of chronic hepatitis B. *Int J Med Sci* 2012;9(1):27-32.

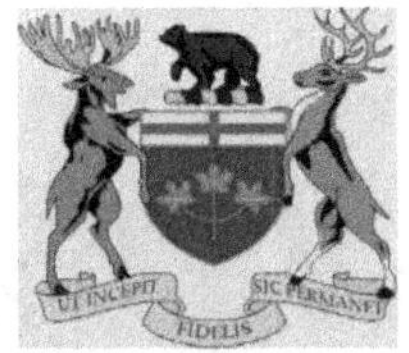

Katz LH, et al. Prevention of recurrent hepatitis B virus infection after liver transplantation: hepatitis B immunoglobulin, antiviral drugs, or both? Systematic review and meta-analysis. *Transplant Infectious Disease* 2010;12:292-308.

Kim B, et al. Validation of FIB-4 and comparison with other simple noninvasive indices for predicting liver fibrosis and cirrhosis in hepatitis B virus infected patients. *Liver Int* 2010;30:546-553.

Kim JH, et al. Virologic response to therapy increases health-related quality of life for patients with chronic hepatitis B. *Clin Gastroenterol Hepatol* 2012;10(3):291-296.

Kim YJ, et al. Possible reactivation of potential hepatitis B virus occult infection by tumor necrosis factor-alpha blocker in the treatment of rheumatic diseases. *J Rheumatol* 2010;37(2):346-350.

Knapp S, et al. A polymorphism in IL28B distinguishes exposed, uninfected individuals from spontaneous resolvers of HCV infection. *Gastroenterology* 2011;141:320-325.

Knapp S, et al. Consistent beneficial effects of killer cell immunoglobulin-like receptor 2DL3 and group 1 human leukocyte antigen-C following exposure to hepatitis C virus. *Hepatology* 2010;51:1168-1175.

Kwo PY, et al. Efficacy of boceprevir, an NS3 protease inhibitor, in combination with peginterferon alfa-2b and ribavirin in treatment-naïve patients with genotype 1 hepatitis C infection (SPRINT-1): An open-label, randomized, multicenter phase 2 trial. *Lancet* 2010 Aug 28;376(9742):705-716.

Lanford RE, et al. The Accelerating pace of HCV Research: A summary of the 15th International symposium on Hepatitis C virus and related viruses. *Gastroenterology* 2009;136(1):9-16.

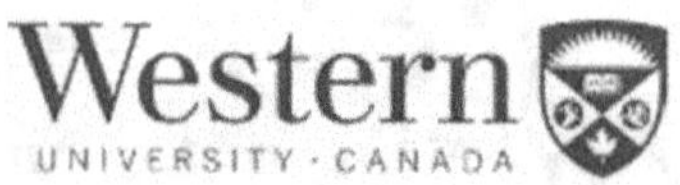

Lange CM, et al. IL28B single nucleotide polymorphisms in the treatment of hepatitis C. *J Hepatol* 2011;55(3):692-701.

Lange CM, et al. Impact of donor and recipient IL28B rs12979860 genotypes on hepatitis C virus liver graft reinfection. *Journal of Hepatology* 2011;55:322-327.

Lee JM, et al. Quantitative hepatitis B surface antigen and hepatitis B e antigen titers in prediction of treatment response to entecavir. *Hepatology* 2011;53(5):1486-1493.

Lee S., et al. Increased proportion of the CD56(bright) NK cell subset in patients chronically infected with hepatitis C virus (HCV) receiving interferon-alpha and ribavirin therapy. *Journal of Medical Virology* 2010;82:568-574.

Levitsky J, et al. Risk for immune-mediated graft dysfunction in liver transplant recipients with recurrent HCV infection treated with pegylated interferon. *Gastroenterology*. 2012;142(5):1132-1139.

Liaw YF. Clinical utility of hepatitis B surface antigen quantitation in patients with chronic hepatitis B: a review. *Hepatology* 2011;54(2):E1-9.

Liu S., et al. Associations between hepatitis B virus mutations and the risk of hepatocellular carcinoma: a meta-analysis. *Journal of the National Cancer Institute* 2009;101:1066-1082.

Lo Re V 3rd, et al. Relationship between adherence to hepatitis C virus therapy and virologic outcomes: a cohort study. *Ann Intern Med* 2011;155(6):353-360.

Lok AS, et al. Chronic Hepatitis B: update 2009. *Hepatology* 2009;50(3):661-2.

Lok AS, et al. Chronic Hepatitis B. *Hepatology* 2007;45(2):507-39.

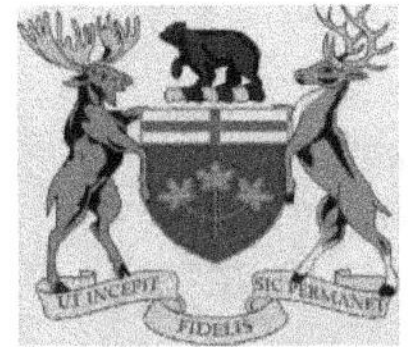

Lok AS, et al. Preliminary study of two antiviral agents for hepatitis C genotype 1. *N Engl J Med*. 2012;366(3):216-224.

Lok ASF. Characteristics of the hepatitis B virus and pathogenesis of infection. *UpToDate*. www.uptodate.com

Lorenz R. Diagnosis and treatment of acute hepatitis C in adults. *UpToDate online journal.* www.uptodate.com

Ly KN, et al. The increasing burden of mortality from viral hepatitis in the United States between 1999 and 2007. *Ann Intern Med*. 2012;156(4):271-278.

Ma H, et al. Quantitative serum HBsAg and HBeAg are strong predictors of sustained HBeAg seroconversion to pegylated interferon alfa-2b in HBeAg-positive patients. *J Gastroenterol Hepatol* 2010;25(9):1498-1506.

Marcellin P, et al. Sustained response of hepatitis B e antigen negative patients 3 years after treatment with peginterferon alpha 2a. *Gastroenterology* 2009;136(7):2169-2179. e1-4.

Marquez RT, et al. Correlation between microRNA expression levels and clinical parameters associated with chronic hepatitis C viral infection in humans. *Laboratory Investigation* 2010;90:1727-1736.

McGilvray I, et al. Hepatic cell-type specific gene expression better predicts HCV treatment outcome than IL28B genotype. *Gastroenterology*. 2012;142(5):1122-1131.

McHutchison JG, et al. Telaprevir for previously treated chronic HCV infection. *N Engl J Med*. 2010;362(14):1292-1303.

McHutchison JG, et al. Telaprevir with peginterferon and ribavirin for chronic HCV genotype 1 infection. *The New England Journal of Medicine* 2009;360:1827-1838.

Medrano J, et al. Modeling the probability of sustained virological response to therapy with pegylated interferon

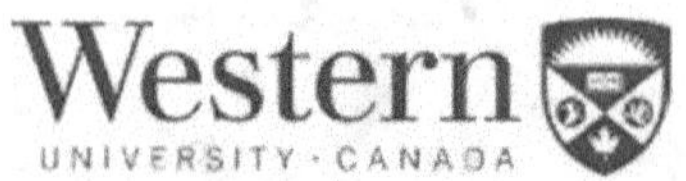

plus ribavirin in patients coinfected with hepatitis C virus and HIV. *Clinical Infectious Diseases* 2010;51:1209-16.

Mino OR, et al. Mallory-Denk Bodies Are Associated With Outcomes and Histologic Features in Patients With Chronic Hepatitis C. *Clinical Gastroenterology and Hepatology* 2011;9:902-909.

Miyagi T, et al. Altered interferon-alpha- signaling in natural killer cells from patients with chronic hepatitis C virus infection. *Journal of Hepatology* 2010;53:424-430.

Negro F. HCV infection and metabolic syndrome: which is the chicken and which is the egg? *Gastroenterology*. 2012;142(6):1288-1292.

Nelson PK, et al. Global epidemiology of hepatitis B and hepatitis C in people who inject drugs: results of systematic reviews. *Lancet* 2011;378(9791):571-83.

Netanya G., et al. Host Response to Translocated Microbial Products Predicts Outcomes of Patients With HBV or HCV Infection. *Gastroenterology* 2011;141:1220-1230.

Okoh EJ, et al. HCV in patients with End-stage renal disease. *The American Journal of Gastroenterology* 2008;103(8):2123-2134.

Omland LH, et al. Increased mortality among persons infected with Hepatitis C virus. *Clinical Gastroenterology and Hepatology* 2011;9:71-78.

Pan CQ, et al. An algorithm for risk assessment and intervention of mother to child transmission of hepatitis B virus. *Clin Gastroenterol Hepatol*. 2012;10(5):452-9.

Pan CQ, et al. Telbivudine prevents vertical transmission from HBeAg-positive women with chronic hepatitis B. *Clin Gastroenterol Hepatol*. 2012;10(5):520-526.

Papatheodoridis G, et al. The EASL clinical practice guidelines on the management of chronic hepatitis B:

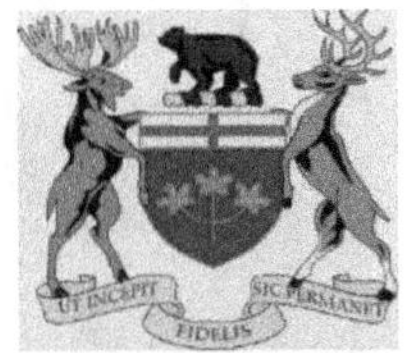

the need for liver biopsy. *Journal of Hepatology* 2009;51:226-7

Papatheodoridis GV, et al. for the HEPNET Greece Cohort Study Group. Virological suppression does not prevent the development of hepatocellular carcinoma in HBeAg-negative chronic hepatitis B patients with cirrhosis receiving oral antiviral(s) starting with lamivudine monotherapy: results of the nationwide HEPNET. Greece cohort study. *International Journal in Gastroenterology* 2011;60:1109-1116.

Parruti G, et al. Rapid prediction of sustained virological response in patients chronically infected with HCV by evaluation of RNA decay 48h after the start of treatment with pegylated interferon and ribavirin. *Antiviral Research* 2010;88:124-127.

Parry J. At last a global response to viral hepatitis. *Bull World Health Organ*. 2010;88(11):801-802.

Patin E, et al. Genome-wide association study identifies variants associated with progression of liver fibrosis from HCV infection. *Gastroenterology*. 2012;143(5):1244-1252.

Pawlotsky JM. Is hepatitis virus resistance to antiviral drugs a threat? *Gastroenterology*. 2012;142(6):1369-72.

Pelletier S, et al. Increased degranulation of natural killer cells during acute HCV correlates with the magnitude of virus-specific T cell responses. *Journal of Hepatology* 2010;53:805-816.

Pessoa SD, et al. Persistence of vaccine immunity against hepatitis B virus and response to revaccination in vertically HIV-infected adolescents on HAART. *Vaccine* 2010;28(6):1606-1612.

Podevin P, et al. Production of Infectious Hepatitis C Virus in Primary Cultures of Human Adult Hepatocytes. *Gastroenterology* 2010;139:1355-1364.

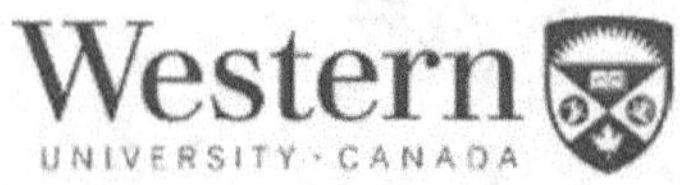

Poordad F, et al. Boceprevir for untreated chronic HCV genotype 1 infection. *N Engl J Med* 2011;364(13):1195-1206.

Poynard T, et al. Liver biopsy analysis has a low level of performance for diagnosis of intermediate stages of fibrosis. *Clin Gastroenterol Hepatol.* 2012;10(6):657-663.

Poynard T, et al. Relative performances of FibroTest, Fibroscan, and biopsy for the assessment of the stage of liver fibrosis in patients with chronic hepatitis C: a step toward the truth in the absence of a gold standard. *J Hepatol.* 2012;56(3):541-548.

Sainz B Jr, et al. Identification of the Niemann-Pick C1-like 1 cholesterol absorption receptor as a new hepatitis C virus entry factor. *Nat Med* 2012;18(2):281-285.

Sandler, N. G., et al. Host response to translocated microbial products predicts outcomes of patients with HBV or HCV infection. *Gastroenterology.* 2011; 141(4): 1220-1230.

Sarasin-Filipowicz M., et al. Decreased levels of microRNA miR-122 in individuals with hepatitis C responding poorly to interferon therapy. *Nature Medicine* 2009;15:31-33.

Scaglione SJ and Lok AS. Effectiveness of hepatitis B treatment in clinical practice. *Gastroenterology.* 2012;142(6):1360-1368.

Sene D, et al. Hepatitis C virus (HCV) evades NKG2D-dependent NK cell responses through NS5A-mediated imbalance of inflammatory cytokines. *PLoS Pathogens* 2010;6(11).

Serfaty L, et al. Insulin resistance and response to telaprevir plus peginterferon α and ribavirin in treatment-naive patients infected with HCV genotype 1. *Gut.* 2012;61(10):1473-1480.

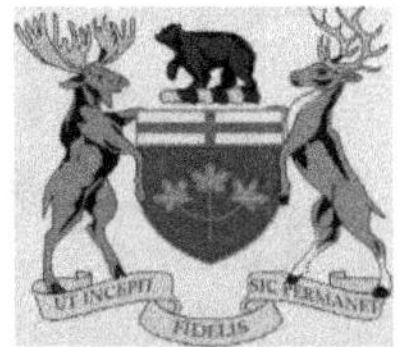

Shamliyan TA, et al. Antiviral therapy for adults with chronic hepatitis B: A systematic Review for the national institute of health consensus development conference. *Annals of Internal Medicine* 2009;150(2):111-124.

Sherman KE, et al. Response-guided telaprevir combination treatment for hepatitis C virus infection. *N Engl J Med* 2011;365(11):1014-1024.

Sherman KE, et al. Sustained long-term antiviral maintenance therapy in HCV/HIV-coinfected patients (SLAM-C). *Journal of Acquired Immune Deficiency Syndromes* 2010;55(5):597-605.

Sherman KE, et al. Telaprevir in combination with peginterferon alfa-2a and ribavirin for 24 or 48 weeks in treatment-naïve genotype 1 HCV patients who achieved and extended rapid viral response: final results of the phase 3 ILLUMINATE study. *Hepatology* 2010;52:401A.

Sherman M, et al. Management of chronic hepatitis B: consensus guidelines. *The Canadian Journal of Gastroenterology* 2007;21 Suppl C:5C-24C.

Shi Z, et al. Lamivudine in late pregnancy to interrupt in utero transmission of hepatitis B virus: a systematic review and meta-analysis. *Obstet Gynecol.* 2010;116(1):147-159.

Simonetti J, et al. Clearance of hepatitis B surface antigen and risk of hepatocellular carcinoma in a cohort chronically infected with hepatitis B virus. *Hepatology* 2010;51(5):1531-1537.

Sonneveld MJ, et al. Polymorphisms near IL28B and serologic response to peginterferon in HBeAg-positive patients with chronic hepatitis B. *Gastroenterology* 2012;142(3):513-520.

Sonneveld MJ, et al. Prediction of sustained response to peginterferon alfa-2b for hepatitis B e antigen-positive chronic hepatitis B using on-treatment hepatitis B surface antigen decline. *Hepatology* 2010;52(4):1251-57.

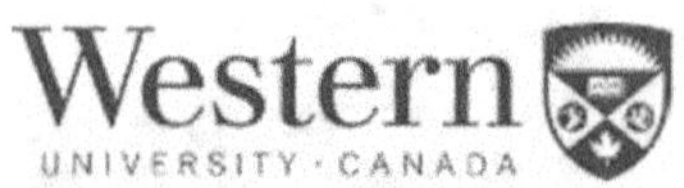

Svicher V, et al. Role of hepatitis B virus genetic barrier in drug-resistance and immune-escape development. *Digestive and Liver Disease* 2011;43:975-983.

Terrault N. Benefits and risks of combination therapy for hepatitis B. *Hepatology* 2009;49:S122-8.

Teshale EH, et al. The two faces of hepatitis E virus. *Clinical Infectious Diseases* 2010;51:328-334.

Tseng TC, et al. High levels of hepatitis B surface antigen increase risk of hepatocellular carcinoma in patients with low HBV load. *Gastroenterology*. 2012;142(5):1140-1149.

Van Bommel F, et al. Long term efficacy of tenofovir monotherapy for hepatitis B virus monoinfected patients after failure of nucleoside/nucleotide analogues. *Hepatology* 2010;51:73-80.

Wasley A, et al. The prevalence of hepatitis B virus infection in the United States era of vaccination. *The Journal of Infectious Diseases* 2010;202:192-201.

Welsch C and Zeuzem S. Will interferon-free regimens prevail? *Gastroenterology*. 2012;142(6):1351-1355.

Wiseman E, et al. Perinatal transmission of hepatitis B virus: an Australian experience. *The Medical Journal of Australia* 2009;190(9):489-92.

Woo G, et al. Tenofovir and entecavir are the most effective antiviral agents for chronic hepatitis B: A systemic review and Bayesian meta-analyses. *Gastroenterology* 2010;139:1218-1229.

Wursthorn K, et al. Natural History: The importance of viral x, liver damage and HCC. *Best Practice & Research Clinical Gastroenterology* 2008;22:1063-1079.

Yang HI, et al. Incidence and determinants of spontaneous seroclearance of hepatitis B e antigen and DNA in patients with chronic hepatitis B. *Clin Gastroenterol Hepatol*. 2012;10(5):527-534.

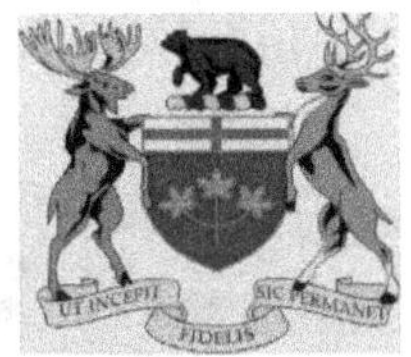

Yang JD, et al. Cirrhosis is present in most patients with hepatitis B and hepatocellular carcinoma. *Clinical Gastroenterology and Hepatology* 2011;9:64-70.

Yoon YH, et al. Alcohol-related and viral hepatitis C-related cirrhosis mortality among Hispanic subgroups in the United States, 2000-2004. *Alcoholism: Clinical and Experimental Research* 2011;35:240-249.

Yuen NF, et al. Three years of continuous entecavir therapy in treatment-naïve chronic hepatitis B patients: VIRAL suppression, viral resistance, and clinical safety. *American Journal of Gastroenterology* 2011;106(7):1264-1271.

Zeuzem S, et al. Efficacy of the protease inhibitor BI 201335, polymerase inhibitor BI 207127, and ribavirin in patients with chronic HCV infection. *Gastroenterology* 2011;141(6):2047-2055.

Zeuzem S, et al. Long-term follow-up of patients with chronic hepatitis C treated with telaprevir in combination with peginterferon alfa-2a and ribavirin: Analysis of the EXTEND study. *Hepatology* 2010;52:401A.

Zeuzem S, et al. Telaprevir for retreatment of HCV infection *N Engl J Med* 2011;364:2417-2428.

Zeuzem S, et al. The protease inhibitor, GS-9256, and non-nucleoside polymerase inhibitor tegobuvir alone, with ribavirin, or pegylated interferon plus ribavirin in hepatitis C. *Hepatology*. 2012;55(3):749-758.

Zhang Y, et al. A proinflammatory role for interleukin-22 in the immune response to hepatitis B virus. *Gastroenterology* 2011;141(5):1897-1906.

Zoulim F and Mason WS. Reasons to consider earlier treatment of chronic HBV infections. *Gut*. 2012;61(3):333-336.

Zoutendijk R, et al. Entecavir treatment for chronic hepatitis B: adaptation is not needed for the majority of naïve patients with a partial virological response. *Hepatology* 2011;54(2):443-451.

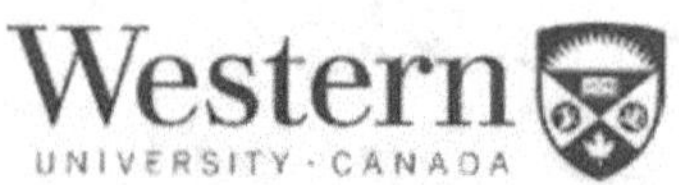

Autoimmune Hepatitis and Variant (Overlap) Syndrome

Bjornsson E, et al. Patients with typical laboratory features of autoimmune hepatitis rarely need a liver biopsy for diagnosis. *Clinical Gastroenterology and Hepatology* 2011;9:57-63.

Czaja AJ, et al. Advances in the Diagnosis, pathogenesis and management of autoimmune hepatitis. *Gastroenterology* 2010;139:58-72.

Dinani AM, et al. Patients with autoimmune hepatitis who have antimitochondrial antibodies need long-term follow-up to detect late development of primary biliary cirrhosis. *Clin Gastroenterol Hepatol.* 2012;10(6):682-684.

Gatselis NK, et al. Comparison of simplified score with the revised original score for the diagnosis of autoimmune hepatitis: a new or a complementary diagnostic score? *Dig Liver Dis* 2010;42(11):807-812.

Gleeson D, et al. British Society of Gastroenterology (BSG) guidelines for management of autoimmune hepatitis. *Gut* 2011;60(12):1611-1629.

Hennes EM, et al. Simplified criteria for the diagnosis of autoimmune hepatitis. *Hepatology* 2008;48(1):169-176.

Ilyas JA, et al. Liver transplantation in autoimmune liver diseases. *Best Pract Res Clin Gastroenterol* 2011;25(6):765-782.

Krawitt EL. Clinical manifestations and diagnosis of autoimmune hepatitis. *UpToDate online journal.* www.uptodate.com 2014

Krawitt EL. Pathogenesis of autoimmune of hepatitis. *UpTodate online journal.* www.uptodate.com 2014

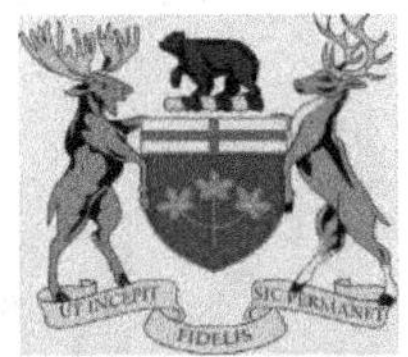

Liberal R, et al. Autoimmune hepatitis after liver transplantation. *Clin Gastroenterol Hepatol* 2012;10(4):346-353.

Liberal R, et al. Pathogenesis of autoimmune hepatitis. *Best Pract Res Clin Gastroenterol* 2011;25(6):653-664.

Lohse A.W. and Mieli-Vergani G. Autoimmune hepatitis. *Journal of Hepatology* 2011;55:171-182.

Lohse AW, et al. Diagnostic criteria for autoimmune hepatitis. *Best Pract Res Clin Gastroenterol* 2011;25(6):665-671.

Loza, Aldo J Montano, et al. Current therapy for autoimmune hepatitis. *Nature Clinical Practice Gastroenterology & Hepatology* 2007; 4(4):202.

Manns MP, et al. Budesonide induces remission more effectively than prednisone in a controlled trial of patients with autoimmune hepatitis. *Gastroenterology* 2010;139:1198-1206.

Manns MP, et al. Diagnosis and management of autoimmune hepatitis. *Hepatology*. 2010;51(6):2193-2213.

Miyake Y, et al. Clinical features of autoimmune hepatitis diagnosed based on simplified criteria of the International Autoimmune Hepatitis Group. *Dig Liver Dis* 2010;42(3):210-215.

Montano-Loza AJ, et al. Risk factors for recurrence of autoimmune hepatitis after liver transplantation. *Liver Transplant* 2009;15:1254-1261.

Montano-Loza AJ, et al. Current therapy for autoimmune hepatitis. *Nature Clinical Practice Gastroenterology & Hepatology* 2007;4(4):202-214.

Montano-Loza AJ, et al. Features associated with treatment failure in Type 1 Autoimmune Hepatitis and Predictive value of the model of end-stage liver disease. *Hepatology* 2007;46(4):1138-1145.

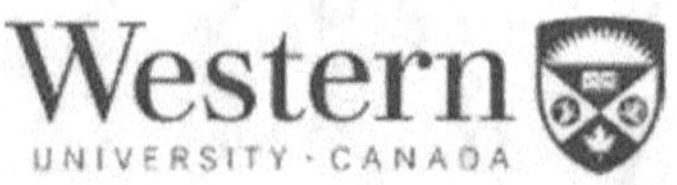

Muratori P, et al. Validation of simplified diagnostic criteria for autoimmune hepatitis in Italian patients. *Hepatology* 2009;49(5):1782-1783.

Qiu D, et al. Validation of the simplified criteria for diagnosis of autoimmune hepatitis in Chinese patients. *J Hepatol* 2011;54(2):340-347.

Silveira MG, et al. Overlap of autoimmune hepatitis and primary biliary cirrhosis: long term outcomes. *The American Journal of Gastroenterology* 2007;102:1244-1250.

Strassburg CP, et al. Therapy of autoimmune hepatitis. *Best Pract Res Clin Gastroenterol* 2011;25(6):673-687.

Vivier E., et al. Innate or adaptive immunity? The example of natural killer cells. *Science* 2011;331:44-49.

Yeoman AD, et al. Diagnostic value and utility of the simplified International Autoimmune Hepatitis Group (IAIHG) criteria in acute and chronic liver disease. *Hepatology* 2009;50(2):538-545.

Zachou K, et al. Anti-α actinin antibodies as new predictors of response to treatment in autoimmune hepatitis type 1. *Aliment Pharmacol Ther* 2012;35(1):116-125.

Drug-induced Liver Injury

Agarwal VK, et al. Important elements for the diagnosis of drug-induced liver injury. *Clinical Gastroenterology & Hepatology* 2010;8:463-470.

Athyros VG, et al. Safety and efficacy of long term statin treatment for cardiovascular events in patients with coronary heart disease and abnormal liver tests in the Greek Atorvastatin and Coronary Heart Disease Evaluation (GREACE) Study: A post-hoc analysis. *The Lancet* 2010;376:1916.

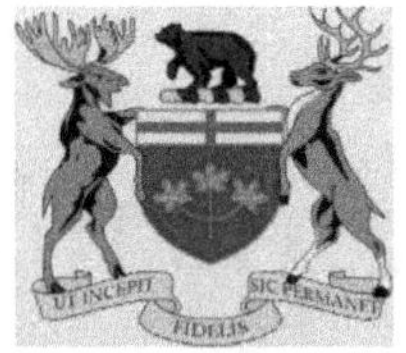

REFERENCES AND SUGGESTED READING

Bader T. Yes! Statins can be given to liver patients. *J Hepatol.* 2012;56(2):305-307.

Bahirwani R, et al. Review article: the evaluation of solitary liver masses. *Alimentary Pharmacology & Therapeutics* 2008;28:953-965.

Chun LJ, et al. Acetaminophen hepatotoxicity and acute liver failure. *Journal of Clinical Gastroenterology* 2009;43(4):342-349.

Daverm TJ, et al. Acute Hepatitis E Infection Accounts for Some Cases of Suspected Drug-Induced Liver Injury. *Gastroenterology* 2011;141:1665-1672.

Fannin RD, et al. Acetaminophen dosing of humans resulting in blood transcriptome and metabolome changes consistent with impaired oxidative phosphorylation. *Hepatology* 2010;51:227-236

Fontana RJ, et al. Standardization of nomenclature and causality assessment in drug-induced liver injury: summary of a clinical research workshop. *Hepatology* 2010;52:730-742.

Fontana RJ, et al. Drug-Induced Liver Injury Network (DILIN) prospective study: rationale, design and conduct. *Drug Saf* 2009;32(1):55-68.

Fourches D, et al. Cheminformatics analysis of assertions mined from literature that describe drug-induced liver injury in different species. *Chemistry Research and Toxicology* 2010;233;171-183.

Gupta NK , et al. Review article: The use of potentially hepatotoxic drugs in patients with liver disease. *Alimentary Pharmacology and Therapeutics* 2008;28(9):1021.

Hunt CM. Mitochondrial and immunoallergic injury increases risk of positive drug rechallenge after drug-induced liver injury: a systemic review. Hepatology 2010;52:2216-2222.

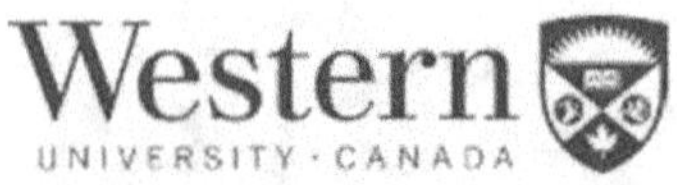

James LP, et al. Pharmacokinetics of acetaminophen-protein adducts in adults with acetaminophen overdose and acute liver failure. *Drug Metabolism and Disposition* 2009;37:1779-1784.

Kimura K, et al. Roles of CD44 in chemical-induced liver injury. *Current Opinion in Drug Discovery and Development* 2010;13:96-103.

Kleiner DE. The pathology of drug-induced liver injury. *Seminars in Liver Disease* 2009;29:364-372.

Lee WM, et al. Intravenous N-acetylcysteine improves transplant-free survival in early stage non-acetaminophen acute liver failure. *Gastroenterology* 2009;137(3):856-864.

Liss G, et al. Predicting and preventing acute drug-induced liver injury: what's new in 2010? *Expert Opinion on Drug Metabolism and Toxicology* 2010;6:1047-1061.

Lucena M, et l. Mitochondrial superoxide dismutase and glutathione peroxidase in idiosyncratic drug-induced liver injury. *Hepatology* 2010;52:303-312.

Reuben A et al. Drug induced acute liver failure: Results of a U.S multicenter, prospective study. *Hepatology* 2010;52:2065.

Senousy BE, et al. Hepatotoxic effects of therapies for tuberculosis. *Nature Review in Gastroenterology and Hepatology* 2010;7:543-556.

Stapelbroek JM, et al. Liver associated with canalicular transport defects: current and futher therapies. *Journal of Hepatology* 2010;52:258-271.

Suzuki A, et al. The use of liver biopsy evaluation in discrimination of idiopathic autoimmune hepatitis versus drug-induced liver injury. *Hepatology* 2011;54(3):931-939.

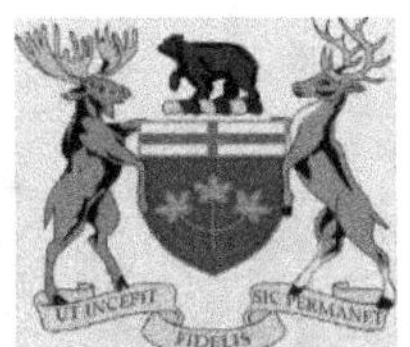

Tujios S, et al. Mechanisms of drug-induced liver injury: from bedside to bench. *Nature Reviews Gastroenterology and Hepatology* 2011;8:202-211.

Uetrecht J. Immunoallergic drug-induced liver injury in human. *Seminar in Liver Disease* 2009;29:383-392.

Wang K, et al. Circulating microRNAs, potential biomarkers fro drug-induced liver injury. *Proceedings of the National Academy of Sciences of United States* 2009;106:4402-4407.

Watkins PB. Biomarkers for the diagnosis and management of drug induced liver injury. *Seminars in Liver Disease* 2009;29:393-399.

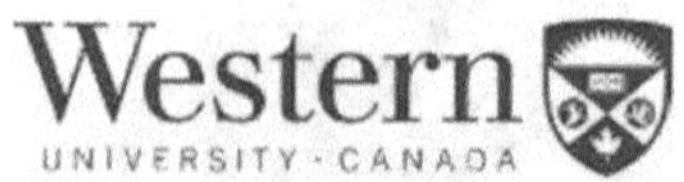

INDEX

Mini_2_Index

Note: Page number followed by f and t indicates figure and table respectively.

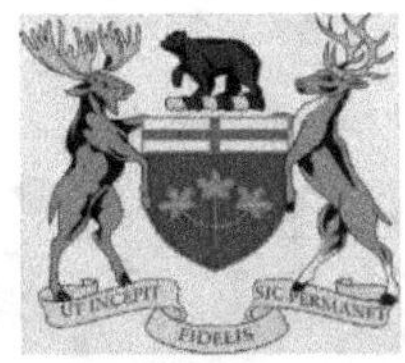

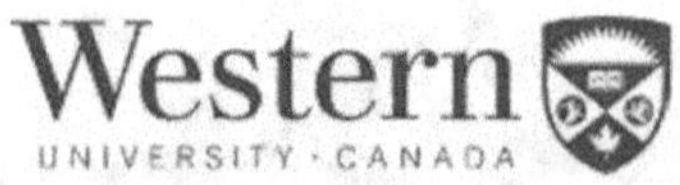
Western
UNIVERSITY · CANADA

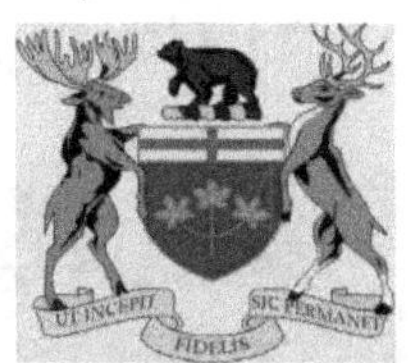
UT INCEPIT
FIDELIS
SIC PERMANET

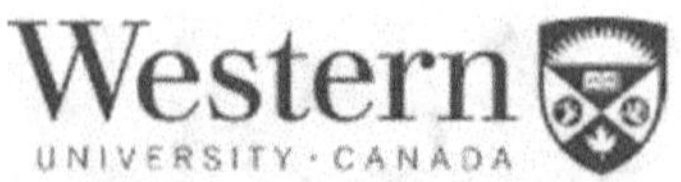
Western
UNIVERSITY · CANADA

B

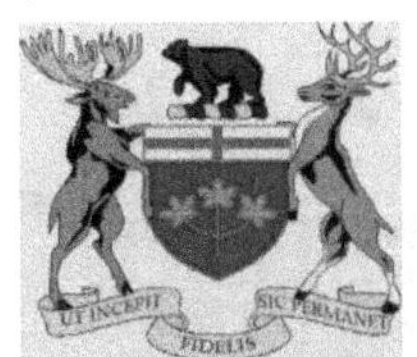

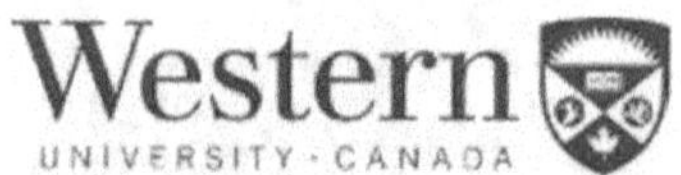
Western
UNIVERSITY · CANADA

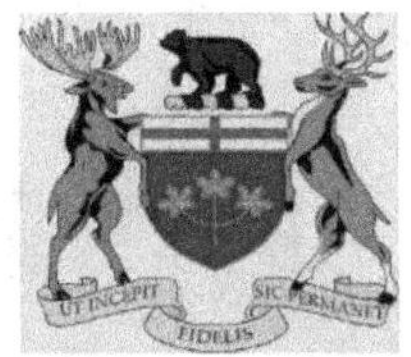
UT INCEPIT
FIDELIS
SIC PERMANET

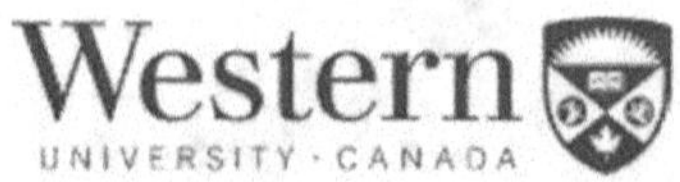
Western
UNIVERSITY · CANADA

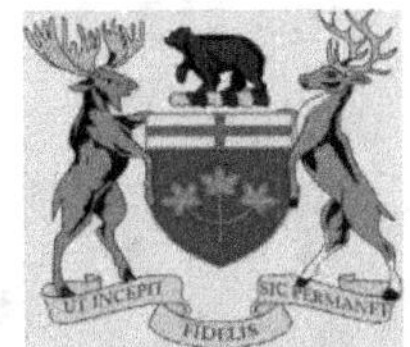
UT INCEPIT
FIDELIS
SIC PERMANET

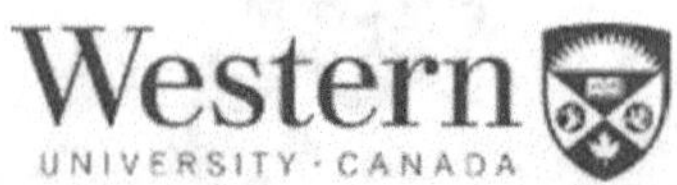
Western
UNIVERSITY · CANADA

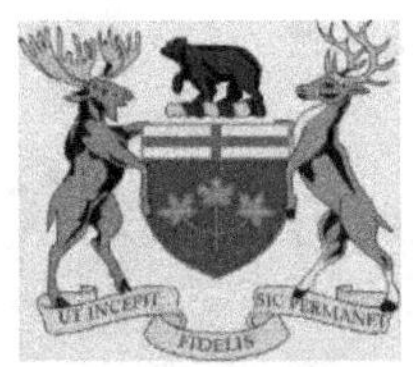
UT INCEPIT
FIDELIS
SIC PERMANET

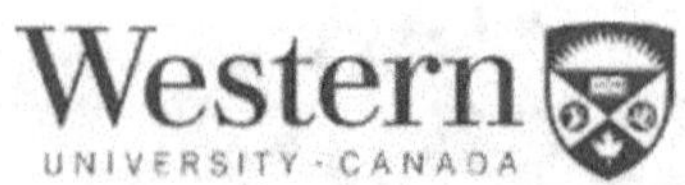
Western
UNIVERSITY · CANADA

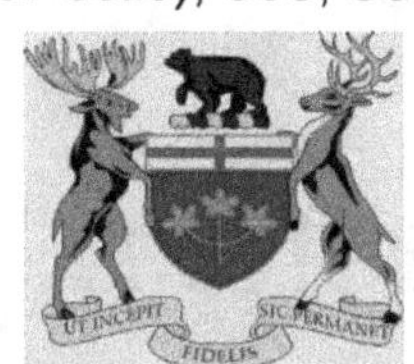
UT INCEPIT
FIDELIS
SIC PERMANET

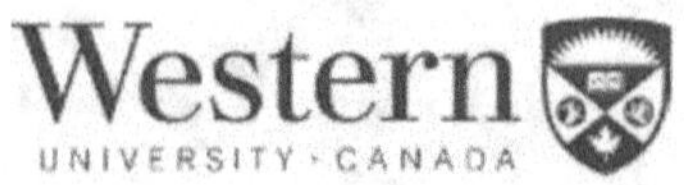
Western
UNIVERSITY · CANADA

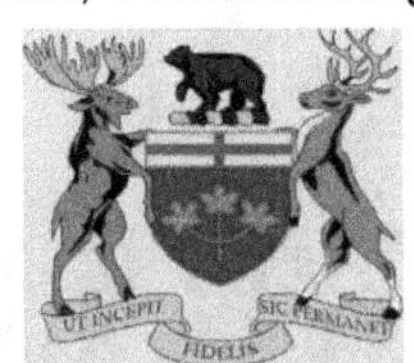
UT INCEPIT
FIDELIS
SIC PERMANET

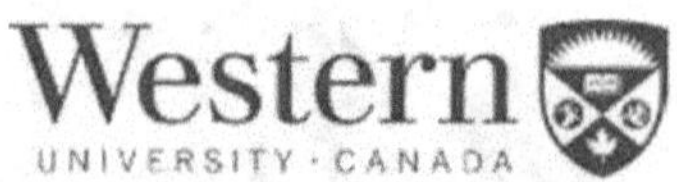
Western
UNIVERSITY · CANADA

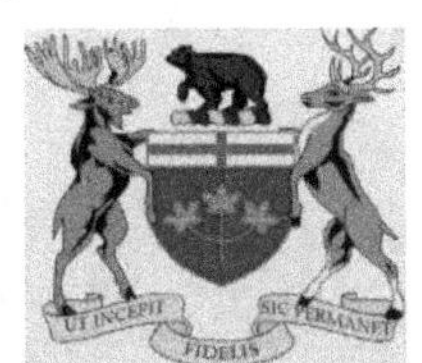
UT INCEPIT
FIDELIS
SIC PERMANET

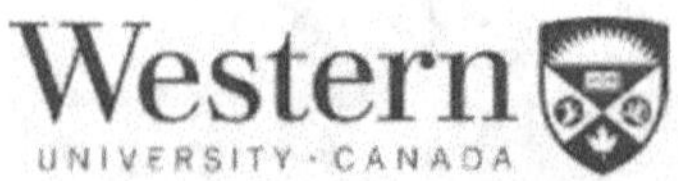
Western
UNIVERSITY · CANADA

F

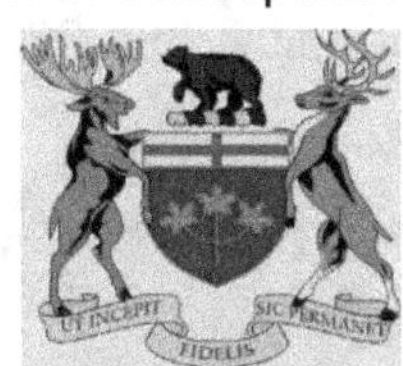

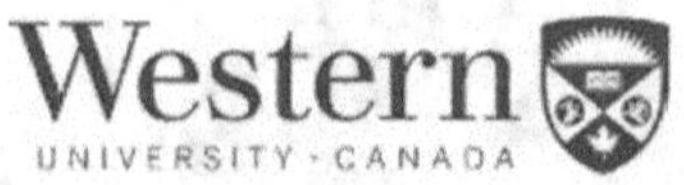
Western
UNIVERSITY · CANADA

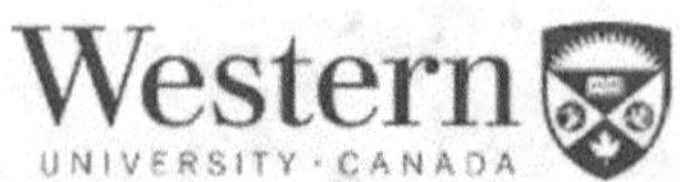
Western
UNIVERSITY · CANADA

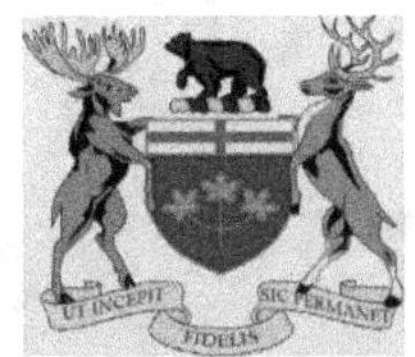
UT INCEPIT
FIDELIS
SIC PERMANET

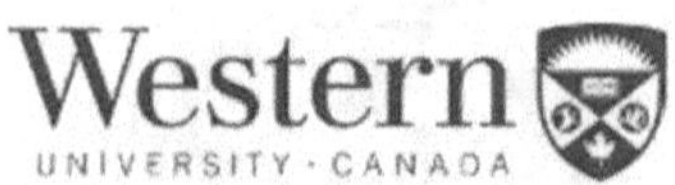
Western
UNIVERSITY · CANADA

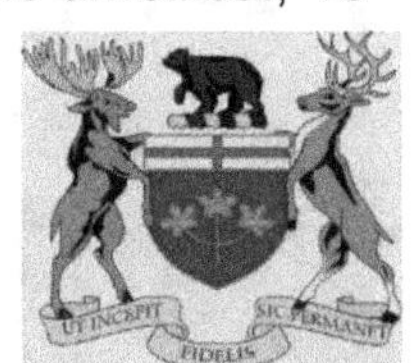
UT INCEPIT
FIDELIS
SIC PERMANET

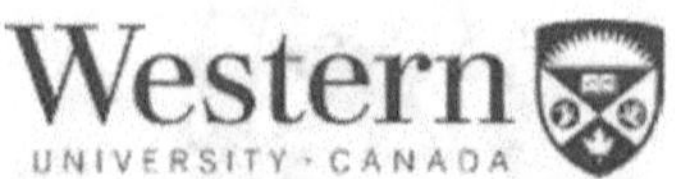
Western
UNIVERSITY · CANADA

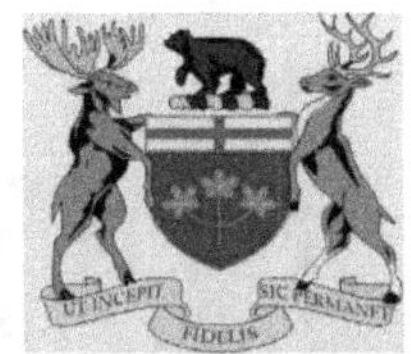
UT INCEPIT
FIDELIS
SIC PERMANET

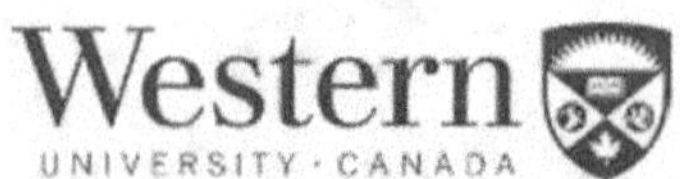
Western
UNIVERSITY · CANADA

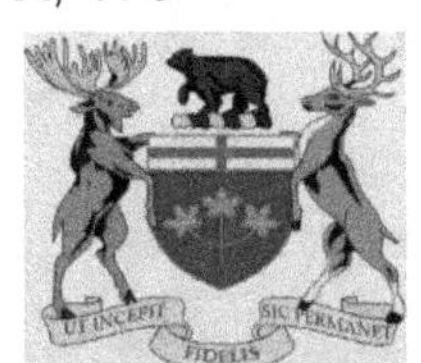
UT INCEPIT
FIDELIS
SIC PERMANET

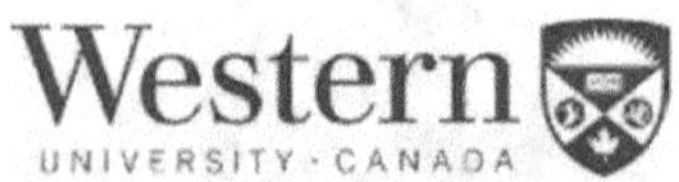
Western
UNIVERSITY · CANADA

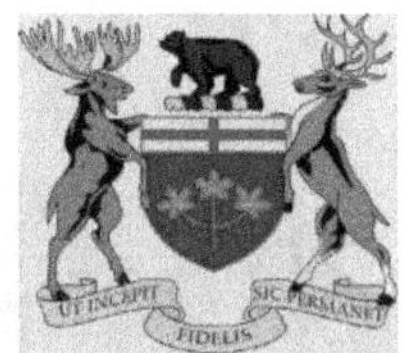
UT INCEPIT
FIDELIS
SIC PERMANET

M

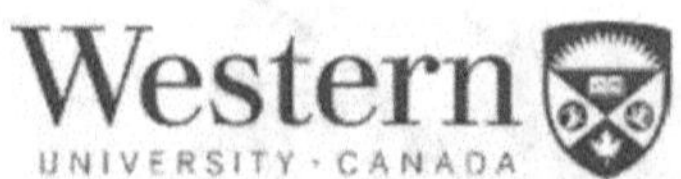

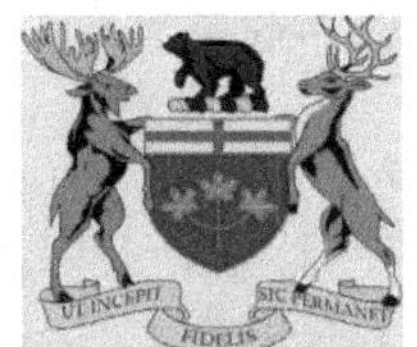
UT INCEPIT
FIDELIS
SIC PERMANET

O

P

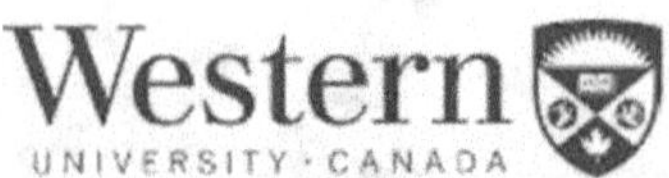

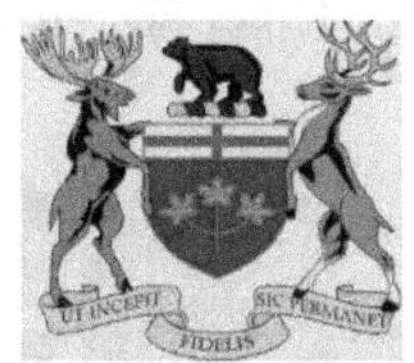
UT INCEPIT
FIDELIS
SIC PERMANET

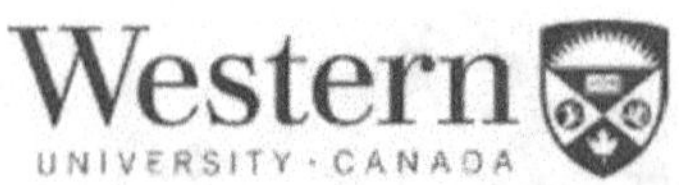
Western
UNIVERSITY · CANADA

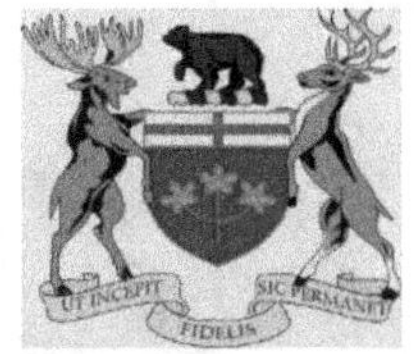
UT INCEPIT
FIDELIS
SIC PERMANET

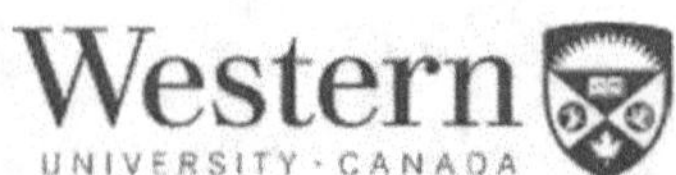
Western
UNIVERSITY · CANADA

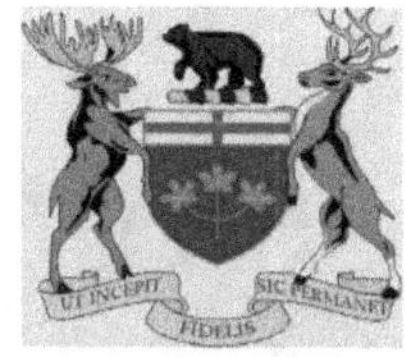

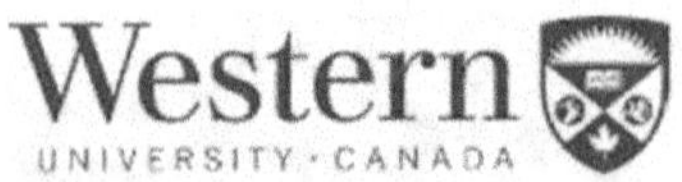
Western
UNIVERSITY · CANADA

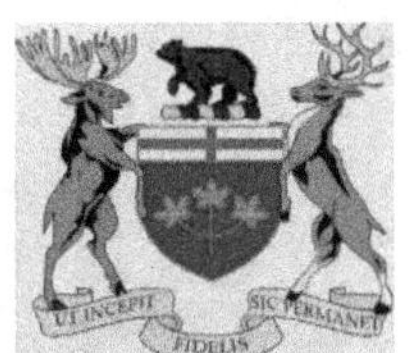
UT INCEPIT
FIDELIS
SIC PERMANET

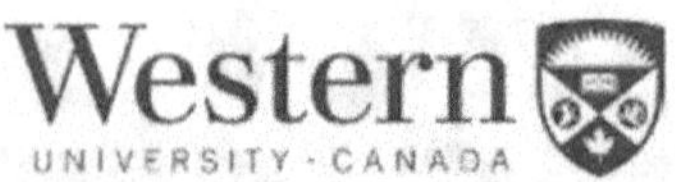
Western
UNIVERSITY · CANADA

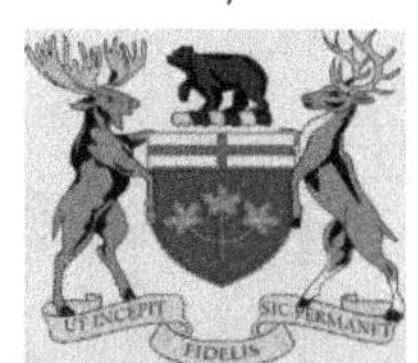
UT INCEPIT
FIDELIS
SIC PERMANET

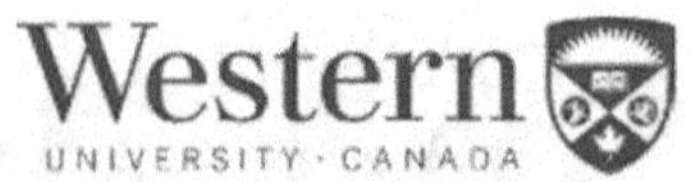
Western
UNIVERSITY · CANADA

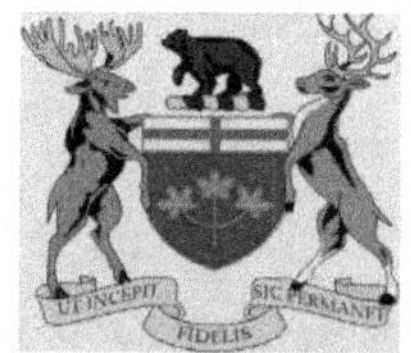

www.ingramcontent.com/pod-product-compliance
Lightning Source LLC
Chambersburg PA
CBHW072300200526
45168CB00014B/7

* 9 7 8 1 5 1 1 6 1 7 6 2 8 *